The Politics of Disease

The Politics of Disease

*An American History
from Columbus to Covid*

DAVID R. PETRIELLO

McFarland & Company, Inc., Publishers
Jefferson, North Carolina

ALSO OF INTEREST
AND PUBLISHED BY EXPOSIT
(AN IMPRINT OF MCFARLAND)

A Brief History of Oral Sex (as David DePierre, 2017)

ISBN (print) 978-1-4766-9110-7
ISBN (ebook) 978-1-4766-4865-1

LIBRARY OF CONGRESS AND BRITISH LIBRARY
CATALOGUING DATA ARE AVAILABLE

Library of Congress Control Number 2022057319

© 2023 David R. Petriello. All rights reserved

No part of this book may be reproduced or transmitted in any form or by any means, electronic or mechanical, including photocopying or recording, or by any information storage and retrieval system, without permission in writing from the publisher.

Front cover image © tsuponk/Shutterstock

Printed in the United States of America

*McFarland & Company, Inc., Publishers
Box 611, Jefferson, North Carolina 28640
www.mcfarlandpub.com*

Dedicated to my Guinevere…

"But sweeter still than this, than these, than all,
is first and passionate Love—it stands alone."

And to everyone who acts shocked when history repeats itself.

Table of Contents

Introduction	1
I. Disease and the Conquest of the Americas	5
II. Inoculation Intrigue	15
III. A Nation Forged in Gout	27
IV. Mosquitos and the Emergence of Political Parties	36
V. Buffalo Fever and the Anti-War Movement	48
VI. "A people so well fed and so clean": Cholera and Jacksonian Politics	56
VII. Presidential Poxes	64
VIII. "The Wretched Refuse": Disease and 19th-Century Immigration Debates	71
IX. Rashes and Reforms	91
X. The Pox of Progressivism: Vaccinations	104
XI. The Pox of Progressivism: Culling the Herd	116
XII. Disease and the Democratic Process	137
XIII. Immigration and Illness in the 20th Century	156
XIV. The AIDS Epidemic?	162
XV. Moon Fever	171
XVI. The "Wuhan" Virus	183
Conclusion	206
Chapter Notes	211
Bibliography	233
Index	237

Introduction

"It's a virus. It's not a political weapon." Despite this statement by then-presidential candidate Joe Biden in October of 2020, the pandemic raging at that time had become perhaps the deciding issue in the upcoming election and one seized upon by both major parties. Yet, the politicization of pestilence was not a new phenomenon. Neither is it an occurrence solely tied to American politics or even the Western world. Disease has a been a constant presence in human society since its formation; this is a truism across the globe and across the human experience. Despite religious differences, geographic determinism, developmental advantages, resource benefits, etc., all civilizations have had to contend with illness. From this common experience has likewise arisen the habit of people using disease to push political ends. Whether its origins and treatments could be explained religiously, naturally, or scientifically, disease has often presented a useful tool for those either in power or seeking to obtain it.

The history of disease in humans stretches back to the Paleolithic Age. Prior to the development of agriculture, roaming bands of hunter-gatherers had to contend mostly with parasites, worms, and bacteria in terms of threats to their health. These have been referred to as heirloom and souvenir diseases, with some existing as holdovers from earlier stages of hominid development while others were acquired during man's movement out of Africa.[1] The migratory nature of human bands, necessitated by their hunting and gathering activities, produced a poor breeding ground for microbes. Man's mobility allowed him to outpace viruses and move away from disease-infested areas. The disease-ridden slums and tenements of the late 19th century and Satanic mills of Blake were unheard of by these early people. At the same time, the movement of man was limited enough to prevent the spread of epidemics over wide areas. In effect, plagues could move no faster at the time than a human could walk and the gaps between human settlements became an epidemiological cordon sanitaire.

The limited population density of the hunting group also helped to negate possible epidemics by producing a dead end for the spread of disease. Most members of the band would undoubtedly become quickly infected, either surviving and developing an increased tolerance, or else the band would be destroyed, taking the disease with it. Likewise, the size of the group and lack of domestication limited the possibility of zoomorphic mutation. Changes in viruses require a larger environment of hosts than early bands of people presented.

The development of disease both paralleled and overlapped the development of advanced society. It is a fundamental truism that the presence of disease necessitates the development of ways to deal with it. Government, communication, science, and law all arise or advance, in part, to deal with pestilence. Conversely, one can see a lack of advancement in primitive society in direct correlation to its lack of disease. Likewise, as society became more settled and more modern, conditions for the rise and spread of disease increased. Advancement produces disease; disease produces advancement.

Man's early encounters with disease were coupled with attempts to resolve the issue. These would often alternate between the natural and the spiritual, with either the application of plants and remedies or the direct appeal to divine powers. The latter method soon became a legitimizing tool for those in power, beginning the politicization of pestilence. Priest-kings in Mesopotamia, pharaohs in Egypt, and the early Shang and Zhou monarchs, among dozens of other examples, saw themselves as the connecting factor between their people and the gods. Disease was largely seen as a personal or divine punishment. This in turn then served as a means by which to protect themselves and their position against the nobles and commoners, as any attempt to overthrow or remove them could be seen as an affront to the gods.

Yet, this belief could become a two-edged sword, as it did in China. Following the rise of the Zhou Dynasty, the concept of the Mandate of Heaven became the dominant political philosophy of the nation for the next 3,000 years. While this was initially an attempt to formalize the right of the Duke of Zhou to take over the title of monarch from the Shang rulers, it later evolved into a general theory on the right of kings to rule. Kings and emperors were seen as receiving their mandate directly from the heavens, but it was entirely dependent upon their virtue as a leader. Under Confucian thought, should the ruler become unvirtuous he could lose the mandate and thus be rightfully resisted or overthrown.

The obvious conundrum, however, was how to tell if the king had actually lost the mandate. Confucian and Daoist scholars opined that this could be discerned through an examination of nature. Due to the monarch's position as the axis between heaven and earth, a disruption in his virtue would manifest itself through famine, natural disaster, and epidemics. Thus, new rulers, once they had seized power, were quick to justify their rebellion by highlighting the various disasters to befall the Middle Kingdom during the previous ruler's time on the throne. The appearance of pestilence or the inability of the leader to successfully confront it, regardless of the era, were challenges to his legitimacy.

This basic formula would find its way into Western political and social thought as well. Regardless of whether disease was seen as natural or divine in either cause or cure, populations looked to leaders to confront them. Part of this undoubtedly emerged from the leaders' own efforts to politicize epidemics. By making disease a state or national issue, communities and individuals began to see themselves as powerless in terms of response. The demands made upon the Church during the Black Death, the Anglo-French belief in the "king's touch" to cure scrofula, and even Parisian riots in the mid–19th century over the government's lack of solution to the cholera crisis all attest to this.

As with all other countries and cultures, America has seen much of its political history, economic development, and social characteristics impacted by pestilence. From the very conquest and settling of the continent, a feat almost entirely completed by disease, onward to the arrival of the pandemic of 2019, there are very few events in the nation's history that have not been caused, catalyzed, furthered, or impacted by illness.

At the same time, the history of the political system of the country has been one of an ever-increasing government, in terms of both its size and grasp. From the administration of Washington to that of Biden, certain groups have pushed for a growth of government. For good or bad, disease has often played a role in this trend. While some have argued for a need to expand state and federal power in order to tackle illness and benefit public health, others have merely used the threat of disease as an excuse to consolidate power and push other agendas. This book seeks to examine both trends and show how pestilence has influenced politics since the founding of the Americas. The politicization of disease is not a new trend but rather one with ancient roots. Yet, it is a phenomenon that has only increased in scope and occurrence over the course of time.

Chapter I

Disease and the Conquest of the Americas

Throughout history, disease has always been a useful means by which to attack "the other." Epidemics and pandemics do not spontaneously generate in a location but instead tend to arrive from elsewhere. Carried by immigrants, traders, armies, or religious processions, contagious disease is usually an external threat. Therefore, it is not surprising to see the origins of disease used as a means by which to smear other nations and people. From the targeting of Jews during the 14th-century Bubonic Plague or Chinese citizens of San Francisco during an outbreak of the same disease there in the 1900s, this practice continues to the present day.

Part of this arises from a traditional belief in the origins of disease. For thousands of years, most civilizations viewed illness as a negative that arose due to some failing on the part of the victim, be it moral or physical. While sickness obviously affected all, it was particularly noticed, mentioned, and emphasized when it struck those who we already viewed as "others" or enemies. The beginnings of this process in American history can be observed in English propaganda against the Spanish, specifically in how the historiography of the conquest of the Americas by the Spanish and the English was portrayed in relation to pestilence. For one, the role of disease was either ignored in order to exaggerate tales of brutality or else depicted as a barbarous tactic, while for the other, outbreaks of pestilence were praised as acts of God or blamed on the primitive nature of the Natives. From the earliest days of the Americas, disease was a useful political weapon.

The Black Legend

Spain has long been a traditional enemy of England, stretching back to at least the period of the Hundred Years' War in the 14th century.

London's traditional alliance with Lisbon early on led to confrontations with Castile, as the various Iberian powers jockeyed for position on the peninsula. These initial disputes though, were seemingly resolved in the early 16th century, as Catherine of Aragon was successively married to Arthur Tudor and, following his untimely demise due to an illness, to his brother Henry VIII. Yet, with her subsequent divorce by Henry and the abandonment of the Roman Catholic church by England, relations between the two began to collapse once more. The concurrent rise of British colonialism in the 17th century thereafter led to over three centuries of conflict between the two states.

Some of the earliest interactions of politics and illness in Anglo-Spanish relations occurred with Catherine of Aragon herself. Medical speculation has always existed as to the causes of Henry's inability to produce an heir with Catherine. While his subsequent failure in his other marriages to likewise produce many surviving children has shifted much of the focus for a cause onto him, initial speculation seems to have been cast on Catherine. This was due to both archaic biological and political reasons.

A letter written by Pope Julius II (r. 1503–1513) early on in her marriage seems to suggest that the young Spanish princess was anorexic. According to the missive, Catherine was prone to excessive fasting under the guise of religious zeal. Julius, while commending the "fervor of her devotion," warned that she "does not have the full power of her own body, and the devotions and fasting ... if they are thought to stand in the way of her physical health and the procreation of children ... can be revoked and annulled by men." According to the pope, her husband had the temporal power to overrule her religious pursuits if they "would stand in the way of the procreation of children."[1] If true, the pope's concerns were not unfounded, as anorexia has been shown to present challenges toward the conception and healthy delivery of infants.[2] Yet, this could also simply have been an attempt to both simply shift the blame toward Catherine, while also showing that it was within Henry's power to correct the issue short of divorce. Though more recent research has tended to place the blame on any number of medical and genetic conditions within Henry VIII himself, questions about Catherine's health have remained popular in English sources and periodicals to the present day.[3]

The religious, colonial, and political differences and conflicts that arose between England and Spain were accompanied by a centuries-long propaganda war. While disparaging one's enemy was certainly not a new phenomenon, the creation of the printing press at this time meant that criticism of Spain became both widespread and permanent. Likewise, the religious component of the conflict produced a visceral reaction between

I. Disease and the Conquest of the Americas

the two parties that went far beyond traditional views of enmity. Catholic Spain became the source of all evil and sin to English audiences.

The charges against Spain became so outlandish and all-encompassing that a name was eventually developed for the practice, the Black Legend. Yet, the smears were so successful that they became accepted facts for many in the Protestant and Anglo-Saxon world for centuries. As one historian has noted, "Their own self-identity came to be linked with blind opposition to the Catholic monarchs and Habsburg dynasty."[4] America's English roots and a reliance on the available English historical sources meant that many of these beliefs became standard for Americans as well.

Some of the more famous charges leveled against the Spanish involved their exploration and conquest of the New World. The source for much of this was the writing of Bartolomé de Las Casas. Though originally a landowner in the New World, he became disillusioned with what he saw as the extreme methods employed by some conquistadors and strove instead for the conversion of the Indians. He returned to Spain in 1515 and began a lifelong campaign aimed at reducing the suffering of Native Americans and pushing for the spread of Catholicism. His *A Short Account of the Destruction of the Indies* detailed numerous massacres and acts of torture committed by the Spanish in the New World and became the authentic text for those who engaged in spreading the Black Legend.

Yet, for all of its inclusion of allegedly accurate scenes of torture and brutality, it makes no mention of the impact of disease upon the Natives. Subsequent research has now demonstrated that 80–90 percent of all Native Americans died within a century of Columbus' landing due to disease, not the brutality of conquest. De Las Casas' omission of pestilence in his widely circulated book reinforced the notion of the Spanish as bloodthirsty brutes. Without disease as the most prominent cause of this population decline, murder remained the only other logical explanation in the minds of the public. Five centuries later, it is still widely read and used in almost all school curricula. An early acknowledgment of the unintended consequence of spreading disease among the Natives may have done much to dismantle centuries of the Black Legend. It is debatable whether de Las Casas' omission was due to lack of knowledge or simply as a means by which to further drive home his thesis.

As for the Spanish themselves, their sources from the time period made frequent reference to the role that disease played in the devastation of the Natives.[5] Perhaps the first of these were letters to Charles V from Vázquez de Ayllón and Hernán Cortés, both writing only a year after the conquest. Bernal Díaz del Castillo, who accompanied the Spanish army that reduced Tenochtitlan, wrote his own history of the time period titled

The Discovery and Conquest of Mexico 1517–1521. In it, he makes reference to the arrival of smallpox in Mesoamerica.

> He happened to have a negro servant with him ill with the smallpox, through whom this terrific disease, which, according to the accounts of the inhabitants, was previously unknown in the country, spread itself through New Spain, where it created the greater devastation, from the poor Indians, in their ignorance, solely applying cold water as a remedy, with which they constantly bathed themselves; so that vast numbers were cut off before they had the blessing of being received into the bosom of the Christian church.[6]

Del Castillo's assessment was shared by numerous other contemporary Iberian writers as well, including Francisco de Gómara. Interestingly, del Castillo claimed that one of his primary motivations in writing a history of the conquest was to correct the errors of Gómara who nevertheless put forward the proposition that at least half of the Aztecs succumbed to the illness. Finally, Fray Juan de Torquemada would write extensively on his own experiences during an outbreak of pestilence in 1576.

> In the year 1576 a great mortality and pestilence that lasted for more than a year overcame the Indians. It was so big that it ruined and destroyed almost the entire land. The place we know as New Spain was left almost empty. It was a thing of great bewilderment to see the people die. Many were dead and others almost dead, and nobody had the health or strength to help the diseases or bury the dead. In the cities and large towns, big ditches were dug, and from morning to sunset the priests did nothing else but carry the dead bodies and throw them into the ditches without any of the solemnity usually reserved for the dead, because the time did not allow otherwise. At night they covered the ditches with dirt.... It lasted for one and a half years, and with great excess in the number of deaths. After the murderous epidemic, the viceroy Martin Enriquez wanted to know the number of missing people in New Spain. After searching in towns and neighborhoods it was found that the number of deaths was more than two million.[7]

Yet, the trend of ignoring the impact of disease upon the decimation of the Natives in favor of blaming purely Spanish butchery continued in most English language history texts that covered the history of the New World. John Campbell's 1762 *An Account of the Spanish Settlement in America* makes no mention of disease as playing a factor in the Spanish conquest of the lands from Mexico to Argentina, nor does the 1789 *The History of South America*. Arthur Help's 1856 work on the conquest of the Americas contains his opinion on the arrival of disease: "I think this cause of the destruction of the Indians (a very convenient one for the conquerors to allege) has been exaggerated."[8]

As late as 1992, 500 years after the arrival of Columbus, a collection of historical essays published under the title *1492: An Ongoing Voyage*,

I. Disease and the Conquest of the Americas

continued to suggest that steel weapons and Native disunity were the biggest problems facing the Natives. For the Spanish themselves, "the greatest problem was fatigue from so much fighting and killing."[9] Interestingly, the author does go on to admit "more Spaniards died in the Conquest years from disease ... than were killed by Indian attacks," but does not make the same claim about the Natives.

Not surprisingly, the British would politicize disease with other national enemies as well. Though their attacks on the Spanish lasted the longest due to centuries of opposition, during times when relations improved or a larger threat surfaced, London's newspapers would focus their attention on the greater threat. Just such an episode occurred during the Great Plague of London. While Daniel Defoe makes mention of Spain's strict quarantine against English ships during the epidemic, he recounts that rumors placed the blame for the outbreak on the French. "Hence it was that this rumour died off again, and people began to forget it as a thing we were very little concerned in, and that we hoped was not true; till the latter end of November or the beginning of December 1664 when two men, said to be Frenchmen, died of the plague in Long Acre."[10] At the time, England was in an uneasy alliance with Spain and the Netherlands against the growing threat of France, culminating in the War of Devolution in 1667, thus it is not surprising to see their pestilence fueled propaganda shifting toward a new target.

Even when it became well known centuries later that smallpox destroyed far more cultures than did Spanish arms, they were oftentimes still held liable for its spread. The historiography of the 1990s began to slowly, and oftentimes begrudgingly, accept the role that disease played in the depopulation of the Americas upon the arrival of the Spanish and others.[11] Yet, it was still viewed through the lens of the Myth of the Noble Savage. As one historian stated, "The Indians who lived in contact with Spanish civilization became dirty because of the disintegration of the moral fiber of their people under the heel of the white man's rule ... the white man's diseases were a far more terrible scourge than even his guns or lash."[12] The transfer of disease along trade routes or through human migration and conquest, a normal occurrence over the past 5,000 years, now became a conscious sin of the Spanish.

This concept was taken a step further by many with the crafting of a legend that the Spanish utilized smallpox blankets to decimate their opponents. As one text stated in 1975, "The conquest of Mexico was accomplished by a 'handful of Spaniards and one Negro with smallpox' whose bedding was given to natives."[13] Historian Adrienne Mayor traced the first occurrence of this story to a Peruvian account written in 1613, which described a black-cloaked Spaniard who presented the Incan ruler with a box, inside of which was "the smallpox plague … which flew out."[14] These tales would proliferate and expand over the years, becoming accepted history by many. In the 19th and 20th centuries, the concept of smallpox being weaponized and delivered by gifts was also occasionally levelled against the United States government. This became the preferred historiography of many on the political left in an attempt to demonize the country's interactions with Native Americans.

Interestingly, the only contemporary documentation which discusses possibly weaponizing smallpox and using it against Natives concerned the English military. In a letter written in 1763, Lord Jeffery Amherst queried Colonel Henry Bouquet whether "it not be contrived to send the small pox among the disaffected tribes of Indians? We must on this occasion use every strategem in our power to reduce them."[15] Bouquet allegedly wrote back committing himself to do just that. Though an outbreak of smallpox did decimate the Natives besieging Fort Pitt that summer, historians are divided as to its actual origins.

The Black Legend was utilized during the 16th through 20th centuries to disparage the Spanish and Catholicism, while at the same time promoting the superiority of the Anglo-Saxon, Protestant settlement of the New World. Later still, it became expanded to include the American push westward and southward. Part of the impetus for the launching of the Spanish-American War was the use of yellow journalism to blame the Spanish for the destructive diseases that were killing hundreds of thousands in Cuba in the 1890s. Modern-day controversies over the celebration of Columbus Day and historical practices of assimilation, as well as left-wing ideological attacks on capitalism, perceived white supremacy, and religious institutions, all rely heavily on the myths and exaggerations associated with these stories.

The White Legend

At the same time that the Spanish were being portrayed as brutal conquerors, the English settlement of the Atlantic seaboard was written of in an entirely different light. While the Indian population of the region had most likely already been heavily depleted over the previous century due to disease and intertribal warfare, there still remained a considerable presence upon the landing of the first English colonists at Jamestown and Plymouth. Disease once more played a pivotal role in the success of European efforts in the region but, in this case, the historiography was presented in a much more positive fashion for purely political reasons.

The three main English attempts at early colonization in the future

I. Disease and the Conquest of the Americas

United States, at Roanoke, Jamestown, and Plymouth, were all both harmed and helped to a degree by disease. While Jamestown and Plymouth saw their European populations decimated by illness, the settlements of New England and Virginia were also aided by the decline in Native populations brought about by the introduction of disease.

Shortly after Walter Raleigh was granted the rights to establish a colony in the New World, he sent out a small expedition to investigate the region. Known as the Amadas-Barlowe Expedition, it sailed in 1584 and made contact with the Secotan Indians of the Roanoke region. The relative success of the mission led to the launching of the Lane Expedition in 1585 for the express purpose of settlement. Yet, despite high initial hopes for the colony, labor disputes, food shortages, and hostilities with the local tribes brought it close to complete destruction. What ended up saving at least a portion of the expedition was disease.

At one point, the colonists began to engage the Secotan Indians in the hopes of acquiring more food and supplies. Though the talks amounted to little, the face-to-face contact between the two would have longer-lasting results. Thomas Harriot would record how, in the aftermath of the English journeys from town to town,

> that within a few dayes after our departure from euerie such towne, the people began to die very fast, and many in short space; in some townes about twentie, in some fourtie, in some sixtie, & in one sixe score, which in trueth was very manie in respect of their numbers. This happened in no place that wee coulde learne but where wee had bene, where they vsed some practise against vs, and after such time; The disease also so strange, that they neither knew what it was, nor how to cure it; the like by report of the oldest men in the countrey neuer happened before, time out of minde.[16]

Panic and confusion gripped the Natives as they sought an explanation to these waves of contagion. Some blamed the English directly while others thought that the colonists were capable of firing "invisible disease bullets." Many of the advisors of Chief Wingina (also known as Pemisapan) urged action be taken against the English, and eventually he relented. Messengers were sent out to various neighboring tribes, and only the quick and preemptive actions of Lane saved his men from complete slaughter. Despite this victory, the English chose to abandon the colony in 1590.

The failed attempt by the English to colonize Roanoke in the late 16th century dampened the desire of those in the British Isles who sought to settle in or profit from the New World. The mysterious and dangerous land across the Atlantic was viewed as the home of whatever terrors the English mind could conceive. Yet, the expedition did succeed in a far greater way than those back in London could have dreamed of. Much as Cortez had laid the foundations for the destruction of the Aztec empire during his first failed visit to Tenochtitlan, so too did the English ensure future success in Virginia on top of the ruins of Roanoke.

The "Roanoke Disease," now tentatively identified as influenza, ravaged the Natives of the region during the 1580s and 1590s.[17] By the time the English returned to the region in the first decade of the 1600s, they encountered a far different environment. The werowance of the Accomac tribe told John Smith during his June 1608 visit "a strange mortalitie … affected a greater part of his people … and but few escaped."[18] The effects of the contagion were magnified by the fact that the region experienced at the same time the worst drought in centuries. Crop failures from 1587 to 1589 would have weakened the local Natives' ability to fend off such diseases as influenza. Leadership of the region likewise became insecure as the local chieftains succumbed to the plague. As well, the damage to the religious beliefs and institutions of the Natives must have been profound as their traditional methods did little to stem the rising tide of deaths. Thus, though Roanoke failed as a colony, it was a necessary failure that allowed for the development of Jamestown.

John Smith, in his 1624 work, *The General History of Virginia, New England, and the Summer Isle*, does frequently reference disease as a characteristic of the Indians in the region. In this case the diseases afflicting them was portrayed as indigenous to the region and as due to their own "primitive" lifestyles and medicinal practices. Interestingly, Smith does reference the emergence of an epidemic in the region following a visit by the English, but this would become viewed in the dominant historiography as a positive and unrelated to what transpired in Spanish America.

The end result of this ambition was finally realized in September of 1620 when 102 passengers boarded the *Mayflower*. Two months later, in November, the Saints (the term used by the Pilgrims to refer to themselves) arrived off the coast of Cape Cod. Landing late in the year and with their food supplies exhausted, the colonists took to raiding Native American graves for corn. Even with these additional supplies, by the spring of 1621, 45 of the original 102 colonists had perished, mostly from disease.

But while Jamestown was largely saved by the perseverance of John Smith and the marital and economic decisions of John Rolfe, Plymouth was preserved, in part, by disease. Unlike their cousins in Virginia, the Pilgrims noticed a distinct lack of Native presence following their arrival. A decade before the English landed at Plymouth, the region of New England was home to an estimated 144,000 inhabitants. The colonists upon landing, though, encountered more graves and bones than actual Natives. To the Puritans this was surely the wrath of God, punishing the Natives for their heathen behavior. As John Winthrop wrote at the time, "The natives,

I. Disease and the Conquest of the Americas   13

they are near all dead of the smallpox, so as the Lord has cleared our title to what we possess."[19]

From around 1616 to 1619 the indigenous people of New England were visited by a pestilence that destroyed their society. It is estimated that much like in other parts of the Americas up to 90 percent of the Natives were exterminated. Only one tribe, the Narragansett, escaped relatively unharmed, with this most likely being due to their practice of burning their dead. The exact pathogen that visited the region has been much debated, with historians and medical experts suggesting smallpox, influenza, diphtheria, and, more recently, leptospirosis as a possible agent of the Natives' destruction.[20]

English fishermen had plied the coast of New England for over a generation, while minor attempts were made to settle both Cuttyhunk and Popham in 1602 and 1607 in search of sassafras (a reputed cure for syphilis).[21] In fact, at the time the Pilgrims landed they reported that they found graves that contained European remains. It is obvious that Europeans had a presence, albeit a small one, in the region of New England for years before the Pilgrims arrived. As has been made evident repeatedly before this point, the presence of Europeans invariably spread disease through the Native communities. These fishermen and proto-colonists laid low the population of New England a decade before the arrival of the Saints, thus paving the way for an easier colonization. The Puritans could rightly claim their success as an act of God.

Perhaps the situation was best summed up by Robert Cushman in 1621:

> They were very much wasted of late, by reason of a great mortality that fell amongst them three years since; which, together with their own civil dissensions and bloody wars, hath so wasted them, as I think the twentieth person is scarce left alive; and those that are left, have their courage much abated, and their countenance dejected, and they seem as a people affrighted. And though when we first came into the country, were few, and many of us were sick, and many died by reason of the cold and wet, it being the depth of winter, and we having no houses nor shelter, yet when there was not six able persons among us, and that they came daily to us by hundreds, with their sachems and kings, and might in one hour have made a dispatch of us, yet such a fear was upon them, as that they never offered us the least injury in word or deed.[22]

The settlement of Plymouth, much like that of Jamestown, was not only burdened by disease but aided by it as well. Disease cleared the region of opposition to both English ventures; bound the colonists more closely together through necessity; and created the prospect of novel cultural, political, and societal evolvements to deal with the various contagions. At the same time, Puritan beliefs trumpeted the decimation of the Natives through disease as a sign of divine providence, epidemiologically confirming that this New World belonged to the English by the grace of God. Lord Byron's similar poetic description of the destruction of the Assyrians by disease nicely sums up the English view of predestined and divine victory. "And the might of the Gentile, unsmote by the sword, Hath melted like snow in the glance of the Lord!"

Nor did the English reliance upon disease as a means by which to push forward its colonies end with the Natives. A smallpox epidemic in the 1630s so decimated the Indians of Connecticut that the colonists were able to quickly overrun the region and deprive the Dutch of a strong foothold there. A similar smallpox outbreak in 1663 would significantly weaken the Dutch position at Ft. Orange, present-day Albany. The arrival of an English invasion fleet the next year would encounter little resistance and seize the entire region between Massachusetts and Virginia with little effort. The Puritans remarked at the time, "The hand of God had gone out against the people of New Netherlands by pestilential infections."[23]

The Spanish were brutal conquerors and butchers who used disease as a weapon to devastate the Natives. On the other hand, the English were lucky enough to move into areas that disease had unfortunately cleared out due to either the primitive nature of the Indians or else the divine will of God. These two separate views of the impact of disease on the early settlement of the Americas would begin a long process of the politicization of pestilence.

Chapter II

Inoculation Intrigue

One of the great historical and political myths to emerge in the politicized history of the past few centuries was that the great waves of smallpox that decimated the Native American populations from the Arctic to Tierra del Fuego somehow bypassed European settlers. In reality, smallpox was an old nemesis in the West, being either endemic to areas or progressing across the continent in periodic epidemics. While still deadly, the majority of Europeans were at least familiar with the disease and had methods by which to reduce its severity, though not without much external and internal scaring. Yet, the Native inhabitants of the Americas were not the only group in the Western Hemisphere to suffer severely from the contagion. Despite living in such an alleged virgin and pristine landscape, the colonists of America tended to succumb to smallpox at higher rates than their European cousins.[1] This was largely due to the irregular nature of outbreaks in the colonies as well as limited access to medicine and doctors. Likewise, many of the settlers contracted the disease at a later age, increasing their likelihood of death. While to many of the Calvinists of New England, perhaps, this was simply the will of God, not all were willing to accept that fate.

Their religious beliefs notwithstanding, the Puritans did seek to take at least some precaution against the pestilence. After an outbreak in 1677 that led to the death of over a thousand in the colony, Boston's town council decided upon the traditional tactic of quarantine, utilizing Deer Island for the purpose.[2] Infected ships would be required to dock there for eight days before coming into Boston proper. However, following subsequent outbreaks in 1690 and 1702, the council abandoned Deer Island in favor of the slightly more isolated Spectacle Island.[3] Yet, considering the proximity of both islands to Boston itself, the allusive nature of the disease, the slow course of communication between ship and port and council, and the lack of direct control over the port, quarantine was a net rather than a wall of protection.

Around 1707, the venerable Cotton Mather was informed by a slave named Onesimus how he had been inoculated in his homeland of Africa against smallpox.⁴ The slave related the details of the method known as variolation, in which material from a smallpox pustule was rubbed into a surgical incision, and proudly recounted the success of the process in his home region. The procedure itself is claimed to have been developed in China before the year 1500 and was widespread in the Middle East by the 1600s. From there it spread along the slave and caravan routes throughout Africa, eventually reaching the Coromantee tribe of modern-day Ghana from which Onesimus claimed membership. The idea that disease could be prevented as well as treated was only just gaining traction in the West and was not accepted by all. The reverend himself had personal reasons for being interested in this matter however, as he had lost two wives to illness and had buried nine of his fifteen children.

Mather was among the earliest group of Westerners to hear about smallpox inoculation. A letter from a Greek physician named Emanuel Timonius that detailed the process made its way around much of Europe in 1714. The *Philosophical Transactions of the Royal Society* for that year states:

> The writer of this ingenious discourse observes, in the first place, that the Circassians, Georgians, and other Asiatics, have introduced this practice of procuring the smallpox by a sort of inoculation, for about the space of forty years, among the Turks and others at Constantinople. That although at first the more prudent were very cautious in the use of this practice; yet the happy success it has found to have in thousands of subjects for these eight years past has put it out of all suspicion and doubt; since the operation, having been performed on persons of all ages, sexes, and different temperaments ... none have been found to die of the smallpox.⁵

Reading this tract in Massachusetts, Mather wrote to London to confirm that he too had heard about the process.

> I am willing to confirm to you, in a favourable opinion, of Dr. Timonius' communication; and therefore, I do assure you, that many months before I met with any intimations of treating the smallpox with the method of inoculation, anywhere in Europe; I had from a servant of my own an account of its being practised in Africa. Enquiring of my Negro man, Onesimus, who is a pretty intelligent fellow, whether he had ever had the smallpox, he answered, both yes and no; and then told me that he had undergone an operation, which had given him something of the smallpox and would forever preserve him from it; adding that it was often used among the Guramantese and whoever had the courage to use it was forever free of the fear of contagion. He described the operation to me, and showed me in his arm the scar which it had left upon him; and his description of it made it the same that afterwards I found related unto you by your Timonius.⁶

II. Inoculation Intrigue

The British ambassador to the Ottoman Empire was first introduced to the process a few years later between 1716 and 1717. His wife, Lady Mary Montagu, subsequently had a Greek physician variolate her own son. After returning to England, she also had a Scottish doctor perform the same procedure on her daughter as well. An epidemic of the disease in England around the same time sparked further discussion of the idea. Having heard of the English outbreak, Cotton Mather went as far as to inform Dr. John Woodward of Gresham College in 1716 that he planned to inoculate his own family and servants against the terrible scourge. It was well understood by this point that an epidemic in one country could quickly arrive in another. Thus, Mather's idea was a preventative measure against what he saw as a certain, future outbreak in the colony.

By the early 1700s, Boston had grown to be a large city. In fact, with over 11,000 souls inhabiting its environs, it was the largest port city in the colonies, with a population almost 50 percent greater than New York City. Therefore, it was very likely hardly noticed by most residents when the HMS *Seahorse* docked in April of 1721. Formerly stationed in the waters off of Barbados, the ship had been part of the British naval effort to protect its profitable sugar trade in the region. A very valuable commodity at the time, sugar heavily impacted colonization, foreign relations, and slavery. The sugar it helped to escort to Boston among various holds was a welcome arrival; the smallpox hidden among the sailors was not.

Once it became known that sailors aboard the ship were stricken with smallpox, Governor Samuel Shute called for a quarantine of the vessel at Spectacle Island. Yet, as many of the sailors had already come ashore, this action was too late. With the arrival of May, eight cases of the disease were reported in Boston, despite the best efforts of local authorities to quarantine the infected. Attempts to cleanse the streets in order to destroy the scourge, proved to be little more effective than the quarantine. Despite all efforts of the town selectman, the sickness continued to spread and, with it, disease's secondary weapons, rumor and panic.

By June, the disease was spreading quickly. In response, nearly 10 percent of the population of the city fled, a typical and age-old response to pandemics. One thousand Bostonians, including the majority of the government, crossed the neck connecting Boston to the mainland, spreading throughout the surrounding area. Obviously, this would serve only to frighten other towns of the region who feared that the disease would spread with the refugees. In response, many other towns and villages began to close their gates to exiles. Trade to and from the port of Boston declined to a trickle as merchants feared to trade with the city and dock workers who stayed inside. Likewise, as traditionally only the wealthy bore the means by which to extricate themselves from an infected town, flight often became a contentious issue between the classes.

Toward the end of summer, the death toll had climbed to 101. Looked at another way, this amounted to 1 percent of the entire pre-plague population of Boston who died in only four months. More Bostonians began to flee, homes fell into disrepair, and basic services began to break down. Yet, the rumor mill that existed and continues to exist in all small towns in America, did not cease to function.

Stories began to spread among the locals of a doctor in town performing smallpox experiments on various persons. Rumor and whisper soon gave way to anger at the thought of the doctor adding to the contagion by purposefully infecting more people. One of the prominent papers of the time, *The New England Courant*, published by James Franklin, spoke out voraciously against the process, adding much fuel to the fire. Yet the truth, when it was learned, proved to be far more disturbing to Boston.

Cotton Mather had never given up the idea of preventative inoculation.

> The grievous Calamity of the Small-Pox has now entered the Town. The Practice of conveying and suffering the Small-pox by Inoculation, has never been used in America, nor indeed in our Nation. But how many Lives might be saved by it, if it were prasticed?[7]

In fact, at the same time in June 1721 that he was preaching obedience to the will of God from the Book of Job to his Boston congregation at the height of the pestilence, he was also writing about quite the opposite. Mather had begun a correspondence with a local doctor named Zabdiel Boylston. Both in letters to the physician and in a series of essays that would eventually become the work *The Angel of Bethesda*, Cotton Mather argued for the use of inoculation both to combat the current smallpox crisis and prevent its reoccurrence. To Mather, though disease was certainly a punishment from God, not using God's gifts (including mental and scientific) to combat it was equally sinful.

Boylston soon acquiesced, deciding to begin the process of inoculation. Using methods recommended by the Royal Society and recounted to Mather by his slave Onesimus, the doctor acquired active *variola* virus to apply to cuts on his patients' bodies. As he himself was naturally immune to the disease, he instead chose three others to begin his experiments. For this, Boylston selected his six-year-old son Thomas, as well as two of his slaves. The inoculation worked perfectly and all three recovered within a week. Boylston had proved that the various accounts of African slaves and the thoughts of Mather and the Royal Society were correct: inoculation could be performed. By mid–July, the doctor had successfully inoculated seven more individuals. Though Boylston had certainly demonstrated the ability to beat smallpox, the question of "should he have" was yet to be answered.

Dr. William Douglass published that same year a pamphlet titled *The Abuses and Scandals of Some Late Pamphlets in Favour of Inoculation of the Small Pox*. It was a general attack on Cotton Mather, seeking to dismantle both his religious and medical arguments for the practice. Douglass accused him and his supporters of "Popish" practices in theology as well as challenged his medical knowledge. "How then can we suppose, a Man of a *Vocation*, which requires all his Time conscientiously to discharge the same, should pretend to a Business of so great Extent? ... To be more or less *Book learned*, is not a sufficient Qualification for a *Physician*."[8] Not surprisingly, one of the publishers of the brochure was James Franklin.

Franklin's newspaper, the *New England Courant*, had only just started publication and, though he offered his pages to both sides to publish reasoned arguments, it quickly became the mouthpiece of those opposed to vaccination. The dispute quickly became a political battle between the Puritan establishment, represented by Mather and Benjamin Colman who published in the *Boston Gazette*, and those duly engaged in medicine, notably Douglass and others. A fiery feud developed as each side lobbed articles, broadsides, and attacks upon the other.

A July 17 article in the *Courant* accused Boylston of being "an undertaker" and "illiterate" and noted the foreign nature of the cure.[9] By August, the paper was accusing Mather and his clique of spreading "false rumors" that were destroying the commerce of the city.[10] Rumors even circulated that Douglass himself had suddenly become stricken with the disease that he had sought to downplay, though Franklin was quick to denounce these claims.

As autumn approached, the death toll mounted and so too did the number of inoculations. By October, 411 men and women had died. Similarly, Dr. Boylston increased the number of people inoculated. Public opinion increasingly turned against the inoculations being used. Many began to see Boylston's actions as either an offense against God's prerogative or possibly a catalyst for the epidemic. An article published a month before stated:

> But Epidemeal Distempers, as they more immediately proceed from a Divine stretched-out Arm, and as sent as Judgments from an angry and displeased God, so they require a different Physic, a different Way of Prevention, Being the greatest Marks of the greatest displeasure, so they call for the greatest Humiliation, the Observation of the strictest Duties of Repentance.[11]

A local parishioner went so far as to throw a homemade grenade into the house of Cotton Mather in November while a minister of Roxbury, a kinsman of Mather, was there to be inoculated. Luckily for the pastor, the zealot's skill in throwing was no better than his science, and the fuse was knocked off as it entered the window. The grenade and its attached note, though, clearly delivered the feeling of much of the public: "Cotton Mather: you Dog, Damn you, I'll inoculate you with this, and a Pox to you."[12] Mather's own thoughts on the matter clearly show his view of both inoculation and its deriders.

> At this Time, I enjoy and unspeakable Consolation. I have instructed our Physicians in the new Method used by the Africans and Asiaticks, to prevent and abate the Dangers of the Small-Pox.... The Destroyer, being enraged at the Proposal of any Thing, that may rescue the Lives of our poor People from him, has taken a strange Possession of the People on this Occasion. They rave, they rail, they blaspheme; they talk not only like Ideots but also like Franticks, And not only the Physician who began the Experiment, but I also am an Object of their Fury.[13]

A similar attack would take place against the good doctor shortly after, with a bomb landing in his parlor where his wife was sitting. Some in the medical community even criticized the nature of Boylston's experiments as well.

By February, the plague had subsided. Over 5,889 persons had been infected, with 844 of them succumbing to death. Three-fourths of all those who died in the Boston region in 1721 did so from the smallpox outbreak. Yet, Boylston's actions were seen by his supporters as a success. In the end he had inoculated 242 individuals, with only six dying from smallpox.

Some embraced the failure of the plague to spread outside of Boston as further proof that variolation was at the least unnecessary or at the most dangerous.

> Who then but Madmen, would have advised Inoculation in the severest Season to those who are like forever to escape the Small Pox? In this Town several Hundreds have escaped, and it is probable many more might have escaped (as was the Case Nineteen Years ago) if Inoculation had not rendred the Infection so universal and intense.[14]

One's view of both the disease and the success of Boylston's treatment became heavily intertwined and politicized.

The plague of 1721 became a religious and political tool in surrounding colonies as well. To the south, the royal colony of Connecticut had been battling with various religious sects for decades, with perhaps one of the most notable being the Rogerenes. Founded in the 1670s by John Rogers, a member of perhaps the wealthiest family in the colony, it quickly moved against many of the practices of the politically dominant Congregationalist church. Among its various beliefs was an anathema to medicine and modern healing practices, instead relying on prayer and the laying of hands.

During the outbreak of smallpox in 1721, Rogers personally traveled to Boston to continue his mission of spiritual healing. Unfortunately for him, this time it failed to work. Rogers himself came down with the disease and soon after traveled back to Connecticut where he died. Governor Gurdon Saltonstall, a staunch opponent of the Rogerenes, used the episode as an excuse to challenge the sect. A strict quarantine was placed around their settlement, forbidding the transit of medicine or doctors as well as the exit of the healthy. This undoubtedly led to additional and unnecessary deaths among the group. Afterward, the government charged the cost for this undertaking to Roger's son, hoping to bankrupt the sect. As a later historian wrote, in 17th- and 18th-century New England, "any deviation from the proclaimed laws of the ruling church was severely punished," and the public fear of smallpox allowed for that to happen.[15]

Further smallpox outbreaks would occur, but so too did inoculation. In 1730, 4,000 were stricken in the Boston area, of which one-tenth were inoculated; in the end only 500 would die. A repeat outbreak occurred in 1752 in which 7,669 were infected either naturally or by inoculation. Of the former, the death toll was around 10 percent, while among those who were inoculated, the death toll was only 1.5 percent. Though subsequent outbreaks would occur from 1754 until 1838, smallpox was never again the scourge that it had been.

Variolation would continue as a method of inoculation until the discovery of cowpox vaccination by Edward Jenner in 1796. It was a risky endeavor, in which recipients would still suffer some of the worst effects of the disease for weeks. In the end, up to 1 percent of those who received the treatment would die. Yet, when compared to the 10–20 percent that would succumb naturally, this proved to be an acceptable risk to many. One of the most famous patients in Boston was John Adams, who traveled to Castle William to be inoculated during the 1764 outbreak. His writings leave for us a detailed account of the process.

> They [the doctors] took their Launcetts and with their Points divided the skin for about a Quarter of an Inch and just suffering the Blood to appear, buried a Thread about (half) a Quarter of an Inch long in the Channell. A little Lint was then laid over the scratch and a Piece of a Ragg pressed on, and then a Bandage bound over all—my Coat and waistcoat put on, and I was bid to go where and do what I pleased.[16]

For many colonial elites, inoculation became a formal social event, in which whole families and cliques would vacation and vaccinate together.[17] At a cost of £3, though, roughly $600 in today's currency, few at the time could indulge in this luxurious and dangerous treatment.

And inoculation was far from a suddenly acceptable practice. Religious qualms, scientific questions, and practical concerns kept it an unpreferred option. These fears proved to be further grounded in the 1760s when a local inoculator, John Smith, set himself up in Roanoke seeking to eradicate smallpox.[18] Residents began to fear the man who had brought "matter enough to infect the world" into their corner of Virginia. Their fears proved justified as Smith's lax practices allowed for some of his patients to ignore their prescribed period of quarantine and mingle freely in Williamsburg. A small-scale epidemic soon erupted, resulting in the death of a handful of individuals. Smith was eventually charged for his crime and his practice shut down.

A similar attempt by two physicians in nearby Norfolk resulted in their business being burned to the ground by angry and mistrustful locals. As late as 1774, an incendiary attack destroyed the new Essex Hospital in Marblehead, and though two men were arrested, they were later broken free by an angry mob. Similar stories abound from various northern and southern colonies, thus fulfilling the ancient aphorism "Medicine is of all the Arts the most noble; but, owing to the ignorance of those who practice it, and of those who, inconsiderately, form a judgment of them, it is at present far behind all the other arts."[19]

In response to these concerns, many local assemblies took action. Charles Town passed a law in 1738 banning the practice of inoculation within two miles of the city. Governor George Clinton followed suit in June of 1747 by eliminating the operation within the city or county of New York, under penalty of prosecution and stiff fines. Numerous petitions were presented to the city councils of Williamsburg and Norfolk in Virginia as well.[20]

Yet, some saw variolation as a necessary evil. Therefore, following various outbreaks, Boston suspended its anti-vaccination laws in 1776, 1778, and 1792. In addition, other physicians slowly began to duplicate the efforts of Mather and Boylston. In 1731, Dr. John Kearsley Sr. of Philadelphia inoculated both himself and his students using variolation and was soon followed by other prominent doctors of that city.[21] Despite his brother's opposition to the practice, Benjamin Franklin also became a vocal proponent of it. The death of his son Francis in 1736 started a flood of rumors that he had been killed by the vaccination process. Franklin himself wrote to several prominent newspapers to denounce the fabrication. "I suppose the Report could only arise from its being my known Opinion, that Inoculation was a safe and beneficial Practice; and from my having said among my Acquaintance, that I intended to have my Child inoculated, as soon as he should have recovered sufficient Strength from a Flux with which he had been long afflicted."[22] Franklin's paper in Philadelphia became a leading voice for the practice.

II. Inoculation Intrigue

In the southern colonies, Thomas Jefferson became a strong supporter of variolation, undergoing the procedure himself in 1766. While overseeing Monticello, he ordered the variolation of his slaves and provided inoculation material to others as well. His acceptance of the process helped to legitimize it in Virginia long before other colonies and states in the region did so.[23] In 1768, Jefferson represented Dr. Archibald Campbell in court, an inoculator whose home had been burned down by opponents after they had forced his patients into local sick houses. Years later, during his presidency, which lasted from 1801 to 1809, Jefferson corresponded frequently regarding the new process of vaccination developed by Edward Jenner in England. As he wrote to George C. Jenner in 1806, "Having been among the early converts, in this part of the globe, to it's efficacy, I took an early part in recommending it to my countrymen."[24] While Jefferson did not use the office of the presidency to provide for the vaccination of Americans, the university he set up certainly did. As early as 1826, the University of Virginia established a dispensary that not only provided free vaccinations to the public but also recommended "students particularly shall be encouraged to be so, as a protection to the institution against the malady of the small pox."[25]

Perhaps the single biggest proponent for variolation was America's first president. As both a young man and a soldier, George Washington had seen the impact that disease could have firsthand. His half-brother Lawrence had told him stories of how in 1741, while he served with the British expedition against Cartagena de Indias, over half of the army died from yellow fever and other diseases. In fact, disease became the largest hindrance to British offensives in the Caribbean during the 17th and 18th centuries. Likewise, Lawrence's own death from tuberculosis in 1752 left George in charge of Mt. Vernon and the family fortune, providing for his ensuing rise in colonial society. During Washington's subsequent military service in the French and Indian War, his bout with dysentery and hemorrhoids kept him initially delayed by the roadside as the Anglo-American force marched to its doom under Braddock at the Monongahela. Finally, while on a trip to Barbados to find relief for his brother's illness, Washington had himself contracted smallpox. Though he ultimately recovered, he understood the devastating impact that disease, especially smallpox, could have on an army of men.

George Washington became a lifelong proponent of healthier and cleaner living. His concern with hygiene can be traced to his youth, as evidenced by his *Rules of Civility* written in his young teens. The collection included numerous recommendations for living a more sanitary life. With the outbreak of the Revolution and his rise to authority over its various forces, Washington was now in a place where he could implement many of those beliefs and ideas.

Most of America's casualties during the Revolution were from disease, either ones that developed and spread naturally or ones that were encouraged by the enemy. Reports and rumors did abound that the English were either using or planning to use biological weapons. Perhaps the two most notorious episodes involved General Gage in Boston and Lord Dunmore in Virginia. In the case of the former, General Washington himself wrote of hearing rumors that the British would use smallpox from an outbreak in the city to sicken the besieging American army.[26] While in Virginia, Lord Dunmore allegedly infected thousands of escaped slaves under the guise of variolation, in order to start an epidemic among the rebels in the state.[27]

The Continental Congress, as well as George Washington, used these reports to push for sanitation reforms within army encampments. General Washington and other commanders issued broadsides calling for a strict adherence to sanitary codes, many of which can be traced back to Biblical injunctions. Some of the recommendations included airing out of bedding, avoiding sleeping on cold and damp surfaces, washing or changing garments frequently, isolating sick soldiers, and digging of necessities far from the main camp. Washington himself looked toward Moses as the epitome of a successful general, "a great army of the Children of Israel ... that continued forty years in their different Camps, under the Guidance and Regulation of the wisest General that ever lived."[28] The management of men and the management of health were becoming inextricably linked within the American military.

Yet, despite his best efforts, disease would still periodically emerge and devastate his ranks. Already a personal proponent of inoculation, Washington became an ardent supporter of the process for his soldiers as well out of tactical necessity. He wrote to the surgeon general, Dr. William Shippen, shortly after the Battle of Trenton:

> Dear Sir: Finding the small pox to be spreading much and fearing that no precaution can prevent it from running thro' the whole of our Army, I have determined that the Troops shall be inoculated. This Expedient may be attended with some inconveniences and some disadvantages, but yet I trust, in its consequences will have the most happy effects.
> Necessity not only authorizes but seems to require the measure, for should the disorder infect the Army, in the natural way, and rage with its usual Virulence, we should have more to dread from it, than the Sword of the Enemy. Under these Circumstances, I have directed Doctr. Bond [Dr. Nathaniel Bond], to prepare immediately for inoculating this Quarter, keeping the matter as secret as possible, and request, that you will without delay inoculate all the Continental Troops that are in Philadelphia and those that shall come in, as fast as they arrive. You will spare no pains to carry them thro' the disorder with the utmost expedition, and to have them cleansed from the infection

when recovered, that they may proceed to Camp, with as little injury as possible, to the Country thro' which they pass. If the business is immediately begun and favoured with common success, I would fain hope they will soon be fit for duty, and that in a short space of time we shall have an Army not subject to this, the greatest of all calamities that can befall it, when taken in the natural way.[29]

When one considers the general view of most Americans and most colonial governments concerning the operation at the time, Washington's order to forcibly inoculate an entire army was revolutionary.

As of 1776, the Council of Safety in Baltimore still forbade the practice among soldiers, largely to prevent an epidemic from spreading among the general population. Boston had only lifted its own ban shortly before the signing of the Declaration, at which opportunity Abigail Adams had herself and the children vaccinated.[30] A few miles away in Marblehead, a riot had broken out three years before after a small inoculation hospital was constructed following an outbreak. Finally, in 1778, Virginia adopted a new law that allowed for, but was heavily regulated by the civil authority, the practice of inoculation.[31] For his own part, General Washington had convinced Martha to undergo the operation in May of 1776 in order to protect her should she spend any time with the perennially unhealthy American army.

Dr. Johann David Schoepf would go on to praise the growing popularity of the practice in America as compared to a continued prejudice against it on the continent: "The almost universal practice of the innoc of smallpox, whereby countless mult. Of children are saved from death, to which the unconq prejudice of our fatherland still continues to offer sacrifice."[32] Increased sanitation when combined with mandatory inoculation programs produced a healthier and more effective fighting force. Without this, winning the Revolution would have been a much more difficult, if not impossible, proposition. The success of Washington's endeavors were soon copied by armies elsewhere as well, most notably by Napoleon who would go on to employ Edward Jenner's newly minted vaccination process to protect his armies from the ravages of smallpox. Due to issues of federalism and the limited scope of federal power, the military largely remained the most popular avenue for pushing inoculation in America. Alexander Hamilton undertook the variolation of soldiers under his command during the Quasi-War with France in 1799, and similar undertakings were done in all subsequent American conflicts.[33]

States and towns in the early republic seem to have only begrudgingly accepted the practice. During outbreaks, local restrictions on quarantines would often be temporarily relaxed but then quickly put back in place after a short while. For example, Boston began a general inoculation campaign in 1792 following an outbreak of the disease. Various contemporary sources record the number who participated as being between 8,000 and 10,000.[34] Four years later, a similar and limited campaign was carried out in Fredericksburg, Virginia.

The practice, though, remained controversial for many. While opponents at the time and since have attempted to portray this as simply due to religious qualms, the reasons are far more nuanced. Religion certainly did play a role for some, especially those who embraced more rigid forms of Calvinism. Yet, at the same time, the Catholic Church worked extensively to bring variolation to Native tribes in South America. For most, opposition to variolation was more practical. While smallpox was certainly fatal to many, the inoculation was not without its risks. Some feared that while variolation was preferred to infection, it was not preferable to avoiding both. Stories frequently circulated of parents whose decision to variolate resulted in the death of a child during a time when a local epidemic was nowhere near their city or town. Washington, in fact, lost his own sister-in-law due to inoculation. Finally, there were legitimate concerns over the reliability of many who practiced the procedure. With little to no regulations of either variolation or the medical field in general, episodes of deaths due to malpractice, contaminated sources, or other events appear in the historical record.

Smallpox and attempts to confront it represent not only some of the first instances of the politicization of disease in America but one that lasted for over two centuries. Opposition to smallpox inoculation would soon be joined by similar resistance to other vaccines as well. Yet, in the 18th century, the federal government and state governments largely avoided mandating or even encouraging the procedure, largely leaving it up to local towns to consider. Only the military became a vehicle by which to push the practice on a larger scale.

Chapter III

A Nation Forged in Gout

Governments and leaders have seized upon disease for millennia to push their own ends. Yet, at the same time, pestilence has often influenced politics as well. Illness has laid low great conquerers, killed kings, decided coups and civil wars, and impacted the shaping of new governments. With disease and medicine impacting every facet of American history, it is not surprising to see it also play a role in the official founding of the country.

The government of the early republic had a higher percentage of medical men in it than in any subsequent period in the nation's history. Eleven of the signers of the Declaration of Independence as well as 5 percent of the members of the first U.S. Congress were physicians. Included among these were Hugh Williamson of North Carolina, an inoculator of smallpox and staunch proponent for federalism; James McClurg of Virginia, a distinguished physician who argued for a stronger, more independent chief executive; and James McHenry of Maryland, who had served as a surgeon in the Revolution and would go on to become secretary of war under presidents Washington and Adams.

At the same time, physicians or not, the Founders themselves were not immune to the diseases that were taking a severe toll on both armies at the time. Perhaps the politician at the time whose career was shaped the most by pestilence was John Hancock. At the age of seven, the death of his father from illness left him under the protection of his uncle, Thomas Hancock. A wealthy and prominent merchant in the area of Boston, Thomas raised and trained John for a future mercantile career. He was educated at Harvard and traveled abroad to England from 1760 to 1761 to expand his business contacts. As his uncle's health declined due to illness in the mid–1760s, John Hancock moved to assume control over the entire business. By the age of 27, he was one of the wealthiest men in the colonies.[1]

The young, wealthy, and flamboyant Hancock soon became a leading political figure in Massachusetts, especially as the economic decisions of Parliament began to impact colonial trade. Over the course of the late 1760s and early 1770s, he served in various positions of power and helped to balance out the more radical thought of Samuel Adams. Yet, by 1774, Hancock began to suffer from gout, a disease that had afflicted his uncle and would impact him throughout his life. His failure to serve in the First Continental Congress, then meeting at that time, was probably due to both his health issues as much as local political ambitions. In fact, using illness to avoid compromising political positions was to become a common tactic for the wealthy merchant.

In Hancock's place, Massachusetts chose James Bowdoin to represent the commonwealth, along with John Adams, Samuel Adams, Thomas Cushing, and Robert Treat Paine. Yet, Bowdoin never departed for Philadelphia, claiming that his wife's health, or perhaps his own, restricted him from doing so.[2] Years later, John Adams would doubt the veracity of these claims, writing that Bowdoin was feigning illness to remain close to the center of power in Massachusetts.[3]

Despite these alleged hopes, the legislature of Massachusetts moved to not only replace Bowdoin with Hancock for the sitting of the 2nd Continental Congress but likewise elected the latter to the office of president of the colony's provincial congress. It was during his journey south to Philadelphia in April 1775 that British officials moved to arrest him at Lexington, thus sparking the beginning of the Revolution.

Hancock was soon after elected to the position of President of Congress, presiding over the body from 1775 to 1777. It was this role, despite later tales and urban legends to the contrary, that resulted in his now famous signature gracing the Declaration of Independence. Yet, Hancock had larger ambitions, with John Adams alleging that he had hoped for a military post in command of the soldiers around Boston.[4] However, his lack of military experience as well as his frequent ill-health doomed these chances, with Washington receiving the position instead.

In late 1777, Hancock asked to step down from his position as president, in part due to his reoccurring ill health, as he was suffering from "a severe Fit of the Gout" at the time.[5] Having overseen both the signing of the Declaration of Independence as well as the Battle of Saratoga, he most likely felt that the time was right for the next step in his rising career. After a brief but disappointing military assignment and several more turns in both the Massachusetts and national legislatures, Hancock was finally elected to be the first governor of Massachusetts in 1780. Hancock was overwhelmingly elected over his seemingly more aristocratic opponent, James Bowdoin, who was disparaged for not attending the First Continental Congress. The latter had actually been suffering at the time from "a long continued Slow Fever," most likely tuberculosis, but this was lost on the voters.[6]

For the next five years, John Hancock oversaw a state that had been financially ruined both before and during the Revolution. Massachusetts possessed the largest state debt after the Revolution, valued at nearly $5,000,000, without taking into account the interest assumed by those who accepted paper from the commonwealth during the war. Hancock and the Massachusetts Assembly not only resisted raising taxes to pay off the amount but did not service the interest for years either.[7] Citizens who served in the war demanded payment, debt holders wanted returns on their bonds, and farmers decried the already high taxes. Hancock proved to be a very uninterested leader, solving none of the economic problems of the state. This was most likely due to the fact that the taxation needed to fund both its debts and needed improvements would have made him unpopular with the masses. He was a politician in the finest tradition of the *populares* of ancient Rome, doling out money to build power and representing the common man in their struggle against the landed interests while paying only lip service to actually needed reforms and actions.

As the situation deteriorated, Governor Hancock, though at the height of his popularity, suddenly announced his resignation in 1785 when he had been expected to run for another term. Claiming to be stricken with a severe case of gout, Hancock retired to private life, paving the way for James Bowdoin and the propertied classes to assume power in the state.[8] A chain of events was then put into place in which the debt holders who now controlled the Assembly pushed through higher taxes to fund the state's obligations. Local farmers rebelled as they were unable or unwilling to pay, and their property was subsequently confiscated. The resulting uprising known as Shays' Rebellion stretched from August of 1786 to June of 1787, and though few were killed, the event dramatically altered American history.

The revolt by the masses of Massachusetts that effectively paralyzed the state for months was employed by some in the political class to demand a stronger central government. One of the roadblocks to this movement had always been General George Washington, and due to this, he became the target of a letter writing campaign by prominent Federalists throughout the nation. Henry Knox's letter of October 23, 1786, represents quite well the way that the rebellion was cast in the public light to frighten reluctant leaders toward the centralization of power:

> The people who are the insurgents have never paid any or but very little taxes. But they see the weakness of government: they feel at once their own poverty compared with the opulent, and their own force, and they are determined to make use of the latter in order to remedy the former ... we shall have a formidable rebellion against reason, the principle of all government, and against the very name of liberty. This dreadful situation, for which our government have made no adequate provision, has alarmed every man of principle and property in New England.[9]

Various other leaders including Alexander Hamilton and James Madison pursued Washington and others until eventually a general convention was called for in Philadelphia to address the unworkable Articles of Confederation.

For his own part, John Hancock not only miraculously recovered from his condition but also was back in the governor's chair the next year, heading Massachusetts from 1787 to 1793. His case of gout, whether real or simply political theater, had paved the road to insurrection that drew Washington and others out of retirement and into Philadelphia to draft what would become the Constitution of the United States.

The need for a stronger union between the states had been always a debated subject among the Founding Fathers. England had long furnished an example of how centralized rule could slowly sap the independence and rights of its people. Yet, the continued economic troubles of the new country, Shays' Rebellion, the Newburgh Conspiracy, continued troubles with both the British and Natives, as well as numerous other issues, had now convinced enough national leaders of the need for a new federal structure. Disease was often employed in the political rhetoric for the troubles then facing the country. Writing to his father in 1787, James Madison noted, "The existing embarrassments and *mortal* diseases of the Confederacy form the only ground of hope, that a Spirit of concession on all sides may be produced by the general chaos or at least partition of the Union which offers itself as the alternative."[10]

At the same time, Alexander Hamilton in *The Federalist No. 21* stated, "It is absolutely necessary that we should be well acquainted with the extent and malignity of the disease."[11] In this case he was referring to what he saw as the three main points of failure for the Confederation government: its inability to enforce any of its decisions or laws, its failure to ensure the safety of the states, and finally its monetary issues. In fact, the collected *Federalist Papers* uses terms such as disease, pestilence, or health nearly two dozen times in making political recommendations.

Even once enough members of the national, political elite had been convinced of the need to change the Articles of Confederation, and had gathered in Philadelphia to begin the process, they did not escape from the impact of illness. Surprisingly, the drafters of the Constitution were largely able to escape the malignant illnesses that often accompanied the summer heat in Philadelphia. Out of those that did fall ill, two cases stand out as influential.

Ben Franklin, who helped craft many of the other compromises of the document, was only able to be present thanks to large cocktails of drugs. The aging Franklin was beset by numerous medical issues, including kidney stones, gout, and psoriasis. Only his frequent consumption of laudanum kept his pain in check, though it also often resulted in his passing out during discussions. Though Madison strongly advised against his drug use, Franklin stated, "he had no other remedy; and thought the best terms he could make with his complaint was to give up a part of his remaining life, for the greater ease of the rest."[12]

Even more important to the future shape of the American government was the nosophobia of Erastus Wolcott and Richard Law. The respected Connecticut politicians had first been selected to join the Continental Congress in 1774 but had turned down the honor due to their fear of contracting smallpox.[13] As previously discussed, the disease was rampant at the time around the country due to the conditions of war. In their place, the colony chose a new slate of representatives, including Roger Sherman. The latter would go on to serve in all subsequent Congresses and would be present at the Constitutional Convention as well. Here, he helped to craft the Great Compromise, which effectively established the country's bicameral legislature.

In many ways the drafting of the Constitution became a less delicate affair than the adoption of the document by the various states. Though the middle states quickly approved the new government, the larger and more important states were more reluctant. By January of 1788, five states, including Delaware, Pennsylvania, New Jersey, Georgia, and Connecticut, had voted for the plan, but Massachusetts proved to be an important holdout. Contemporary observers expected the measure to fail in the Bay State by only a few votes. It was at this point that Governor John Hancock was *again* stricken by the gout and took to his bed, a rather timely occurrence considering his ambiguous position on the Constitution.

Many at the time suspected the political roots of his illness, with Rufus King writing, "Hancock is still confined, or rather he has not yet taken his Seat; as soon as the majority is exhibited on either side I think his Health will suffer him to be abroad."[14] The Federalists quickly pounced on him, hinting at offers of the vice presidency as well as a Bill of Rights.[15] Suddenly with his health partially recovered, Hancock returned to the state house wrapped in flannel and carried on a litter to deliver his voting block to the new government. The measure would pass in February by a vote of 187-168 with the working out of the Massachusetts Compromise by both Hancock and Samuel Adams. In many ways, the U.S. Constitution was both produced and passed by a case of the gout.

Feigning illness for political purposes was certainly not a new tactic. Literature is awash with characters who pretended to be mentally ill to avoid certain situations. Two of the more prominent examples are Odysseus during the Trojan War or Hamlet in Shakespeare's play.

> How strange or odd soe'er I bear myself,
> As I perchance hereafter shall think meet
> To put an antic disposition on[16]

While outside of the realm of literature, many historical figures have committed similar acts. The great Chinese general Bai Qi once feigned an illness in 250 BC to avoid having to lead a campaign for King Zhaoxiang of Qin that he knew was doomed to failure. In the year 325, Pope Sylvester I declined to attend Emperor Constantine's call to join the Council of Nicaea, claiming he was ill. Napoleon Bonaparte claimed illness in 1795 to avoiding having to command troops in the War in the Vendee, a position that he saw as a demotion and a conflict, which he disagreed with. Likewise, Mao Zedong is rumored to have used a diagnosis of malaria in 1929 to withdraw from the public eye at a time when his reputation had been heavily damaged due to the failed Autumn Harvest Uprising. As late as the 1990s, a private doctor claimed that Russian president Boris Yeltsin faked several medical episodes and conditions in order to keep his opponents off balance.[17]

Hancock's pestilence theater was therefore not a unique episode in human history but a time-honored practice among generals, politicians, and workers. Likewise, he would not be the last American leader to practice it. While many politicians have gone to great lengths to hide illnesses, a topic that will be covered in depth in a later chapter, several have embraced disease to make connections with the public. Perhaps the first to do so was Dwight D. Eisenhower.

Though a popular choice for the Republican nomination in 1952, Ike certainly wasn't the healthiest. His warrior image was only skin deep, with Crohn's Disease, advanced heart disease, and several other issues plaguing him. In traditional fashion, the several episodes of minor and severe illness that confronted him in the late 1940s and early 1950s were adroitly covered up. Yet, on September 24, 1955, Ike suffered a massive heart attack while visiting his in-laws in Denver. After he complained of chest pains around midnight, his physician, Dr. Henry Snyder, was called to the residence. Arriving an hour later, he administered oxygen, amyl nitrate, papaverine, and morphine to stabilize Ike. The next day, the president again complained of chest pains and, after examination with a portable electrocardiograph, was driven to a local hospital. After almost twenty-four hours of suffering, the president walked to his own limousine and was then driven to Fitzsimmons Army Hospital, where an analysis revealed that Eisenhower had suffered a left anterior myocardial infarction and bore a scar on his heart the size of an olive.[18]

In stark contrast to previous administrations, especially that of the recent Roosevelt, those of the Eisenhower White House spoke openly

III. A Nation Forged in Gout

about the president's condition. Vice President Nixon and the entire executive team were quickly notified, and the press was allowed access to the hospital.[19] There seems to have been no adverse reaction from American citizens to the news, as polls taken in October of that year on whether Ike should run again recorded that well over 55 percent approved.[20] As part of the campaign to win over the nation, Nixon insisted on employing civilian doctors as well as army medical staff. He stated, "We cannot overlook the fact that many people in the country might have more confidence, however unfounded, in a civilian specialist of national reputation."[21] For this reason, the military brought in renowned cardiologist Dr. Paul Dudley White of Massachusetts General Hospital.

Though the public seems to have taken the heart attack in stride, Wall Street was not as kind. On Monday, September 26, only two days after the incident, the New York Stock Exchange opened and then abruptly collapsed, with the Dow Jones losing 6.5 percent of its value, an estimated $14 billion, its worse loss since 1929. The president's heart attack had put an end to the economic miracle that had begun roughly in 1942 and had continued largely unabated until this time. It was exactly these fears that had driven several previous presidents, most notably Grover Cleveland, to go to extreme ends to cover up illnesses.

Subsequent presidents, most notably Bill Clinton and George W. Bush, have undergone minor medical procedures and been fully open with the American public, but it would take President Donald Trump before the country was again confronted by a major health scare. In early October 2020, the White House announced that Trump and his wife had both tested positive for Covid, also known as the Wuhan Virus. Though initially his diagnosis seemed positive, by Friday afternoon it was announced that he was being taken to Walter Reed Medical for oxygen and treatment.

Beyond simply communicating this information to help inform the public and ally fears, Trump made sure to demonstrate his health by walking to and from the presidential helicopter. This was similar to what Ike had done seventy years before, delaying his release from the hospital until he was healthy enough to walk out under his own strength. Trump also used Twitter to post videos assuring the public of his condition. In a message he delivered three days later, on October 5, the president told Americans, "Don't be afraid of Covid. Don't let it dominate your life. We have developed, under the Trump Administration, some really great drugs & knowledge. I feel better than I did 20 years ago!"[22] Trump would return to the White House later that night and in subsequent days touted his returned health and the great medical solutions available to confront the disease. While many in the media at the time were pushing a much more "doom and gloom" view of the pandemic, Trump continuously tried to prevent the nosophobia, which he saw as crippling the country. His own diagnosis with the disease became a useful public example of how recovery was assured for the vast majority of those who fell ill, even one with several comorbidities.

Another man whose political choices were driven by his own personal illness was George Washington. The choice of the Revolutionary hero for the office of president was largely a foregone conclusion but who would follow him was much more of an unknown. Among those who feared what would occur should he eventually retire, some pushed for crowning the former general as a hereditary monarch. Once more, disease would help to shape the politics of the new nation.

George Washington had contracted both smallpox and tuberculosis as a young man. Though he was able to fight off these conditions, they seem to have left his body permanently scarred in the shape of infertility. Washington and his wife never had any children but, based upon the four children that she had during seven years of marriage to her first husband, the fertility of the future first lady seems reasonably established. It seems then that the "stallion of the Potomac" was actually a gelding. While many theories have been put forward to explain this, Washington's infertility was most likely caused by the smallpox and/or tuberculosis that he had contracted in his late teens. Numerous studies have shown that both can lead to sterility, especially genitourinary tuberculosis or tuberculosis epididymitis.[23]

The importance to history of Washington's sterility arises from what it possibly prevented. James McHenry once opined to the first president, "You are now a king under a different name."[24] Yet he was far from the only one to make such a statement or take it to its logical conclusion. In fact, in May 1782, General Lewis Nicola wrote a letter to Washington from Newburgh, New York, that strongly suggested the establishment of a monarchy to be headed by the latter: "This war must have shown to all, but to military men in particular, the weakness of republicks ... but if all other things were once adjusted I believe strong argument might be produced for admitting the title of king."[25] Several of the Founders were noted fans of monarchy, including Gouverneur Morris, Alexander Hamilton, and Nathan Gorham. As one historian has pointed out, the Declaration itself never specifically condemned monarchy, only the unjust reign of George III.[26]

Washington himself was appalled at the notion however, writing to Nicola that "no occurrence in the course of the War, has given me more painful sensations than your information of there being such ideas existing in the Army as you have expressed, and I must view with abhorrence, and reprehend with severity.... You could not have found a person to whom your schemes are more disagreeable."²⁷ Yet the thought must have lingered in the minds of some, as one of drafts of the president's First Inaugural Address from early 1789 contained a firm denial on his part of any desire to found a dynasty. Washington went so far as to cite his lack of children as evidence of this.²⁸ Had a monarchy been established, upon the death of Washington in 1799 a rather messy battle might have commenced between his nephews and his adopted children and grandchildren from Martha Washington.

The Founding Fathers were both impacted by pestilence and used it to further their own ends. Disease not only helped to lay low the British army in many theaters and ensure an American victory, it also contributed to the shaping of the national government that emerged from the conflict.

CHAPTER IV

Mosquitos and the Emergence of Political Parties

Science and politics have long been invariably linked. Priest-kings of the earliest civilizations would utilize reasoned observations of the natural world to inform their religious role as guardians of farming, curers of illness, and allayers of natural phenomenon. Yet, as there was only one king in a nation and science tended to evolve and progress at a glacial pass, there was little conflict between the two. This began to change in the 17th century as political parties emerged in various governments and the Scientific Revolution led to competing theories and camps. It became almost natural that the divides in economic thought, social thought, and political thought would also embrace scientific thought as well. For America, the impetus for this was the yellow fever epidemic of 1793.

The roots of this, at least in the Anglo-Saxon tradition, can be traced to the days of the English Civil War in the 17th century. Just as the political forces of the nation were splitting into supporters of Parliament or the king, scientific forces were separating into partisans of Paracelsus and Galen. The conflict between the two scientific ideologies mirrored many of the same arguments and concerns as the political war. Likewise, both Charles and his Parliamentarian adversaries would latch on to their respective scientific camp for their own benefit. Adherence to a political ideology at the time usually meant adherence to a distinctive scientific one as well.

To fully understand the scientific split at the time, one must appreciate the differing theories that were naturally competing with each other. Medical thought before this time had been largely shaped by Galenic thought. Named after Galen of Pergamon, a Greek who practiced medicine in the second-century Roman Empire, it was the dominant theory for nearly 1,500 years. Based largely off of his personal observation and practice of dissecting animals, Galen formulated what became known as the Humor Theory. He theorized that the human body was composed of four fluids: blood, yellow bile, black bile, and phlegm. Any changes in behavior or health therefore represented an imbalance in this system. Galen prescribed bleeding, enemas, or vomiting as ways to then rebalance the system. His ideas became largely unquestioned by centuries of medical men, and the profession began to favor an almost Scholastic appreciation of him over empirical observation.

The Galenic system was first successfully challenged by Theophrastus von Hohenheim, better known as Paracelsus, in the early 16th century. A Swiss scientist, Paracelsus developed a rival theory based upon his own practice of observation. Heavily influenced by astrology and alchemy, he promulgated the *Tria Prima* of sulfur, mercury, and salt. Believing that disease was caused by poisons introduced from the outside and localized to particular organs, he favored utilizing natural and inorganic materials to help produce cures. As opposed to Galen's principle of contrariety, which favored a cure that was opposite in nature to a problem, Paracelsus promoted the principle of similitude, which sought to find a cure that resembled the problem, also known as the doctrine of signatures. His theory of "like cures like" would rely heavily upon substances that could often be toxic themselves, most notably opium, mercury, and feces. The expression *sola dosis facit venenum* is often attributed to him and his focus on noxious cures. Yet, what endeared him more to the Puritans of England was his insistence on the connections between science and religion. To him, the role of science was to better understand God and medicine itself represented a divine mission. Just as the Puritans sought to employ the most stringent codes of morality and focused on godliness to embrace God, so too did Paracelsus strive to find dangerous cures and embraced toxins to battle toxins.

The Royalist forces in England appreciated the traditionalism of the Galenic system and its disconnection from religion. On the other hand, Calvinist Parliamentarians naturally gravitated to what they saw as not only the "new" method of medicine but one which saw itself as divinely commissioned and harsh in its cures. Thus, despite the wealthy and educated background of much of the College of Physicians in London, its members tended to side with Parliament during the Civil War. While some had attempted to explain this as a product of their desires to standardize and elevate the profession to aristocratic levels, their adherence to Paracelsian thought certainly played a role as well.[1] Similar political-medical alliances would emerge during America's battle with yellow fever during the late 18th century as well.

While today yellow fever is commonly thought of as a tropical ailment, prior to the work of Dr. Walter Reed and others, as well as nearly a century of land reclamation, it menaced much of the American continent.

From the 1600s to the 1900s, outbreaks raged from Boston to Miami and as far west as Texas. Originating in eastern or central Africa, the disease was carried west with the Atlantic slave trade, reaching the Americas at least as early as 1647. It was a debilitating illness with a fatality rate of between 20 and 50 percent, which was spread by the *Aedes aegypti* mosquito.

The dates for when yellow fever first arrived in the future United States are subject to debate. An outbreak in Barbados in 1647, which spread to the Yucatán and Cuba by the next year, was noted by the authorities in Massachusetts who put in place a quarantine. Despite ships journeying between the two locations, and John Winthrop recording "an epidemical sickness was through the country ... a special providence from God appeared for not a family, nor but a few persons escaping it," it is unknown if it struck Boston.[2]

The first truly identifiable epidemic of the disease in America occurred in New York City in 1668. Yellow fever had been reported in Cuba over the two previous years, making it likely that the disease was carried north by ship to New York. By the early fall, many residents of the city were dying of the mysterious illness. A local minister wrote, "The Lord begins to deal in judgment with his people. He has visited us with dysentery, which is even now increasing in virulence. Many have died of it, and many are lying sick. It appears as if God were punishing this land for its sins."[3] Unable to combat the scourge medically, Governor Francis Lovelace, the brother of the famous Restoration era poet, proclaimed a day of humiliation for the citizens of the colony. "A Fast bee kept throughout this Government to deprecate Gods afflicting hand from us, & to imprecate his Blessing upon the Governor & Government."[4] With the arrival of the first frost, the disease all but disappeared, though Philadelphia seems to have been visited by it during the next summer.

Boston saw a similar outbreak in 1693. Much like the outbreak in New York City a generation earlier, this one was brought north from the Caribbean. An English naval force had been sailing in the region earlier in the year under Adm. Francis Wheler, attempting to take Martinique. With disease ravaging his crew, he was forced to end the expedition and withdrew to Boston. While he hoped to refit and lead a colonial assault on Quebec, he instead unleashed a yellow fever epidemic upon the city that killed many.

Outbreaks only worsened in frequency and severity as the 18th century progressed. This was caused by both increased trade between colonial ports and the Caribbean as well as the rapidly expanding population of the American cities. Epidemics in Charleston in 1699 and 1706 killed an estimated 7 percent and 5 percent of the city respectively, while one in New York in 1702 resulted in the loss of perhaps 10 percent.

IV. Mosquitos and the Emergence of Political Parties

Public health measures of the time generally called for the employment of quarantines, the cleaning of streets, and the reliance upon divine intervention to stem epidemics. Yet, as the vector for yellow fever was through mosquitos, it appeared to spread in different ways than traditional plagues. This inability to confront the illness often led to strife both in the political and scientific worlds.

The Founding Fathers had hoped to create a nation that was not plagued by the political parties that had so damaged both ancient and contemporary republics. In his *Federalist No. 10*, Madison lamented that political factions led to "the instability, injustice, and confusion introduced into the public councils, [which] have, in truth, been the mortal diseases under which popular governments have everywhere perished."[5] Yet, despite the best wishes and constitutional safeguards of the Founders, these developments became inevitable both due to practical reasons as well as the personalities of Jefferson and Hamilton. Washington's wish in his Farewell Address to avoid political parties went completely unheeded by those around him. Every proposed law, national discussion, and international event became fodder for the developing parties, and the yellow fever epidemic of 1793 proved to be no different.

The roots of this epidemic lay in the ongoing bloody rebellion in Saint-Domingue. The outbreak of revolution in France in 1789 inspired similar actions in several of its colonial possessions. The island of Saint-Domingue was home to various discontented groups, including wealthy planters, poor whites, free people of color, and slaves. A revolt by the last of these groups in August 1791 soon gave rise to a multisided war of brutality, whose horrors were only compounded by the presence of yellow fever on the island.

After almost two years of warfare and tens of thousands of deaths, French refugees began fleeing north to the United States. By July, thousands had reached Philadelphia and were greeted by a welcoming populace who had even raised $12,000 to help the newest émigrés. Yet, hidden in the hulls of the various hulks that had transported the French to America was another immigrant that had not visited Philadelphia in more than thirty years—the yellow fever virus.[6] The summer of 1793 had been particularly hot in the region, drying up many brooks and creeks and turning the area around the Delaware River into a stagnant marshland, the perfect breeding ground for mosquitoes.

Reports at the time stated that the first identifiable victims were all connected to a brothel or boardinghouse on Water Street near the wharves. Over the course of only a few days, two French sailors, an Englishman, an Irish woman, and the establishment's owner and his wife all fell sick and died. Due to the nature of the establishment, their perceived intemperate lifestyles, and the general filth of the neighborhood, the news was not shocking to most and appears to have gone unnoticed by the majority of the capital's population. The doctor who initially responded to the sickness was Isaac Cathrall, who the next year wrote a book on his experience. To him, the disease was perhaps related to yellow fever but seemed to be something new and far more dangerous.[7]

Notice of the disease began to be taken toward the end of August, following the sickness and death of several notable members of the city. Dr. Benjamin Rush, a renowned physician and a signer of the Declaration of Independence, began to attend to a growing number of well-off patients, including Catherine Le Maigre, the wife of a prominent merchant who had opened his house to refugees from the Caribbean. Her death on August 20 pushed Rush to demand a meeting with the city's mayor.

Rush informed Matthew Clarkson that the illness was most certainly yellow fever, a disease that he had previously seen as a medical student in the 1760s. The first move by Rush, other doctors, and the city's politicians was to locate and eliminate the perceived vectoring agent. In this case, Drs. Benjamin Rush and John Foulke hypothesized the cause to be a rotting pile of coffee that had been left on the docks of Water Street by the *Amelia*. This was clearly in keeping with the miasma theory of the time and was held to be true by almost everyone, including Thomas Jefferson who wrote, "A malignant fever has been generated in the filth of the docks of Philadelphia."[8] Under this initial miasmic theory, Rush recommended that Clarkson order the cleaning of streets and neighborhoods along the waterfront, which the mayor quickly agreed to. Unfortunately, this would have done little to deter yellow fever, perhaps only increasing the pools of water in which the mosquitoes that carried the illness could breed.

Conditions worsened with each passing week, and, as is customary with such events, various theories and folk remedies arose. Women and boys took to smoking tobacco, as it was thought the smoke would drive away the miasma causing the yellow fever. Some individuals resorted to consuming or wearing garlic, while others avoided barbers and hairdressers, and some began to practice self-bleeding as a means to remove the illness. Pedestrians bypassed sidewalks and used the streets instead, and handshaking become a dangerous rarity. Yet, nothing could abate the spreading disease. The local papers reported that the mayor called for the formation of a committee to help the poor and borrowed $1,500 from the Bank of North America for that express purpose. They also carried stories about a local woman who died in the street with her infant still suckling at her breast.

By mid-September, Philadelphia was grinding to a halt. Churches, coffeehouses, and the city library had all closed, and three of the four

IV. Mosquitos and the Emergence of Political Parties

newspapers had stopped printing. Mayor Matthew Clarkson's much celebrated committee of twenty-six men, which was raised to deal with the crisis, also faced insurmountable problems when four of its members refused to attend and four died of fever. Rush and those that remained soon turned toward experimental techniques.

As most believed that the contagion was transmitted person-to-person, it became increasingly difficult to find nurses to man the hospitals and quarantine sites. Prospective nurses were even offered exorbitant salaries but none accepted.[9] Dr. Rush recalled that during an outbreak of yellow fever in Charleston in 1742, local slaves had died at a much lower rate than whites. Therefore, he published an article in a local paper under a pseudonym calling on blacks in Philadelphia to offer their services as nurses. The local black churches under Absalom Jones and Richard Allen responded, "confiding in Him who can preserve in the midst of a burning fiery furnace, sensible that it was our duty to do all the good we could to our suffering fellow mortals."[10] Much valuable service was rendered to the community, more often than not out of genuine altruism than profit seeking. Yet, despite the best efforts and intentions of the black community and the hypothesis of Dr. Rush, 240 black nurses and assistants would succumb to the yellow fever, a figure on par with whites when one compares their percentage as part of the local population.[11] Even the quarantine centers and hospitals soon began to collapse. Of the seven individuals housed at one such center at Rickett's Circus, two were dead by the end of the month. A servant girl had to be pressed into service to remove one of the bodies, while the other was left to rot for over 48 hours, "crawling with maggots and in the most loathsome state of purification."[12]

As the city had replaced New York City as the national capital under the Residence Act of 1790, the entire federal system began to falter. Though Congress had not been in session since June, the president and many other notables were present during the outbreak. Alexander Hamilton, the secretary of the treasury, was taken ill and soon began to miss cabinet meetings. On September 7 Dr. James Hutchinson, the port physician and an opponent of President Washington, succumbed to the disease. Writing to his secretary of war, the president advised, "I think it would not be prudent either for you or the Clerks in your Office, or the Office itself to be too much exposed to the malignant fever, which by well authenticated report, is spreading through the City; The means to avoid it your own judgment under existing circumstances must dictate."[13]

On September 10, under pressure from his wife and others, President Washington finally decided to abandon the city: "The house in which we lived being, in a manner blockaded, by the disorder and was becoming every day more and more fatal."[14] Withdrawing to General Howe's former Revolutionary headquarters in Germantown, the president queried his cabinet as to his ability to relocate Congress as well. Vice President John Adams was already out of the city, and his official residence of Bush Hill had been turned into a makeshift hospital that soon became "a great human slaughterhouse where numerous victims were inoculated at the altar of riot and intemperance."[15] Many Southern leaders, including both Jefferson and Madison, worried about the effect of the outbreak on the construction of the new national capital along the Potomac River. This move had been an integral part of Southern acceptance of Hamilton's economic plan, but reoccurring malignant fevers could lead to Northern leaders demanding a more temperate location.

Beyond the role of the disease in the debate over the placement of the capital, its treatment became a political issue. As the various doctors battled to control and defeat the yellow fever, a clear divergence emerged between the two political parties then forming in the nation. Treatment methods both reflected party allegiance and defined political philosophy. Rush's cures came to be seen as a democratic approach to the illness, while others reflected the ideology of the Federalist Party.

Benjamin Rush remained at the center of the epidemic as it raged from August to October 1793, working in conjunction with the city government and administering treatments directly to patients. Rush relied largely on bloodletting and the application of various purgatives to treat the illness, methods previously used by Dr. John Mitchell who had dealt with a comparable outbreak in Virginia in 1741. "I had attended less to the effects of purging in producing this change in the pulse. Dr. Mitchell in a moment dissipated my ignorance and fears upon this subject."[16] Still more evidence of this was given to Dr. Foulke by a French military surgeon who "had for many years bled the recruits from France, as soon as they arrived, and thereby assured them from a seasoning by the yellow fever."[17] Apart from bloodletting, Rush recommended the use of jalapeno, camphor, and mercury as purgative agents. In essence, his treatment procedure called for the draining of the classic humors from the body in order to rid it of the yellow fever. The whole body was to be the focus, rather than individual components, in an effort to correct a perceived imbalance in the system.

An alternative viewpoint on treatment was offered by other physicians, notably Drs. Edward Stevens and Adam Kuhn. These practitioners preferred the use of quinine bark, wine, laudanum, and cold baths to battle the illness. As Kuhn was a professor of *materia medica* at the Medical School of the College of Pennsylvania, it is not surprising to find him recommending these various medicines rather than more traditional bloodletting and attacking precise components of the disease rather than broadly attacking the body itself. To Kuhn and Stevens, the individual's own body was the surest method by which to combat illness once outside interfering forces were removed. The physician should focus on individual members and allow the larger whole to continue unabated.

Rush's focus on bloodletting was seen as truly democratic in that it was open to all members of society. Regardless of wealth or position, any person could partake in the practice. Philosophically, the act of purging an excess of the humor could be seen as a metaphor for Rush's political view of the purging power of frequent elections.[18] Minister Timothy Dwight even referenced the notion a year later in a letter to Oliver Wolcott where he warned of "the yellow fever of politics," urging the latter "to use doctor Rush's remedies."[19] Likewise, Rush and his fellow Republicans pushed for improvements to the sanitation of the city, moves that would both eradicate disease as well as improve the condition of the masses. As part of this, the city council of Philadelphia voted to acquire five water carts to help regularly reduce the filth of the city's streets. Finally, the Republican view of disease treatment was more accepting of experimentation. Rush himself wrote frequently of attempting to employ the methods of various doctors and theorists, including Kuhn and Stevens. "I published the next day an account of the ill success which had attended the use of the remedies recommended by Dr. Kuhn, in my practice, and of the happy effects of mercurial purges and bleeding."[20] Once again, this was in keeping with Rush's view of the democratic experiment then unfolding in the nation. "A new order of things is rising in medicine as well as in government.... Human reason cannot be stationary upon these subjects ... the lancet, shall be considered among the most efficient articles of knowledge, and rights of man."[21] Medical experimentation seemed to parallel the belief in federalism as well as the notion of individual self-rule.

Federalists and their physicians focused their attention around much more expensive and rarer treatments to counter symptoms. Quinine bark, laudanum, and wine became the standard prescribed remedies, items that in and of themselves tended to be priced too high for consumption by the lower classes. In the early 19th century, the cost of Peruvian bark rose an astronomical tenfold as it moved from the forests to Lima for sale, with these costs only increasing exponentially as it worked its way closer to Philadelphia.[22] Even more cost prohibitive, however, was the need for a trained and knowledgeable doctor to administer the treatments. The treatment of the Hamilton family exemplified this factor. Alexander Hamilton and his wife had abandoned the capital city as their conditions worsened. Sending their children to Albany, they themselves withdrew to Fair Hill, some two and a half miles from the city. Luckily for the Hamiltons, they were soon visited by Dr. Stevens, one of Alexander's boyhood friends from St. Croix. Having a certain amount of experience in dealing with the disease while in the West Indies, Hamilton's doctor proceeded to prescribe Peruvian Bark, aged Madeira, cold baths, and laudanum to help combat the illness. In addition, both Kuhn and Stevens pushed for the consumption of fresh fruit, the frequent changing of linens, and the introduction of fresh air into the rooms of those infected. After recovering within five days' time, Hamilton was so convinced by the doctor's skill that he penned a letter to the College of Physicians in Philadelphia recommending that it follow Stevens' approach to dealing with yellow fever. The Federalist commitment to employing more expensive methods and consulting authority stood in sharp contrast to the Republican focus on the individual as did their philosophical reliance on the body itself to fight the causative agent of the disease rather than combat it through outside efforts.

The flight of the Hamiltons was mirrored by that of thousands of other families, including Governor Thomas Mifflin who left after finding a dead body on the steps of the capitol building. By the end of September, a general exodus had begun from the city.

> The removals from Phil began about the 25th or 26th of this month; and so great was the general terror, that, for some weeks, carts, waggons, coachees, and chairs were almost constantly transporting families and furniture to the country in every direction. Many people shut up their houses wholly; others left servants to take care of them. Business then became extremely dull. Mechanics and artists were unemployed; and their streets were the appearance of gloom and melancholy.[23]

An estimated 17,000 individuals fled Philadelphia for surrounding areas. As was usually the case, those who left tended to be of the wealthier classes. Jefferson lamented to James Madison, "Every body, who can, is flying from the city, and the panic of the country people is likely to add famine to disease."[24] As can be expected, withdrawal from Philadelphia tended to be contingent upon the financial ability to do so. This was seized upon by Jefferson and his followers, worsening the rift between Federalists and Republicans in the city. Jefferson went so far as to accuse the secretary of the treasury of faking the illness, proclaiming him as "timid in sickness" as he was in war. Dr. Rush even publicly blamed Hamilton's support for Stevens' cure for the deaths of hundreds. He did attempt to re-create Stevens' methods, in a fashion, by throwing buckets of cold water on patients and injecting quinine directly into their bowels, but the results were not promising.[25]

Republican contempt for the methods of Kuhn and Hamilton was no doubt influenced by fears that the onset of yellow fever would turn many in the government away from the construction of a new capital even deeper in the south. This move had been an integral part of Southern acceptance of Hamilton's economic plan, but reoccurring malignant fevers could

IV. Mosquitos and the Emergence of Political Parties

lead to Northern leaders demanding a more temperate location. Likewise, a concern for the common man led them to develop early methods of urban sanitary improvement, a plank in the party platform that would expand significantly during the cholera pandemics 40 years later. Interestingly, despite their ideological pronouncements, it appears that the elites of both parties frequently employed both methods when they themselves became sick. "Some others (probably most or all now) bleed & purge but either inadequately, or counteract their effects by then giving bark and laudanum!"[26] Politics always faded before the prospect of death.

Roadblocks and patrols soon began to show up on the various roads leading from Philadelphia as surrounding communities began to isolate the diseased city. Those who had not left by early September would oftentimes find themselves forced to remain in the confines of the region. Reports from the city, though horrible in their own truth, were quickly exaggerated as they traveled farther afield. Tales of hundreds of deaths per day grew to thousands as they reached Maryland. Surrounding towns and cities soon began to more actively protect themselves from the spreading pestilence of Philadelphia. On September 11, New York City required the registration of all persons from Philadelphia to track their condition and movement. Soon after, the governor of New York prohibited all ships from the diseased city from sailing past Bedloe Island and hired physicians to inspect all vessels. By September 17, all trade was stopped from Philadelphia, and, following reports of secret landings in New York City by sickened merchants, a night watch was put in place and all citizens were entreated to report anything or anyone suspicious. Yet, New York was not alone in its isolation of Philadelphia.

By mid–September, both Trenton and Lamberton, New Jersey, cancelled all ferry service across the Delaware and positioned militiamen at roadblocks to stop foot traffic as well. Most towns in Maryland followed suit over the next few days, restricting trade, travel, and communication. As the month progressed most other states would impose similar restrictions, Virginia on September 17, Massachusetts on September 18, Rhode Island on the 21st, North Carolina on the 28th, and South Carolina and Georgia in early October. By November, the sheer amount of roadblocks and armed men patrolling the roads and countryside seemed to evoke memories of the Revolution.

Those that remained in the city began to rally around the efforts of the mayor and his Committee of 26, as most of the town council had fled.[27] Clarkson's committee began to organize a modern hospital to replace Bush Hill, which would consist of over 140 beds. Separate rooms were established for the sexes and depending upon a patient's condition. Each patient was afforded clean sheets and pillows and was visited twice a day by a French physician who had experience confronting the disease in Haiti. Victims dined on meals of broth, rice, bread, boiled beef, prunes, and cream of rice, all washed down with porter, claret, water, centaury tea, and lemonade. Within two weeks, the city had managed to carry out most of the reform measures, yet deaths continued to mount. Of the over 1,000 people admitted to the hospital, 500 would never come out. In fact, one-third did not survive two days in the facility. Worse yet, an additional $5,000 had to borrowed by the city from the Bank of North America to fund the hospital reorganization.

The Committee soon began to appropriate more power to itself to fight the plague. Closed houses were forcibly opened to be aired out and cleaned, lime was deposited in privies, and the bedding and clothing of the sick was burned. By November, a lack of compliance on the part of many citizens led the committee to hire assistants to carry out the regulations or else arrest citizens on criminal charges.

Some help did arrive from the outside world in the form of medicine, supplies, and donations. In addition, many towns offered asylum to those who fled Pennsylvania, including Woodbury, Springfield, and Elizabeth in New Jersey, Elk in Maryland, and Wilmington in Delaware. Yet, it was not until the onset of winter that life began to return to normal in the nation's capital.

The costs of the yellow fever epidemic were severe. It is estimated that around 5,000 people in the city of 50,000 died during the outbreak. Among these victims were a disproportionate number of doctors, clergy, maids, men, and the poor. Carey records 10 physicians who were killed and suggests that some became sick three or four times during the epidemic.[28] The disease fell especially hard upon the poor who represented seven out of every eight victims. Much of this resulted not from unsuccessful medical treatments but instead the inability of the poor to flee the city.

The disease did produce some positive results, especially in the field of public health management. For example, Philadelphia created a permanent Board of Health in 1798. It possessed the power to levy taxes upon citizens in order to fund the fighting of disease. One of its first acts was the construction of the Lazaretto, a quarantine site located 10 miles south of the city at Tinicum. Likewise, all ships destined for Philadelphia were required to be inspected and quarantined if necessary. To assist in the process a hospital and public warehouse were constructed as well. The Philadelphia Board of Health would successfully run the Lazaretto until 1893 when the state assumed responsibility for the quarantine of shipping arriving in Pennsylvania.

In the end, despite the enormous loss of life and the fact that the economy and the workings of the government did falter, they did not fall.

IV. Mosquitos and the Emergence of Political Parties

The epidemic nearly led to the removal of the government to the north or further west, moves that would have drastically altered the course of the nation toward civil war. Yet the outbreak and its associated different methods of treatment did help to further divide the political parties then forming in the nation. The Federalists exemplified themselves as the party of tradition, privilege, consistency, and means, while the Republicans would embrace the common man, political change, and government solutions. These differences became exacerbated, no doubt, due to the fact that yellow fever was not spread from person to person, nor did any of the cures actually serve to defeat the illness. It was to be a combination of both parties' ideas, the Federalists' focus on new and expensive methods, experienced physicians, and quarantine, as well as the Democrat-Republicans' focus on improvements in public sanitation that would eventually help to revolutionize medical treatment over the next two centuries. Yet, this outbreak was to expose and develop the basic, fundamental philosophical differences between the two political parties for the next two centuries. One party focused on combating symptoms, attacking the whole body politic at once through a method that was accessible to all in an attempt to correct a bodily imbalance, while the other attempted to find and cure the root cause, striking at precise issues rather than by employing broad strokes, a difference that continues to this day.

The fight between the left and right that emerged over the yellow fever epidemic of 1793 would continue with almost every epidemic for the next two centuries. Debates over quarantines, government mandates, vaccinations, and methods of treatment would come to characterize the extreme politicization of disease. Yet, as shown here, this is hardly a new phenomenon. Revolutionary poet Philip Freneau satirically memorialized the political debates over the pestilence at the time in a verse that would be apropos two centuries later.

> Doctors raving and disputing,
> Death's pale army still recruiting—
> What a pother
> One with t'other!
> Some a-writing, some a-shooting.[29]

Chapter V

Buffalo Fever and the Anti-War Movement

"How many were destroyed by diseases in the crowded prisons of the *John*. How many were poisoned by the pestilential atmosphere of the *Scorpion*. How many were suffocated in the scuttled holds of the *Strombolo*."[1] Doctor Benjamin De Witt, a member of the esteemed Jeffersonian Republican family in New York, spoke these words in 1808 while delivering a funeral oration for the dead being interned in a new monument in New York City. He was part of an elaborate spectacle being put on by Tammany Hall to further inflame public opinions against the United Kingdom. Death from disease, a subject historically glossed over in military annals, now took center stage in an effort of pure, political propaganda.

In the middle of September 1776, the British military occupied Manhattan. For the next seven years, New York was an occupied city. Due to its location amidst the other colonies and its port facilities, it quickly became a depot for the tens of thousands of captured American rebels. Following the devastating fire of 1776 that destroyed large sections of the city, and with the number of prisoners increasing almost daily, buildings, churches, and warehouses were quickly requisitioned and were soon filled to overflowing. Conditions in these buildings became notoriously terrible but worse was yet to come.

The British command decided to moor a series of ships in Brooklyn Harbor for use as prison vessels. These would eventually include the *John*, *Scorpion*, *Strombolo*, *Hunter*, and the infamous *Jersey*, a former hospital ship that was now fulfilling a far different purpose. Housing over a thousand soldiers at any given time, the *Jersey* included men captured from campaigns as far afield as Halifax and St. Augustine. Disease ravaged the prisoners held below deck, with typhoid, dysentery, yellow fever, smallpox, and scurvy recorded by those who survived.

> The heat so intense (the hot sun shining all day on deck) that they were all naked, which also served the well to get rid of the vermin, but the sick were

eaten up alive. Their sickly countenances and ghastly looks were truly horrible; some swearing and blaspheming; some crying, praying and wringing their hands, stalking about like ghosts and apparitions; others delirious and void of reason, raving and storming; some groaning and dying, all panting for breath; some dead and corrupting. The air was so foul at times, that a lamp could not be kept burning, by reason of which three boys were not missed until they had been dead three days. One person only is admitted on deck at a time, after sun-set, which necessarily occasions much filth to run into the hold, and mingle with the bilge water.[2]

The death toll aboard the *Jersey* could reach over 10 a day. British guards would approach the hatches in the morning demanding the prisoners "turn out their dead."[3] As they were often refused permission to come above deck at night to relieve themselves due to fear of escape, excrement would pile up for feet around the hatches by morning. When combined with the lack of good food, poor ventilation, lack of medical care, poor sanitation, and the various preexisting conditions brought aboard by the prisoners, disease spread rapidly. As one prisoner wrote:

At the time I was on board, there were about 1,100 prisoners, no berths to lie in, or benches to sit on; many were without clothes. Dysentery, fever, pleurisy, and despair prevailed. The scantiness and bad quality of provisions, the brutality of the guards, and the sick pining for comforts they could not obtain altogether furnished the cruelest scene of horror ever beheld.[4]

Estimations for how many men were killed aboard the prison ships range from a low of 10,000 to far higher numbers. Two to three times as many men were killed here, off the coast of Brooklyn, than in any other theater of the war. Out of those that died, almost all succumbed to disease. While illness tended to be the largest cause of death in all conflicts prior to the 20th century, it represented almost the entirety of casualties on the prison ships. As Philip Freneau recounted at the time shortly after his own capture and imprisonment:

> Convey'd to York, we found, at length, too late,
> That Death was better than the prisoner's fate;
> There doom'd to famine, shackles and despair,
> Condemn'd to breathe a foul, infected air
> In sickly hulks, devoted while we lay,
> Successive funerals gloom'd each dismal day[5]

Disease was a topic usually omitted from most accounts of war prior to the modern era. Stories of battles highlighted deaths, wounds, casualties, and massacres but tended to gloss over sicknesses or those who died due to pestilence. This historiographical omission was most likely due to a combination of factors, including an ignorance of the nature and impact of illness, a miasmic view that associated it with filthiness or immorality, and a desire to provide glorious, battlefield deaths to soldiers rather than ones in hospital cots. Yet, the experience of the prison ships allowed for the topic of disease to be seized upon as a means by which to push anti–British sentiment. In this case, the conditions on the hulks were not the fault of the American soldiers and sailors but instead could be used to disparage the English. With the prevalent and rising political tension between the two countries after the Revolution, it was only a matter of time before politicians did just that.

One of the many divergent issues between the Federalist and Jeffersonian Republican parties of the early republic period was in the field of foreign relations. Hamilton and his followers tended to be Anglophiles, favoring closer diplomatic and economic relations with the United Kingdom. On the other hand, Jefferson and his party were much more pro-French and looked toward the Continent for relations. Following the victory of Jefferson in 1800, the government began to pursue a much more anti–British foreign policy. This coincided with England's ongoing war with Napoleon, in which they aggressively attempted to restrict American trade with Europe.

During the time period from 1801 to 1812, the British encouraged and aided Native American attacks on the American frontier and kidnapped thousands of sailors under a policy known as impressment. These assaults on American ships increased dramatically around 1803 and were a major source of anger among Republicans in coastal cities and communities. The culmination of these attacks on the new country's ability to operate freely and openly on the high seas came in June 1807. On the 22nd of that month, the British HMS *Leopard* attacked and boarded the smaller American warship USS *Chesapeake* right off of the coast of Virginia. The practice of impressment had reached a much more aggressive level. President Jefferson himself wrote, "Never, since the battle of Lexington have I seen this country in such a state of exasperation as at present: and even that did not produce such unanimity."[6] On the national level, what followed was Jefferson's infamous Embargo Act of 1807, which effectively destroyed foreign trade. These and other moves slowly brought the United States toward war with the United Kingdom, a conflict that would finally erupt in 1812.

Shortly after the *Chesapeake-Leopard* Affair and the passage of the Embargo Act, Republicans moved to seize upon and incense the anti–British sentiment at the time. As early as 1803, Congressman Samuel L. Mitchell of New York had petitioned Congress for federal money to help allay the cost of constructing a proper burial vault and monument for victims of the British prison ships. Throughout the time period from 1776 to the turn of the century, locals had periodically recovered bodies, skeletons, or partial remains that washed up on the shores of Wallabout Bay in Brooklyn.

V. Buffalo Fever and the Anti-War Movement

As the poet Philip Freneau, himself both a Jeffersonian Republican and a former prisoner aboard one of the ships, famously wrote,

> Each day, at least three carcases we bore,
> And scratch'd them graves along the sandy shore;[7]

A local shipbuilder by the name of John Jackson had gathered up the remains for years as they washed ashore. Jackson had begun a small shipbuilding industry in Wallabout Bay during the war. By 1801, he had received a federal commission to build the New York Naval Shipyard and produce warships for the country. The necessary expansion of his property and operation only exposed further human remains in the area. Both he and many of his men were also staunch proponents of Tammany Hall, openly sharing their stories of finding thousands of remains with local Democrat-Republican leaders. Yet, Mitchell was unable to procure any promises from Congress, and the victims of the *Jersey* and other prison ships continued to be unceremoniously deposited around Wallabout Bay.

Benjamin Romaine, a longtime sachem at Tammany Hall, saw political promise in the issue, and began a longtime campaign to construct a proper monument for the deceased. As part of this, he wrote to President Jefferson to express Tammany's support for a more aggressive attitude toward England as well as an appeal to remember the victims of the prison ships.[8] In January of 1808, only a few months after the Chesapeake affair, the Jeffersonians of New York's Tammany Hall formed the Wallabout Committee to both design a monument and push for state funding. The state, under Republican governor Daniel Tompkins, would eventually respond by allocating $1,000 for the purpose.

The Tammany Society undertook an involved project to construct a tomb for the remains and ceremoniously reinter them. On April 13, 1808, a procession moved from the old ferry in Brooklyn, down Main Street, Bridge Street, York Street, and Jackson to the waterfront of Wallabout Bay in modern-day Vinegar Hill. Leading the march was a company of U.S. Marines, followed by various local Tammany officials and dignitaries. The gathered Republicans ceremoniously laid the cornerstone for the burial vault and then stood in a moment of silence. "It was a moment big with patriotic, and exalted, and enthusiastic feelings. It seemed that the recollections and sensibilities of America were concentrated—and that the debt of gratitude to the memory of 11,000 of her brave but unfortunate defenders which it belonged to a nation to discharge, was about to be cancelled."[9] Orations were delivered and testimony was read that specifically highlighted the terrible conditions of the ship, being "infected with contagion ... pregnant with putrid fever and deadly with nauseous contagion."[10]

The entire ceremony was both solemn and outrageously vindictive against the English.

The corner-laying ceremony was followed a month later by a formal reinterment of the bones of the victims. On May 26, a massive funeral procession was held to deposit the remains, accompanied by guns, trumpeters on black horses, various military officials in ceremonial costume, soldiers, bands, clergy, the entire Tammany delegation, the mayor and governor of New York, various trade unions, and finally as many citizens as wanted to join the march. In short, it was a massive political march during an election year.

The presidential election of 1808 was a contest between the Republican James Madison and his Federalist opponent Charles C. Pinckney. Jefferson's Embargo Act had largely crippled foreign trade and turned much of New England and New York against him. Many in the party feared that Pinckney could ride this issue to the presidency, especially if he carried New York. As Morgan Lewis lamented in a letter to James Madison in September, "The prevailing Opinion that the Embargo was producing a Change in the public Sentiment ... would give a Chance for a federal President."[11] Madison's choice of George Clinton of New York as well as Tammany Hall's exaggerated performance and erection of the Prison Ship Memorial can all be seen as efforts to tilt the state into the Republican column.

Part of this was clearly driven by trends in local state elections that had been occurring. In April 1808, shortly before the erection of the memorial, Jefferson's party lost six house seats in the state to Federalists. This completely reversed the steady gains that the Republicans had been making for nearly 20 years, and represented the first time since 1789 that the two parties were essentially tied in representation. In the 1st Congressional District, which at the time covered Kings and Queens counties as well as the rest of Long Island, the Republican candidate only managed to win by 18 votes out of 4,200 votes cast.

Yet, following the Tammany performance, Madison and Clinton carried most of the electoral votes of New York and easily beat Pinckney with 122 electoral votes to his 47. Likewise, during the next congressional election in 1810, Republicans reclaimed three House seats and Ebenezer Sage of the 1st Congressional District this time coasted to victory with nearly 95 percent of the votes. What followed was four more years of anti–British sentiment and legislation as well as a slow walk toward the War of 1812. It does become an interesting historical question of whether the Republicans were pushing for war, electoral victory, or both.

Once war was officially declared, casualties followed a similar path to what had occurred during the American Revolution. Bravery on the

V. Buffalo Fever and the Anti-War Movement

battlefield mattered little when the vast majority of deaths were caused by illness. It has been estimated that three-quarters of all American deaths in the conflict came from viruses and bacteria, as opposed to bullets and bayonets. Diseases such as pneumonia, typhus, influenza, dysentery, and various other conditions took lives, crippled armies, ruined offensives, and directed the course of the conflict.

From the earliest days of the republic, the free press quickly became dominated by the emerging political parties. Newspapers had viciously promoted their candidates and attacked others, debated political laws and issues, and pushed agendas and ideas. Now, with the first major war to occur in the country breaking out in 1812, Federalist and Republican journalists quickly moved to either praise or demonize the conflict. As one historian recounted, "In fact, papers were published whose sole purpose was to oppose and ridicule the war."[12] The outbreak of disease among the soldiers became an unlikely, but ultimately understandable, source of confrontation between the two. Federalist papers saw illness as a way to embarrass President Madison and his administration. Much as with the Republican politicization of the prison ships, in which they blamed the British for causing the conditions that resulted in disease decimating the pure and innocent soldiers, the Federalists sought to place the blame for deaths in this war solely on the White House. At the same time, Republican papers worked hard to downplay all allegations of diseases erupting along the front. At the same time, both sides blamed the other for politicizing the issue. The most serious example of this came with the outbreak of the "Buffalo Fever" over the winter of 1812–1813.

The initial and obvious plan for the campaign against British Canada involved an advance from New York. This would follow the traditional invasion routes that had been used for over a century by the English and colonists during wars with the French. Following the failure of the American army at Queenston Heights in October of 1812, the military moved toward building up and training units in upstate New York for a spring offensive the next year. The massive camps that sprung up in the region became a breeding ground for bacteria and viruses from across the country.

Among the various diseases then visiting the soldiers in upstate New York, which included measles, typhoid, and dysentery, several more ambiguous and deadly outbreaks occurred. The most famous of these was the Buffalo Fever outbreak of 1812–1813. The exact nature of the disease as well as its very existence became the subject of debate among rival political newspapers at the time. Several New England Federalist papers reported its presence in November of 1812 and claimed that infections were crippling the military and preventing victory. The *Washingtonian* of Windsor, Vermont, carried articles that stressed the suffering of soldiers at Burlington and Plattsburgh, pointing out that no funds or supplies were being provided to them and bodies were either being left unburied or else placed in shallow graves. The *New England Palladium* carried an article in December that said "the dead were thrown into a hole in the sand barely deep enough to admit of their being covered."[13] The *Portland Gazette* even strongly hinted that disease was a prime cause of the army's failure at Queenston, lamenting "what excellent providers for an army, our War Hawk's are."[14]

In response, Republican papers sought to correct or downplay the news. The *Enquirer* of Richmond published a letter from James Mann, a U.S. Army surgeon, which not only cleared the soldiers of any blame but praised the government's response as well. Though Mann admits "one third of the men had been seized with the measles," he points out that it is a "disease subject to no human control."[15] Likewise, he went on to state that the subsequent fever, which struck the gathered armies in New York and which proved to be so fatal, was due to the weakened state of those who had contracted measles. "The disease for several days was alarming, in consequence of the many sudden deaths," but this "was not owing to any inattention on the part of the government, or neglect of the officers."[16] The paper itself went on to vouch for the views of Dr. Mann by stating that its own reporters had visited the camps and seen the men well cared for and bodies buried properly.

Federalist papers, though, continued to track its progress and rage about the conditions faced by American soldiers in the field. On January 4, 1813, the *New York Evening Post* reported, "The fever which has made such dreadful havoc among our soldiers and cities continues to rage."[17] The disease had now apparently escaped from the overcrowded camps of the Hudson and Mohawk Rivers and entered the cities of upstate New York. By January 13, the *Evening Post* had begun to refer to the plague as the "Buffalo Fever."[18] Other papers soon began to carry death announcements for citizens, citing the Buffalo Fever as the cause of their demise.[19]

Republican apologists and army surgeons continued to respond to these criticisms in various periodicals. Dr. Benjamin Waterhouse, perhaps the earliest proponent of Jenner's smallpox vaccine in the country, wrote a lengthy rebuttal to Federalist claims in the *Richmond Enquirer* on January 14, 1813. The Boston physician identified the cause of death for the "but little over an hundred men" as measles and complications from it, discrediting the entire presence of a "Buffalo Fever."[20]

Despite this, the sickness continued to rage in the towns of the region, being reported endemic at Herkimer on February 2.[21] By early February, the *New York Evening Post* reported that over two dozen members of the

State Assembly had taken ill, and two had died, Aaron Olmsted and Josiah Bartlett. The paper's editor opined, "I have no doubt an adjournment of the Legislature will take place, probably to New York."[22] Over the next week, an additional member, Nathaniel Medbury, died as well. Talk of having to relocate the state government would have brought back memories of the yellow fever epidemic of a generation before and been used as political fodder by the Federalists. A move by the Republicans to relocate the legislature would be interpreted as both an admission of the severity of the situation as well as be perceived as flight in the face of danger. As the *Baltimore Whig* lamented in mid–February, "The disasters in war were occasioned ... by cowardly or treacherous officers."[23]

Over the next few weeks, though, the disease seems to have run its course and subsided. The Assembly stayed in Albany and death rates dropped as the spring approached. As April progressed and the St. Lawrence River thawed, General Dearborn was even able to undertake a raid on Canada that burned the town of York (Toronto) to the ground. Disease would continue to devastate both the American and British armies and dramatically contribute to the relative stalemate of the conflict, but its failure to impact the general public on a large scale most likely contributed to its disappearance as a talking point from newspapers by the middle of 1813.

> We are happy to have it in our power to state, that the sickness among the soldiers in this town has abated ... from the public prints you would be induced to believe that the troops have been intirely destroyed by sickness, disease, etc ... the fact is they have wanted for nothing ... while they were sick for a time, health is now perfectly restored.[24]

Proof of the ability of Republicans to downplay the outbreaks is shown by the fact that Governor Tompkins won reelection in 1813 with 52 percent of the vote, only 2 percent less than what he achieved in 1810. This came despite the wave of elections that removed most Republican governors and legislators from power that same year.

The events leading up to the War of 1812 and the conflict itself presented the first major opportunities for the politicization of disease on a national level. The conflicts between Federalists and Republicans during the yellow fever epidemic of 1793 now spilled over into the press. While one side sought to proclaim the outbreak of a general epidemic due to the malfeasance of the government, the other sought to downplay any tales of illness and praise its own response. Yet in the end, disease was an immense force in the war, much as it had been in all conflicts. Similar battles over disease by a politicized press would occur in subsequent wars as well.

Chapter VI

"A people so well fed and so clean": Cholera and Jacksonian Politics

The Jacksonian era is often looked at as a time of modernization for the United States. The country experienced tremendous change in terms of its economy, politics, technology, demographics, and societal norms. The Industrial Revolution dramatically transformed the Northeast, the nation began its steady push westward across the Mississippi River, cities began to grow and spread, and reform movements emerged to address issues in prisons, mental asylums, and public schools. The United States that emerged from the Jacksonian Era was a far different country than that of only a generation before. Yet, these advancements were not without their critics and not without their associated negative results. Early industrialization brought with it urbanization and all of the problems normally associated with cities. Chief among these in the 1830s and 1840s was disease.

The 19th century saw the emergence of a new disease on the world stage, cholera. Though the illness had been endemic for perhaps centuries in India, it had most likely never escaped from the confines of the subcontinent. Caused by the bacterium *Vibrio cholera*, the disease caused massive dehydration and was frequently fatal. Cholera could be found in some of the rivers and streams of India and spread due to unsanitary drinking water and waste disposal systems. Due to both its vectoring agents as well as the speed with which it consumed its host, the pestilence tended to not make it beyond the boundaries of India. Yet, this suddenly changed with the onset of the 19th century.

The British takeover of India, the various wars of imperialism that plagued the continent, and the advent of clipper ships, steamships, and, eventually, railroads helped to transport cholera far beyond its traditional environment. Multiple pandemics then followed between 1817 and 1896, which touched every part of the planet. Tens of millions of lives were lost over the course of the century, with profound changes also taking place that impacted the politics, economy, and society of the entire world.

VI. "A people so well fed and so clean"

Though the first pandemic, which raged from 1817 to 1824, never reached Europe, it did excite interest among the general public. At the time, the disease was often seen as little different than dysentery, and the two terms were frequently used interchangeably. By and large, however, the general assumption was that cholera would never reach Europe and the Americas, not solely because of any particular geographic barrier but due to the cleanliness of the people. As James Fenimore Cooper would opine, "I should not think it will prove a very bad disease among a people so well fed and so clean."[1] Not only the Mediterranean and Atlantic but also the tenets of miasma theory would protect the West.

These beliefs began to be shattered, however, in the early 1830s, as the second pandemic reached both places. Deaths quickly topped 6,500 in the UK and 100,000 in France, with over 3 percent of the city of Paris succumbing. While Americans followed these developments in the press, most hoped that the cordon sanitaire of the Atlantic, as well as the perceived superior cleanliness of the population, would provide ample protection.

Newspapers, especially those with a more Whig bent, followed the path of the pandemic in Europe very closely in 1831, reporting almost daily on case numbers and deaths. Yet, despite this, very few called for any sort of active preparation should the disease cross the ocean. Those that did, such as the *Rhode Island Republican*, suggested focusing on the quarantining of ships arriving in American ports.[2] As 1832 dawned, and the bacteria creeped closer to America, other papers began to join in the chorus. An op-ed featured in the *Phenix Gazette*, in February of 1832, urged President Jackson to demand from Congress that "some measures may be pursued, that some barrier may be raised, to prevent the approach of this cruel disease."[3]

The politicization of the disease was early on confined more to its use as a pejorative for the rule of "King Andrew." The same *Gazette* used the term in January of 1832 to describe the vitriolic temper of the president. "His pains are in no measure abated but daily increase, until they have arrived at a point approximating to non-endurance, and he 'roars' terribly."[4] A few weeks later, the pro–Jackson *Plattsburgh Republican* harshly criticized another paper for using the same term, calling it "disgraceful."[5] In late May, Vice President Martin Van Buren was in Paris, visiting with the nation's leaders. An American newspaper opined as to the dangers of the "little Magician" contracting the disease, specifically the impact it would have on the Jackson administration.[6] One must appreciate that in the era of miasmic thinking, the implication being presented was that Van Buren was a member of the poor and intemperate who were subject to the illness.

Democratic newspapers overall tended to downplay the threat posed by cholera. One such periodical, the *Phenix Gazette*, referred to the illness in May 1832 as pure "humbug."[7] A few months earlier, the *Plattsburgh Republican* argued, "Imagination is the thing to be afraid of," proposing that the nearly constant reports of the disease in Whig periodicals were causing the most damage to the nation.[8] Yet, as the year wore on and public interest in the contagion faded, even the anti-administration newspapers began to lose interest in the contagion. An article carried in the Richmond-based *Constitutional Whig* quoted Parisian officials as saying, "The cholera is a grave disorder. It is however more alarming when expected than dangerous when it actually exists."[9] Likewise, an article in the *Phenix Gazette* a week later reassured Americans that the disease would only strike the poor and unclean.[10]

Yet, this all began to change with the onset of June 1832. Early in that month, cholera finally arrived in the New World. Tradition assigns its origins to the ship *Constantia,* which docked in Montreal in June. Though this may have been the initial vector for the bacteria, additional sailings certainly brought it to other ports as well. Based upon the spread of the disease and its chronology, it is almost certain that cholera infected vessels docked at New York City, Philadelphia, and New Orleans during the summer of that year. Likewise, coastal trading ships carried the illness between ports as did those people fleeing the disease by land. Overall, a conservative estimate based on available death totals per state would place the ultimate casualties of cholera at some 16,000–18,000 Americans, with two-thirds of those cases occurring in New York and Louisiana alone.

Though the initial panic over cholera in Canada soon subsided, responses to the pandemic quickly diverged along party lines as it took hold in New York City and other areas. Initially, reports of victims were often couched by both sides in the fact that the victims were immigrants or else led intemperate lives.[11] This trend of victim shaming had as much to do with miasma theory as it did with politics and would see repetition with subsequent diseases, most notably AIDS in the 1980s, as well as during the pandemic of 2020. Because of the rapidly increasing death tolls, quarantines and restrictions on immigration seemed to be the proper course of action to many. This view was particularly favored by National Republicans and Whigs who sought to separate the sick from the healthy and exclude the former from the nation. Though utilized for centuries to combat epidemics, internal quarantines were viewed by many Democrats as an affront to personal liberty, while politically the party could not afford to alienate the Irish or slow immigration.[12]

Despite this, many prominent Democratic politicians thoroughly embraced the tactic. Most notable among this group was perhaps Walter

Bowne, the mayor of New York City. Several months before the announcement that cholera had reached Canada, Mayor Browne had preemptively declared a total quarantine of the city with regards to ships arriving from Europe and Asia.[13] With the arrival of news that the disease had crossed the Atlantic, this quarantine was turned into a general embargo against all shipping.[14] These tactics harkened back to the approaches of Jefferson in dealing with the impressment tactics of the English and likewise produced visceral responses from Whigs who saw it as destroying their businesses.

Governor Enos Throop of New York did attempt an external quarantine by blocking the approaches from Canada, seeking to stem the flow of disease into the state from that direction as early as July 4, 1832. A few weeks later, Dr. Lewis Beck was dispatched from Albany to the Canadian border to study the progress of the disease. His groundbreaking study showed the steady march of the illness down the various canals of New York and toward the city. While his discovery predated that of Dr. John Snow's by a generation, Beck did not speculate as to the microorganismal nature of the disease. Apart from scientific limitation, he may have been hampered by fears of damaging the economic backbone of the state or of increasing animosity toward the Irish.[15] Overall, he argued that the disease was not contagious, largely based upon data that those who were caring for victims were not themselves acquiring the illness.[16] In response, Democratic administrations tended to focus on using the power of government to improve the conditions of the poor, including the cleaning of streets and the improvement of public sanitation within those afflicted areas.

Class distinction became even more apparent as those who possessed the means to do so began to abandon the cities for long vacations in the countryside, informally establishing quarantines in most urban areas. Yet, this tactic only further exposed the divide that existed within Jacksonian Era urban society. As one newspaper reported at the time, "The roads, in all directions, were lined with well-filled stagecoaches, livery coaches, private vehicles and equestrians, all panic-struck, fleeing the city."[17] In keeping with the fact that his Log Cabin persona was largely a political veneer, Jackson himself recommended to his adopted son, Andrew Jackson Donelson, that he "remove ... into the country if the disease should appear to seize all persons, those of regular as well as those of irregular habits."[18] Overall, flight and separation were the approaches favored by National Republicans and the wealthy of both parties.

The Irish likewise became a natural target for many due to both their status as immigrants and their perceived low class and intemperate nature. Newspapers frequently cited the Irish as victims of the plague due to their "imprudent" lifestyles.[19] With the then current miasmic thinking, it was considered that the Irish largely brought the disease upon themselves.

With the disease arriving in the middle of the Second Great Awakening, a religious revival of Protestantism across the nation, the influx of hundreds of thousands of Catholic immigrants was viewed with loathing and religious opposition by many. Some communities went far beyond simply blaming the Irish and openly targeted them for their role in spreading the contagion. The most notable of these episodes occurred in late July or early August 1832 when 57 Irish immigrants were massacred at the Duffy's Cut stretch of the Philadelphia and Columbia Railroad in Pennsylvania.

The use of violence against those who were perceived to be the prime spreaders of illness was certainly not a new phenomenon. In 1793, during the yellow fever epidemic that raged in Philadelphia, the city of New York formed street patrols to make sure that refugees from that stricken metropolis were not arriving in Manhattan. The lower classes and immigrants often became targets for these men, in part due to fear that they were breeding grounds for the arrival of contagion. A combination of nosophobia and classism led to a series of assaults and confrontations, all of which culminated in the Whorehouse Riots.

For two nights in October 1793, local New Yorkers attacked and razed a collection of brothels in lower New York City. The attack first erupted against two establishments owned and operated by Mrs. Carey and Co. near Chatham Row. The mob was widely reported to be an army of the lower class, as one contemporary paper stated, "Boys, apprentices and Negroes as well as Sailors, formed a great proportion of the persons concerned in the shameful riot Monday and Yesterday evening." The men besieged the building for hours, even receiving musket fire from the inhabitants. After burning the home to the ground, the mob moved on to Canvas Town, a den of scandal and sin that had grown out of the ashes of the great fire of 1776. Homes were destroyed and buildings lit alight, before a citizen militia on horseback rode into the area to clear out the mobs.

Though massive loss of life was avoided and only a few buildings were ultimately destroyed, the causes of the riot stand out as particularly interesting. The initial impetus for the uprising was given at the time as a reaction to the acquittal of a gentleman accused of rape. Stories spread that the victim had been forced into prostitution, thus making the brothels a target. The larger zeitgeist of the time appears to have been a concern over the yellow fever epidemic then spreading through Philadelphia. Armed, agitated, and active groups were present within the city and needed only a slight spark to conflagrate into a general riot. Incidentally, not all residents of the city were opposed to the actions of the mob, with many praising their attacks:

> The Citizens of New-York are greatly obliged and much indebted to the vigilance and conscientious care which the Corporation and Committee, who

VI. "A people so well fed and so clean"

act in conjunction for the preservation of health, have uniformly manifested. Hitherto we have acted on general terms. We now invite the Gentlemen's attention to Duke and mill-streets, where proper subjects present themselves for minute investigation. Let us take a view of the ruins and avenues that lead to and from the same, and then determine whether or not such places claim the attention of those who are invested with authority—Remedies there are and redress expected. The exposed state of some dwelling houses, and yards adjoining the ruins is unsafe, being liable at any time to the inroads and interruption of evil-minded persons.[20]

These concerns over the role that immorality and imprudence were playing in helping to spread the disease were also seized upon by some of the religious institutions of the day. "It is, indeed, a very solemn spectacle to see sick persons carried through the streets in such vast numbers.... Great fear and much excitement prevail almost amidst all classes of people. The cholera! The cholera! ... Oh that his fear might lead the wicked inhabitants of this city to humble and unfeigned repentance."[21] In June, shortly before the announcement that the disease had entered Canada, the Dutch Reform Synod of New York wrote to President Jackson, asking for a "general observance of a day of fasting, humiliation, and prayer, that if it please God that our country may be preserved from the attacks of the pestilence."[22]

President Jackson's reply, written shortly afterward, harkened back to Jefferson's Danbury Letter of 1802. Though he acknowledged "the efficacy of prayer," the president doubted the constitutional wisdom of proclaiming a day of fast.[23] Yet his opponents were quick to point out that Washington, Adams, and Madison had all proclaimed days of fasting, making this hardly an unprecedented or unconstitutional act.

Henry Clay quickly seized upon the incident, combining it with the president's dissolution of the U.S. Bank to produce a formidable platform.[24] In Congress, Clay introduced a resolution two weeks after Jackson's letter, requesting the president to set aside a day of fasting and prayer in order to implore God to "avert from our country the Asiatic scourge which is now traversing and devastating other countries."[25] The Democratic Senate approved the measure the next day by a vote of 30 to 13, with almost half of the president's party breaking ranks to support the bill. The overwhelmingly Democratic House moved to amend the legislation to remove the need for Jackson's announcement, but Clay and his allies quickly moved to oppose it.

Democratic newspapers were quick to attack Clay for this maneuver, citing his hypocrisy in both religion and in concern for an official day of fasting. "These Pharisees wish for long prayers, to injure General J. and defeat his election; but they disclaim and reject praying and fasting, to avert the Cholera. It is not the Cholera that makes them so pious; it is a hope to steal a march on the old Hero."[26] Clay himself was rather agnostic about his religious beliefs and was well known at the time for his "drinking and carousing," yet nevertheless, he was openly embraced by the religious forces of the Second Great Awakening in response to his stance on the day of prayer and fasting.[27]

The disease disrupted campaigning, stifled voices, and even led to the deaths of several candidates and party leaders. The most notable of these was probably William H. Maynard, a state senator from New York. The latter had been organizing a trip to Ohio in June 1832 when he was stricken with the illness. Maynard was an influential member of the Anti-Masonic Party and was hoping to travel to the state to cement an alliance between the two main anti–Jacksonian parties. Unfortunately, his death reduced these prospects. Stronger support from the Anti-Masonic Party would have allowed Clay and his party to win New Jersey, Vermont, and possibly Ohio as well. As Clay himself lamented in a later October letter to James Brown, "The Ohio Election has gone against us … owing, as it is said, to the want of arranging a proper concert between the Anti Masons and N. Republicans."[28]

As the election grew closer, some pro–Jackson newspapers began to report Henry Clay's death from cholera. A minor illness experienced by the senator while attending his daughter's wedding in Louisville in the fall of 1832 was soon magnified by newspapers to show that Clay had perished due to cholera. Clay had to take the unprecedented step of informing his friends that he was in fact very much alive: "You may probably hear that I caught the pestilence, and have been long since dead and buried. You are authorized to contradict, most positively, such a report if you should hear it."[29] Clay himself utilized the disease as a foil for his attacks on the terrors of Jacksonian Democracy: "Jacksonism! It is worse than the Cholera, because it has been more universal, and will be more durable. The Cholera performs its terrible office, and its victims are consigned to the grave, leaving their survivors uncontaminated. But Jacksonism has poisoned the whole Community, the living as well as the dead."[30] One reader wrote to the *Corrector* in New York in September that by not voting for Jackson an acquaintance of his was cured of the disease.[31]

Democratic newspapers likewise used the contagion to critique Clay and his supporters. The *Plattsburgh Republican* announced in September 1832 that the four greatest terrors confronting the nation were "cholera, the comet, Clay, and creditors."[32] At the same time, the *Rhode Island Republican* opined that Clay himself was as destructive as the disease. "The preventative to the first is to be found in the intelligence, purity, and independence of the people—the remedy against the second, is in their cleanliness, temperance, and care."[33]

VI. "A people so well fed and so clean"

Though the disease damaged the American economy and certainly affected several local races, its impact on the national contest between Clay and Jackson was less clear. Apart from the loss of Kentucky and South Carolina, the former due to the fact that it was Clay's home state and the latter due to the president's actions during the Nullification Crisis, the Democrats won more states than in 1828, even making advances into New England. This was possibly due to a number of factors, including the relatively late arrival of cholera during the election cycle, increased voter turnout in cities, driven in part by Irish immigration, and the fact that Clay seemed unable to use the pestilence to turn enough public anger against Jackson and the Democrats. The latter point had much to do with the political landscape of the time in which local and state government were still seen as the primary vehicles by which to tackle public health issues rather than the federal government. Nevertheless, disease was now a highly politicized component of national life. Politicians and their parties used its arrival, spread, and containment for their own political ends, a trend that would only accelerate over the next two centuries.

CHAPTER VII

Presidential Poxes

Battles developed between the political philosophies over how best to tackle pandemics that struck the nation. Yet, at least during the 19th century, these episodes were largely seen as falling under the responsibilities of individuals or, at best, the state. The federal government, and specifically the White House, was seen as having no major role, apart from setting aside days of prayer, in the confrontation of epidemics. Yet, this did not stop the parties from using the appearance of disease to attack their opponents in office.

Many cultures have historically viewed the arrival of disease as a sign of natural or divine displeasure. This anger could be directed against the society as a whole but more usually was viewed as a sign of a loss of favor by the leader. Indeed, the outbreak of an epidemic became one of the most common signs for the Chinese of the loss of the Mandate of Heaven. These episodes frequently then led to internal rebellion, attempted coups, and even the downfall of dynasties. Though early on American presidents largely played no role in either the arrival or management of disease, the chance to paint them as responsible was too much for politicians to ignore.

Disease was often used as a label to attack entire political parties and movements. Some of the earliest examples of this occurred during the Jeffersonian era. Federalists feared not only Jefferson's actions but also the dangerous philosophies that were then arriving from France. Newspapers frequently reported on the excesses and horrors of the French Revolution during the 1790s and, though they had largely passed by the time Jefferson was elected thanks to the coronation of Napoleon, Federalists still played up the dangers. A letter to the editor of the *Alexandria Daily Advertiser* from November 1804 discusses the "French political disease" of the Jeffersonians. The author went on to claim that the Republicans were eliminating what they saw as the warts of the legislative process, Article 2 of the Constitution, and elections. He finished by stating that they carried their creed "hanging around their necks like *goiters* … proud of their deformity."[1] Similar accusations that "the political head is diseased" were lobbed at

Jefferson in 1808 as Anglo-American relations deteriorated and war seemed inevitable.[2]

Jefferson's allies hurled similar attacks against their opponents. The Federalists were accused of having "again overshadowed the land and filled it with political disease."[3] Likewise, as the Second Party System crumbled in the 1830s and 1840s, disease was frequently used as a metaphor to describe its newly emerging parties. An 1837 article in the *Madisonian* referred to the Locofocos faction of the Democratic party as a diseased appendage.[4] Likewise, an editor of the *Mississippi Democrat* encouraged his readers not to fear the newly emerged Whig party as it was merely composed of the diseased parts of the Democratic party, which had sloughed off.[5] Similar language was used to describe the decline of the party as well, with one writer referring to it as a "diseased" death.[6]

Perhaps the most famous example of disease being used to target an individual politician involved President John Tyler. While every president from Washington to Harrison had produced a certain level of hatred among the opposite party, none was more universally loathed at the time then Tyler. When General William Henry Harrison ran for the office of presidency in 1840, the Whig Party felt that it needed a southerner to effectively balance out the ticket. With few southern Whigs available, the party eventually settled on Senator John Tyler of Virginia.

Tyler was far from a traditional choice, however. From the start of his political career, he had been a staunch Jeffersonian, arguing for an extremely limited federal government. A vibrant supporter of the War of 1812 and of free trade, he was far removed from the Federalist Party platforms of the time. Yet, the rise of Andrew Jackson soon saw Tyler growing at odds with his own party. The Democrats began to embrace the idea of a stronger, centralized government. At the same time, Jackson's own power grabs were viewed with increased apprehension by the Virginian. By 1833, he found himself siding more often with Clay and the Whigs than his own party. What followed was a predictable resignation after the Democrats took power in Congress in 1836.

Tyler was nominated for the vice presidency in 1836 by the Whigs, during a messy election that involved multiple candidates. When 1840 arrived, and Harrison was chosen to be the only standard bearer for the party, Tyler was once again considered a good compromise candidate for the second position. The party's inventive electioneering, which focused heavily on free alcohol, advertisements, catchy songs, mythological histories for the main candidate, and little to no platform, swept "Tippecanoe and Tyler Too" into the White House in March of 1841. Tyler would have most likely enjoyed a quiet four years on his farm had not President Harrison succumbed to pneumonia only a month after his inauguration.

Yet, Tyler was hardly a caretaker president or a Clay-style Whig and quickly moved to both exert himself and veto much of the party's legislation. What followed was an acrimonious four years, the mass resignation of his cabinet, the override of his veto, and an attempt at impeachment. When an epidemic erupted in New England, it became only natural to associate it with Tyler as well.

An outbreak of influenza struck the area of New England around the early summer of 1843. While this would have perhaps gone unnoticed outside of the immediate area, the presence of Tyler at its epicenter, as well as the general opposition to him at the time, soon made it a political tool. President Tyler was touring New England during the summer of that year, culminating in his arrival in Boston for the unveiling of a monument to the Battle of Bunker Hill on June 17. While local newspapers did periodically carry stories of the disease, it became national news when Tyler's attorney general and acting secretary of state, Hugh S. Legare, contracted it and died on June 20.

A few days later, on June 24, the *US Gazette* out of Philadelphia referred to the disease as the "Tyler Grippe," the latter term being a common name at the time for influenza. On June 28, the pro-administration *Daily Madisonian* lambasted the rival paper's editor for his choice of words. Yet, this derision seems to have merely exposed more readers and journalists to the term.[7] An advertisement even appeared the next day in the *New York Daily Tribune*, recommending bathing at Vandervoort's Sea Water Baths in Brooklyn to prevent against Tyler's illness.[8]

The disease was used to attack the character of Tyler, with a Democratic paper out of Virginia describing him as "sniveling, snuffling, and sneezing as is the gentleman of this name now on a visit to this city—a namesake of him in a guise, even less pleasant."[9] One Northumberland, Pennsylvania, newspaper stated, "The prevailing epidemic, the 'Tyler Grippe,' has not neglected us in its visitations, and left us almost as prostrate, physically, as its great namesake is in a political point of view."[10] That year, Henry Clay, who was also stricken with the disease, commiserated with a friend who had likewise been afflicted, "I sympathize with you in your suffering under the Tyler Grippe. I too have had it, and I found it as mean & insidious as its detestable name implies."[11]

The *Alexandria Gazette* carried an article in late July that laid out the history of the disease and its philosophical connections to the president. "It is a disease the least sympathetic, the most relaxing, the most contemptible, and the most harassing, which, without being dangerous, ever afflicted a community; thus occupying in physic the same position which Tylerism does in politics."[12] This particular outbreak of influenza was hardly deadly in comparison to cholera, yellow fever, or other disorders in the century, and this perhaps allowed both parties to focus their attention on the faults of the president instead.

Nor was the disease confined solely to the occupant of the White House but was also applied to those who fell under Tyler's patronage. Martin Van Buren, though an opponent of Harrison in 1840, held some views in common with Tyler and was accused by several papers of having been stricken with the Tyler Grippe.[13] A New York newspaper from July 1843 labeled the three biggest threats facing the country as "the locusts, the Tyler Grippe, and the Tyler influence, as exhibited in the bestowal of public office."[14] When the *Richmond Enquirer* made attacks a few months later against John C. Calhoun for siding with Tyler on several matters, the city's *Daily Whig* accused its editors of "having the Tyler grippe."[15]

Though the epidemic was reported to have crossed the Mississippi by the first week of August, newspapers in that region likewise tended to focus on using it as a means by which to defame the president rather than seeing it as a cause for alarm. Periodicals even carried songs and poems that used the expression to lambast the White House.

> But quick; as if his muse was piqued,
> Or seized with the Tyler Grippe:
> Convulsed; quite from his canoe, he leaped;
> And vowed the Mashine to whip.[16]

Reports of the "Tyler Grippe" died out with the epidemic by the late fall of 1843. But as the next year brought a hotly contested political contest for both the White House and Congress, its metaphorical usage quickly returned. Despite Tyler's own hopes at renomination, neither of the two parties seriously considered running him. Clay, despite advancing age and ill health, saw 1844 as his last chance to win the presidency and quickly sidelined Tyler. A popular Whig song ran at the time:

> Says he (Clay), of late I've been unwell,
> And therefore kept me in my cell,
> But since I've heard of Henry Clay,
> The Tyler grippe has passed away.[17]

As election results began to trickle in, a Maryland-based Whig newspaper lamented, "Oh! A pain struck—we think it is the Tyler grippe, and we fear Dr. Clay *can't* cure it this fall."[18] In a similar vein, after the final victory of Polk in the 1844 election, a newspaper reported that "the Tyler grrippe … was only shaken off on the 4th of March."[19]

The term would continue to surface periodically over the next few decades. The return of cholera in 1857 prompted one newspaper in Iowa to reference the 1843 Tyler grippe.[20] The *Richmond Palladium* in 1867 recommended referring to the outbreak of an upper respiratory fever that year as the "Johnson grippe," due to the fact "he being a cuzzen to that extinguished Virginian *vice* president."[21] Likewise, an 1871 eruption of influenza produced similar references.[22]

Though the vast majority of those who remembered the Tyler presidency were no longer alive, the term itself was resurrected in 1889. In that year, a particular dangerous outbreak of the disease erupted in Europe and references soon began to be made to the Tyler grippe.[23] After writing that the Whig party had been responsible for connecting the disease to the former president back in 1843, a Democratic-affiliated paper out of Pennsylvania was quick to opine, "The two most decided epidemics have followed the election of a Harrison to office and the Democrats may make the most of it."[24] Despite these predictions, little political hay was made of it. The term once more reemerged in a few sources in 1918 with the onset of Spanish influenza, more as a historical reference than a political attack.

Nor was Tyler the only such victim of political disease-labeling. In fact, during a visit by George Washington and his entourage to Boston in 1789, they were stricken with a local epidemic of illness, which many at the time dubbed the "Washington influenza."[25] Some papers around the time of the Spanish influenza pandemic, when referencing the history of the term "Tyler Grippe," also made reference to the "Jackson Itch."[26] Yet, there appears to be little to substantiate these claims, as periodicals from the Jacksonian era bear no reference to any such disease connected to Andrew Jackson. Though a scalp disease can be found in advertisements from the time referred to as "barber's itch" or "Jackson itch," there is no evidence of it being named after the president.

On the other hand, Grover Cleveland did become the target of a minor attempt to paint him in the same epidemiological light as Tyler. As early as March 1885, the *Evening Capital* of Annapolis carried an article that proclaimed the arrival of "the Cleveland Grip," justifying it with "for surely Mr. Cleveland has a strong grip upon the heads and hearts of the people."[27] Yet, apart from a reprinting of the same article by other papers, the term did not catch on.

A few years after the press associated Tyler with the outbreak of an epidemic, there were some minor attempts to do the same with President Zachary Taylor. The latter's victory during the 1848 election had surprised many and pleased few. Concerns over his views on slavery and his Whig agenda left many in both parties unhappy. While he was hardly the pariah that Tyler was, both parties did occasionally issue powerful rebukes of his actions and policies.

Taylor's presidency was also contemporaneous with the second visit of cholera to America. As early as May 1849, while the cholera pandemic raged across the nation, many expressed concern over the health and safety of the new president. While Taylor wasn't particularly unhealthy, at the age of 64 he nevertheless was the second oldest inhabitant of the White House up to that point. The only man to be elected at a more advanced age was William Henry Harrison, who had died shortly after taking office. A newspaper at the time quoted an encounter between the president and someone recommending that he stay in the White House to avoid the disease: "Give yourselves no uneasiness gentlemen, Fillmore is no Tyler."[28]

Opposition newspapers were far less supportive. A Democratic editor wrote in mid–August, "We are happy to find that Taylorism, like the cholera, is rapidly disappearing, and will soon cease to be dangerous. It reached its most violent point last fall, since which time it has been gradually losing ground."[29] Politically, at least, the newspaper was accurate; a sizeable number of local and national seats had been lost since Taylor's inauguration to the Democratic Party.

Due in part to this fact, at the height of the pandemic, in the late summer of 1849, the president undertook a multistate tour, delivering speeches and greeting dignitaries. His itinerary began in Baltimore on August 8, had him traversing most of Pennsylvania for the rest of August, and arriving in Buffalo by early September. Initially, Taylor was then set to travel throughout New England as well. The goal of this entire tour was to buttress support for his party for the upcoming midterm elections of 1850.

Despite initial reports of its success, tragedy soon struck. A newspaper reported on August 18, that President Taylor had been struck with cholera while visiting Carlisle, Pennsylvania. "He was on Monday taken with vomiting while receiving friends at the court house. The diarrhea was stopped, but the symptoms were very bad."[30] It is unclear whether the president actually contracted cholera or simply a similar gastrointestinal issue. Taylor's condition seems to have been serious, as he struggled to continue his itinerary. After viewing Niagara Falls and finally reaching Buffalo on September 5, it was announced that he was returning home because "business calls."[31]

Regardless of the actual nature of the illness, various periodicals began to refer to the entire undertaking as "Taylor's Cholera Tour." First pushed by a newspaper in late September, the name stuck and was utilized over the course of the next several months.[32] The obvious implication here was on the impropriety of Taylor having developed the disease as well as his lack of foresight in visiting a stricken area. As previously discussed, cholera was seen at the time as a disease of the intemperate, both in terms of body and morality. Taylor's sickness was therefore labeled "cholera" for purely political reasons. Though the term seems to have finally gone out of fashion in December, it was resurrected by the *New York Herald* the next year for a brief story on European relations.[33]

Though President Taylor survived the episode, he would ultimately succumb to a gastrointestinal disease the next year, dying in July 1850. The exact nature of his demise has been hotly debated ever since, with some once again pointing toward cholera. In 1859, a company was even running ads that purported to offer cures for Taylor's demise from the disease.[34]

Interestingly, the entire Know Nothing Party became the frequent target in the 1850s of disease-themed attacks in the media. The *Bedford Gazette* carried an article in April of 1855 that stated that joining the party was like an illness: "No one has it twice. It is like the measles in this respect."[35] Around the same time, a South Carolina newspaper featured a supposed lament of a former party member in which he begs to be stricken with smallpox, whooping cough, and neuralgia rather than be struck down by "Know Nothingism a second time."[36] Some even developed a disease to specifically assign to those who joined the party. Termed Know Nothing Monomania, it was said to be the cause of their beliefs and platform.[37]

Though the tactic of associating disease with a particular politician seems to have faded as the 19th century wore on, it was briefly resurrected in the 21st century. In July 2020, several months after the initial peak of the coronavirus pandemic that circled the globe, Speaker of the House Nancy Pelosi referred to the disease twice as the "Trump virus."[38] Once again, though, the nomenclature did not widely catch on and was only occasionally employed by political opponents or web denizens. Pundit Mehdi Hasan used it in September 2020 to attack what he saw as the failure of Trump to successfully confront and contain the virus. "Fine, let's call it the Trump virus.... Put it this way: if you wanted to spread the coronavirus, if you were trying to get people to get the virus, what would you do differently that Donald Trump's already not doing right now?"[39]

Part of this move away from at least politically labeling epidemics during the 20th century may come from both an increased knowledge of their origin and spread, as well as the recognition that ultimately it was usually foreign sources that led to the outbreaks of disease in America. This latter point would instead lead to increased stigmatization against foreign nationals and immigrants as well as efforts to restrict their arrival.

CHAPTER VIII

"The Wretched Refuse": Disease and 19th-Century Immigration Debates

Due to its often-foreign nature, disease has always been associated with "the other." Illness was rarely endemic to an area but instead would arrive and spread periodically with the movement of humans. While this certainly included merchants, explorers, diplomats, and soldiers, it was the immigrant who historically received the most attention. That is not to say there was not validity to these concerns, as mass movements of people, particularly those facing poverty, famine, and pestilence in their homelands, were more likely to bring disease with them. Yet, even in the absence of confirmed incidents of illness being brought to America, miasma theory and nativist beliefs used the concern to help demonize those arriving in the country. With immigration being a divisive issue historically, the debates over migrants and disease quickly became political.

The Germans

One of the first episodes of this occurred in 1755 in Pennsylvania. For several decades, tens of thousands of Germans had been arriving in Philadelphia. They represented the first large-scale immigration to the American colonies of a people from outside the British Isles. As such, opposition to their arrival did emerge in certain segments of Pennsylvanian society. Some of these Germans sought to escape religious persecution at home, some were looking for economic opportunity, and some were only recently released prisoners. Many departed from Europe already infected with disease, while thousands of others contracted illnesses during the miserable trip across the Atlantic. Ships were purposefully overbooked, passengers were crowded into tight quarters with very little food or water, and medical aid was non-existent. It's impossible to determine the exact number of persons who perished during the crossing, but some historians have actually posited that the percentages were either comparable or slightly worse than those experienced at the same time on slave ships plying the Atlantic.[1] One such ship that reached Philadelphia at the time, the *Love and Unity*, saw only 34 of its original 150 passengers survive.[2]

Nor did arrival in the Americas suddenly mean the end of these horrors. Studies have shown that the sickness rate among those who disembarked in Philadelphia ranged from 1 to 11 percent during the 1720s–1750s.[3] Many of these would later succumb to their illnesses while others would spread them among the local population. This was often worsened by the fact that many German immigrants were unable to find employment upon landing, despite earlier promises from recruiters back home. Instead, they would wander the streets, lacking housing or proper nutrition.

In 1754, an outbreak of typhus erupted in Philadelphia, which largely came to be blamed on German immigrants. Interestingly, it seems to have been a far worse experience for the new arrivals, as their mortality rate that year has been reported at 104.6 per 1,000 while that of the general population was only at 34.1 per 1,000, only a slight jump above the 32.4 per 1,000 of the previous year but down substantially from its height in the 1740s.[4] Overall, from 1738 to 1756, recent arrivals experienced a death rate nearly twice that of residents.[5]

The response from the colonial government was one of concern over general public health. In December 1754, Governor Robert Hunter Morris requested that the Assembly pass a measure to limit the importation of sick persons. Yet, despite initial hopes among those in the capital, the crafting of the legislation proved difficult. Considerations over the role of the government in limiting trade, even the trade of humans, as well as anti–German sentiment in some areas, led to a prolonged struggle between Morris and the legislature. In a reply to Morris dated May 15, 1755, the Assembly accused him of removing useful components from the bill to satisfy the interest and greed of those council members who have a financial stake in the importation of Germans.

> We could wish he had been pleased to have exercised his own Judgment upon this our Bill, without referring the Consideration of it to a Committee of his Council, most of them such, as we are informed, who are, or have lately been, concerned in the Importations, the Abuses of which this Bill was designed to regulate and redress.[6]

The Assembly's letter then goes on to attack the immigrants themselves, claiming that they were "afflicted with such secret and loathsome Diseases at the Time." The more recent arrivals were seen as

> a great Mixture of the Refuse of their People, and that the very Gaols have

contributed to the Supplies we are burdened with ... and do become very frequently common Beggars from Door to Door, to the great Injury of the Inhabitants, and the Increase and Propagation of the Distempers they have brought among us.⁷

Morris himself was convinced that the Assembly was merely playing politics by refusing to meet with the council and took extreme umbrage at their suggestion that he had "no Regard for the Health or Safety of the Inhabitants of this Country; in doing which I cannot think you have paid a proper Regard to Truth." As more vital debates over the duty of the colony to support the British offensive against the French in Ohio at the time soon arose, the row over immigration subsided with little action to improve public health. Despite this, Benjamin Franklin, a leading adversary of Morris and a well-known opponent of German immigration, chose to reprint a piece by Scottish physician John Pringle later that year.⁸ Originally written several years before, Franklin hoped to further prod the governor into action to tackle the connected issues of immigration and disease.

With us, since the late Practice of scumming the Gaols in Germany to make up Freights, the Ships are observed to come in more unhealthy, as the Sickness may now be brought on board as well as produced on board. It is said that several of our People lost their Lives last Year by purchasing Dutch Servants out of sickly Ships.⁹

The Germans were to be the first in a long line of immigrant groups targeted for their actual or perceived connection to the arrival of disease in America.

The Irish

The English have long associated disease with the Irish as a way to denigrate that particular culture. At the start of the Tudor conquest, Edmund Spenser frequently employed the metaphors of disease and contagion when addressing the problems of Ireland in his 1596 *A View of the Present Situation in Ireland*. Two centuries later, in Jonathan Swift's *A Modest Proposal*, the pestilential nature of the Irish is highlighted as one of the major problems confronting that nation. Much as with their derogatory view of the Spanish, these beliefs and attitudes were brought over to America as well. Well before the potato blight and associated famine even hit Ireland, newspapers periodically discussed the perceived pestilential nature of the Irish. An article in an 1827 paper reported disease as rampant on the island, with English trade being their only saving grace. "If it were not for the steamboats which convey the Irish to England, typhus fever and disease ... would soon do the business of the plague among that unfortunate people."[10] A few years later, the *Times of London* referred to the people of that nation as "the diseased and helpless Irish."[11]

With the onset of the potato blight in the 1840s, which decimated the crop of much of Ireland and other parts of Europe, attention turned once more to the microbial condition of the Irish. This was clearly augmented by the beginnings of the mass Irish immigration to America, which occurred around 1845. Newspapers carried frequent stories regarding the situation in Ireland, most out of general public curiosity but with some doing so in order to establish a portrayal of the Irish in the minds of the public. Those who emigrated from the island certainly did suffer from illness but more often than not presented a far greater threat to themselves than the citizens of America. It has been estimated that nearly one-quarter of all Irish immigrants perished from disease on the aptly named "coffin ships" during the journey across the Atlantic, a number that was once again worse than the experience of slaves on the Middle Passage.

The *New York Herald*, which was well known in the mid-19th century for its anti-Catholic and anti-Irish bias, began to publish frequent articles that depicted the Irish as a pestilential people. In one piece, published in June 1847, the paper condemned the idea "to saddle Irish destitution on the Saxons and send ragged wretchedness in shoals across the channel, to foster and spread disease and contagion around."[12] Other papers who leaned in similar political directions carried stories in the same vein. The *Northern Galaxy* out of Vermont reported in June 1847 as well that Liverpool was only receiving "Irish destitution and disease."[13] Stories like this arose as Irish immigration to America was reaching its height.

As previously mentioned, the emergence of cholera in 1849, which was possibly brought over by the Irish, made them a further target for certain groups. The *Hillsdale Whig Standard* of Sandusky, Ohio, directly blamed both the Irish and German immigrants who lived in the town for having produced and spread the disease.[14] A Louisiana newspaper in 1850 recounted the commonly held belief about the illness and trope about the Irish: "Disease in almost every instance is brought on them by intemperance."[15] These beliefs were also utilized by defenders of slavery at the time, who claimed if the institution was abandoned, the nation would be overrun instead by the diseased Irish.[16] Attacks on the Irish were frequent, with disease offering yet another angle for hatred against them when combined with economic concerns and religious bias. The murder of the Irishmen at Duffy's Cut as well as the Philadelphia Riots of 1844 stand out as some of the most damning examples of this. Nor were all of these associations between the Irish and disease unfounded. For instance, in 1849

VIII. "The Wretched Refuse"

in Boston, a clear preponderance of cholera cases and deaths occurred in their neighborhoods.[17] Though this was no doubt augmented by the attitudes and policies of the native population that led them to live in overcrowded and unsanitary areas.

One of the results of this was the formation of an entire political party devoted to ending the influx of Irish Catholic immigration to America. The roots of this movement can be found in the American Republican Party, which organized in New York City around 1843. It was largely a one issue party, focusing on limiting immigration from Catholic nations, particularly Ireland, and increasing the requirements to obtain citizenship. The group proved to be moderately successful in New York and Philadelphia and, by 1845, had changed its name to the Native American Party. Another similar group, the Order of the Star Spangled Banner, formed in 1849 in New York as well. All of these would eventually amalgamate into the American Party by the 1850s.

Better known historically as the Know Nothings, from the supposed answer of its members whenever they were asked about their clandestine meetings and doings, this was a potent third party in the antebellum era. Though anti-Irish and anti-Catholic views dominated their agenda, they also represented a populist labor/proto-socialist viewpoint. As can be expected, they employed disease frequently in their portrayal of immigrants, particularly the Irish. One candidate, during an 1847 address in Fayette, mentioned "cities are filled to overflowing with poor, diseased, and degraded immigrants."[18] As early as 1846, future secretary of war Simon Cameron, at that point the head of the Philadelphia Board of Trade and a member of both the Democratic and Know Nothing parties in succession, petitioned the Senate for legislation to restrict the immigration of diseased persons to America.[19]

George D. Prentice, the founder of the *Louisville Daily Journal*, utilized the paper to push Know Nothing ideology in Kentucky. Almost daily he harangued his readers to rise up against the "most pestilent influence of the foreign swarms."[20] His articles have been credited with helping to spark the Bloody Monday riot of 1855, which left dozens of Irish and Germans dead or wounded and hundreds of properties destroyed. Occurring on election day, they helped to sweep the Know Nothings into power and led to a mass exodus of recent immigrants from the state.

The Know Nothing Party scored impressive victories in Massachusetts and elsewhere in the early 1850s. Not surprisingly, it emerged strongest in the states that saw the quickest growth of Catholic populations at the time, including Maryland, New York, Massachusetts, and Louisiana. The group was even successful in halting construction of the Washington Monument in 1855 due to its concern that marble gifted by the Vatican and other Catholic nations had been employed. Its height was arguably reached in 1855 when it held 51 seats in the House of Representatives, stood as the main opposition party to the Democrats and even managed to place its own candidate, Nathaniel P. Banks, in the Speaker position. In 1856, it formally nominated former president Millard Fillmore for the presidency as well. Though not a Know Nothing himself, he accepted the decision and campaigned largely on a platform of national unity, ignoring the growing debate over slavery. The Know Nothings managed to carry the state of Maryland and its electoral votes and scored an overall 870,000 votes across the nation. This represented an astounding 22 percent of all votes cast that year, the best showing for a 3rd party until 1912 and the second best in American history overall.

The Chinese

The distance of China, as well as the exotic nature of goods that flowed from there to the West, had always produced in the minds of many a distorted image of the region. This was not a habit unique to the Western mind, nor was it confined to simply an understanding of East Asia. Similar stereotypical views developed in China regarding countries that surrounded it, in Europe with regard to sub-Saharan Africa, and between the early American settlers and the Natives. What is interesting here, however, is that the while the vast majority of these views were one-sided and static, some embraced an odd dichotomy of extremes. Rousseau's description of the Natives of the Americas as noble savages fit nicely into this category. China likewise presented a strange collection of extremes to Westerners: a land of barbarity and advancement, of filth and longevity of life. Its perception by Europeans changed due to time, events, and politics, particularly due to issues of illness. Historically, numerous diseases began in the region of China before traveling across the globe to strike Europe and the Americas and, while these mechanisms may not have always been clearly understood by Americans, the immigrant status of the Chinese and their perceived exotic nature led them to be connected to disease by some groups.

Many of the early founders of this country wrote in praise of China, specifically concerning its health and its medical expertise. Of these, perhaps none wrote more about the country than Benjamin Franklin. Evidence exists that Franklin had even read the works of Confucius as early as 1724.[21] Writing in the *Pennsylvania Gazette* in 1737, he excerpted a passage on the Chinese philosophy: "This is what Confucius proposed to the princes, to instruct them how to rectify and polish first their own reason,

VIII. "The Wretched Refuse" 77

and afterwards the reason and person of all their subjects."[22] Nor was Franklin the only one to be influenced by the East Asian thinker. Inventories from the home of George Washington show that he had copies of Louis Le Comte's *Travels through China*. This book from 1738 served as the standard work on China for most Westerners during the 18th century.

Yet, what seems to have impressed Franklin most about the land of China was its scientific advancements, particularly those that concerned medicine. The Philadelphian frequently commented upon the silk industry of the nation as well as its inventions, including the compass.[23] In several of his letters and journals, he pointed out the advanced state of Chinese medicine and medial theory.

> The Eastern Physicians agree with the Europeans in this Point; witness the Chinese Treatise, entitled *Tchang seng*, i.e., *The Art of procuring Health and long Life*, as translated in Pere Du Halde's Account of China, which has this Passage. 'As of all the Passions which ruffle us, Anger does the most Mischief; so of all the malignant Affections of the Air, *a Wind that comes thro' any narrow Passage*, which is cold and piercing, is *most dangerous;* and coming upon us unawares, insinuates itself into the Body, often causing grievous Diseases. It should therefore be avoided, according to the Advice of the ancient Proverb, as carefully as the Point of an Arrow.' These Mischiefs are avoided by the Use of the new-invented Fire-places, as will be shewn hereafter.[24]

He also wrote about the pay of physicians in China. Franklin noted, "A Silversmith and his Apprentice earn 6s. 3d. in 22 Days."[25] By comparison, a physician making a four-mile visit was compensated at the rate of 30 *d*. This would have taken the silversmith 9 days to earn, showing the value of physicians in the region.

Likewise, Franklin commented on the wealth of the faraway country, as well as the way in which it cared for its own people. Writing in 1769, he pointed out, "Hence it is that the most populous of all Countries, China, clothes its Inhabitants with Silk, while it feeds them plentifully and has besides a vast Quantity both of raw and manufactured to spare for Exportation."[26] He also marveled at the Qing method of effectively using census data to feed and care for the population in times of illness and famine.[27] In this light, China represented an advanced nation, one from which the fledgling United States could learn much.

Yet, at the same time, Franklin also slipped into some of the popular beliefs concerning the "diseased East." While unaware of the origins of influenza from the region, he did point out in an entry in *Poor Richard's Almanac* written in 1750 his belief that bedbugs originated in China. "*Bed-Bugs*, by some called *Chinces*, because first brought from China in East-India Goods, are easily destroy'd, Root and Branch, by boiling Water, poured from a Teakettle into the Joints, &c. of the Bedstead, or squirted by a Syringe, where it cannot well be poured. The old Ones are scalded to Death, and the Nits spoilt, for a boil'd Egg never hatches. This done once a Fortnight, during the Summer, clears the House. *Probatum est.*"[28] While in reality, tales of bedbugs stretch back to at least the plays of Aristophanes in the West, they most likely have coexisted with modern human across the globe throughout history. The tendency to blame China for disease in this case places Franklin well within that standard dichotomous view of the East.

The Jacksonian era saw an explosion of purported Chinese medicines and cures. This occurred as part of the larger rise of patent medicine and medical quackery that characterized the movement west and anti-elitism of the era. One of these items that appeared frequently in newspapers in the antebellum era was Dr. Lin's Celestial Balm of China. First appearing around 1842, it promised to be "a positive cure for the piles, and all external ailings—all internal irritations brought to the surface by friction with this Balm; son in coughs, swelled or sore throat, tightness of the chest, this Balm supplied on a flannel will relieve and cure at once. Fresh wounds or old sores are rapidly cured by it."[29] An advertisement in a Rhode Island newspaper that same year nearly filled an entire column and recommended Dr. Lin's as a cure for any conceivable health problem.[30] The supposed Oriental nature of the product was further pushed by its label's imagery. The front of the product contained an engraving "of a Chinese sage sitting in an elaborate chair; one servant held a parasol over his worthy head while another brought a bottle of the Balm."[31] This particular product seems to have run its course in the marketplace rather quickly. By 1846 only a few scattered newspapers in North Carolina continued to advertise it. The last mention of it seems to have been in *The Southerner* in August 1860.

Another similar nostrum was Dr. Drake's Canton Chinese Hair Cream. This product, apart from once again containing Eastern imagery, was also advertised with the following slogan.

> Our distant brothers, the Chinese,
> Long fam'd for their refreshing Teas,
> Produce a *Cream*, so rich and full,
> That clothes with hair the baldest *skull*.[32]

Other purported Chinese cures included Carey's Chinese Catarrh Cure, which was produced by Carey and Son of Waverly, New York. It is perhaps ironic that this purported cure for catarrh, a term often used interchangeably with influenza at the time, was said to originate in the land often held to be the origin of the illness. Yet others were Bryan's Oriental Dentifrice and Joseph Burnett's Oriental Tooth Wash. The latter began appearing in newspaper ads in the 1850s and was produced in Boston. It promised to be a general cure and treatment for almost any tooth or mouth issue. Major papers continued to promote the medicine until the 1870s. Burnett himself was a young druggist who made his living selling both the tooth wash as well as cocaine for the growth of hair.[33]

A final patent medicine that claimed Oriental roots was Dr. Lin's Temperance Life Bitters and Chinese Blood Bile. First appearing around 1840, this product was sold as an accessory to the age-old practice of purging in order to encourage digestive health. An 1841 advertisement in a newspaper from Mississippi stated, "Why do the Chinese live to such immense ages and still retain the powers of youth or middle age? Because they purify the blood. The Chinese Blood Pills—so called because they work upon and cleanse the Blood—are the standard remedy."[34] Combining both an East Asian origin story as well as being purportedly made by a Chinese doctor, Dr. O.C. Lin, these Blood Bile pills represented a prime example of the medical fascination with China. The actual purveyor of the medicine was Comstock and Co. out of New York, which most famously marketed Dr. Morse's Indian Root Pills during much of the 19th century.[35]

The other half of America's dichotomous view of China arose later in the 19th century. Earlier fascination with the Far East was replaced in some circles with fear and condescension as immigration from China increased. In 1852, an estimated 25,000 Chinese were living in the United States. Over the next thirty years, this number grew to 300,000, accounting for 10 percent of California's total population. As with all large immigration waves in American history, the mass arrival of people from China produced visceral reactions among some groups, especially those on the West Coast. Apart from traditional economic fears, this hostility was compounded by the perceived alien nature of Chinese culture, religion, and language. Therefore, whenever outbreaks of disease occurred in the nation, especially in the states and territories that bordered the Pacific, the Chinese were quickly blamed.

Cholera had been the great scourge of the early 19th century. Under the current miasmic theory of contagion, it was assumed to largely affect the filthy and intemperate. Thus, in the 1850s, when the disease once more appeared in the Americas, its Chinese victims became the focus of many periodicals. In October of 1851, a newspaper from the capital reported "a disease has broken out among the Chinese population of California resembling cholera. The dysentery is also very prevalent."[36] Though the exact nature of the disease that afflicted the Chinese at this time is unknown, as was whether or not it was also spreading to the local white population, the paper's decision to report upon it as a Chinese-only illness speaks volumes. A month later, the *Alexandria Gazette* carried a report from San

Francisco: "Our city continues to be very healthy, with the exception of a disease among the Chinese which is confined exclusively to them, and was reported to be cholera ... fostered by their manner of living."[37]

Though how the disease spread was still unknown, already by the time of the first outbreak most had recognized India as its origin. Yet, this did not stop many from rewriting the biological history of the illness. In a lengthy article published in 1856, the Hawaiian-based *Polynesian* newspaper laid out a supposed origin for cholera. "This terrible malady manifested itself first in China, then spread to the other countries of Asia, and afterward reached Europe."[38] Claiming to have received the report directly from eyewitnesses in Shandong province, the author goes on to expound upon its beginnings. In 1820, "a mass of reddish vapor was noticed one day upon the surface of the Yellow Sea ... the Chinese were seized with terror." The paper went on to describe the various magical and primitive means by which the locals tried to assuage the spirits assumed to be associated with the phenomenon. "These red vapors spread ... and wherever they passed men found themselves suddenly attacked by a frightful disease, which in a moment deranged the entire organization, and changed a living man into a hideous corpse." Claiming this to be the origin of cholera, the author then traces its path through Asia and Europe. Interestingly, the article was immediately followed by one that announced the formation of a vigilance committee to monitor Chinese vices in the area.

This anti–Chinese origin story for the pestilence was soon parroted and spread by other periodicals as well. In 1867, the *Weekly Caucasian*, a pro–Democratic Party newspaper out of Lexington, Missouri, carried a similar article. In this case, the author detailed an alleged Chinese cure for the disease as well but cautioned against using it. "I would seriously debate the question between their cure of cholera and death before submitting to their treatment."[39]

Smallpox was still a major cause of death in China during the 1800s, a century in which pestilence decimated the Qing Empire. In fact, Tongzhi, the 18-year-old Chinese emperor, succumbed to the disease in 1875. This is even more interesting when one considers that China itself had been the birthplace of the practice of variolation centuries before.

Beginning in the 1870s, newspapers made frequent references to Chinese victims of the dreaded disease. Arriving ships that held smallpox-stricken Chinese aboard were pointed out ostensibly as a way to alert the public.[40] One such outbreak occurred in 1873 in San Francisco following the arrival of the *Colorado* with several stricken passengers aboard. Likewise, in 1876, shortly after the death of the Tongzhi emperor from the disease, smallpox once more arrived in California. In a predictable fashion, recent Asian immigrants and residents of Chinatown were blamed for its spread. "It is the opinion of medical men that were it not for the filthy habits of the Chinese and the impossibility of dealing with the disease in their quarter there would be little or no fear of it becoming epidemic."[41] Chinese arrivals were blamed for importing the disease, their "filthy" living conditions were attacked for allowing it to spread, and they were often accused of hiding victims and even corpses. "During the progress of their explorations they have unearthed about one hundred convalescent cases of small-pox which the Chinese had secreted in their midst."[42]

The smallpox arriving from China was seen by some as a distinct variety. This was due in part to the fact that it seemed to largely only affect them, as well as the need to paint negatively all that came from the country. One newspaper article, written in 1873, suggested weaponizing the variety for use against the Modoc Indians. "The entire squad of the Modocs should be invited to Washington at Government expense. The Chinese variety is sure shot."[43]

Local governments relied upon the fumigation of Chinese passengers and their environs, forced vaccination, and the adoption of local public health ordinances specifically aimed at negative stereotypes of that population. One example would be the Cubic Foot of Air rule adopted in Portland in June of 1873. "Directed at the Chinese," the ordinance sought to combat the overcrowding that accompanied the Chinese settlement in the city.[44]

Another illness at the time that became associated with the Chinese was leprosy. This ancient malady was given new life with the influx of Chinese into America. By 1860, newspapers were already reporting "frequent cases" of the disease among Chinese immigrant communities in Australia.[45] Not surprisingly, Hawaii became the first territory to deal with the issue of leprosy arriving on its shores. As early as 1860, laws were being passed to "restrict the Chinese leprosy."[46] The presence of so many sufferers from the affliction in Hawaii, in fact, led to the establishment of a leper colony on Molokai that would exist for a century. Much like with cholera, the origins and history of the illness were soon rewritten to present as a product of East Asia. During an anti–Chinese meeting in San Francisco in 1861, Alfred Buetell claimed, "Leprosy, too, came from China."[47]

Upticks in Chinese immigration following the ending of the Civil War raised concerns: "The Chinese leprosy, which prevails in the Sandwich Islands, it is feared will reach San Francisco."[48] By 1873, reports were spreading that Chinese immigrants with the disease "are to be found in public places, and there is danger that the plague may spread."[49] Once again, much like with cholera and smallpox, the lethality of this "version" of the disease was exaggerated. "Chinese leprosy, and that you know is much worse than the leprosy of the ancients."[50]

Hundreds of articles ran in newspapers in the 1870s, detailing the spread of the infection in San Francisco thanks to Chinese immigrants. The perceived spread of the disease by touch was also used to attempt to push the Chinese out of the cigar-making industry in California, opening up more jobs to whites.[51] Likewise, lepers themselves were used to push the public toward banning Chinese immigration. A doctor from California named C.C. O'Donnell brought two Chinese victims of the disease to Philadelphia in 1884 to display them for the general public.[52]

Disease and, more often, fear of it eventually emerged as one of the main arguments put forth by those who wished to permanently end Chinese immigration. Newspapers at the time carried frequent articles that laid out the horrors associated with the arrival of migrants across the Pacific. An 1878 article in the *Canton Advocate* cited disease as the next biggest problem associated with the Chinese after opium. "John Chinaman disregards all sanitary laws in this city.... Living as they do in the very heart of the city, surrounded by a populous, wealthy and intelligent community, their willful and persistent disregard of sanitary laws is the means of sending forth the deadliest of poisonous exhalations to contaminate the atmosphere and endanger the health of everybody who lives in the metropolis."[53]

A few years later, an article in the *Daily Astorian* mentioned pestilence as the most serious problem of Chinese immigration. "The different race of people who have settled this continent brought something, either a particular trait, physical development, or talent which has been added to the general stock. The Chinese ... bring contagious disease."[54] Hundreds of other examples populate newspapers, speeches, and books that existed at the time.

These political attempts to utilize the issue of disease to target the Chinese were largely centered in California. Much as the anti–Irish movements were to be found in the cities along the Northeastern coastline where they settled, the parties that targeted the Chinese arose where that group tended to land. California had historically passed several laws aimed at restricting the arrival of Chinese people to the state. The first such piece of legislation was passed in 1850 and placed a tax on all foreign miners. In 1854, the California Supreme Court ruled that Chinese persons could not serve as witnesses in court against Americans. A further move came in 1858, when the state moved to restrict the access of the Chinese to schools and hospitals. Finally, in 1870, they prohibited the entry of any Chinese person who was not proved to be of upstanding moral character.

Yet, these acts did little to temper the anti–Chinese sentiment that existed at the time and was largely grounded in economic and epidemiological concerns. In 1877, Denis Kearney capitalized on these fears by

VIII. "The Wretched Refuse" 83

forming the Working Man's Party of California. Modeled in part on the Know Nothings, this was a nativist, pro-worker political party. Its heyday came in 1879 with the election of Isaac Smith Kalloch as mayor of San Francisco. Kearney frequently used disease to reference his hatred of the Chinese. In one interview with a local newspaper, he referred to several Chinese opponents as "almond-eyed lepers."[55]

These moves in California, most of which violated the preexisting, Republican-negotiated, Burlingame Treaty of 1868 with China, did not go unnoticed by the federal government. In 1875, California Representative Horace Page helped draft and push through Congress the Page Act, which aimed at reducing the importation of forced labor and prostitutes from China. Some of this was pushed on the grounds of helping the Chinese themselves from being taken advantage of by human traffickers, while fears over the spread of venereal diseases also played a role.[56] In fact, the American Medical Association claimed at the time that the Chinese carried "distinct germs," which would wreak havoc on American bodies.[57] In 1879, Ambassador George Seward began negotiations with the Qing government to prohibit the arrival of criminals, prostitutes, diseased persons, and contract laborers to America. President Hayes saw this as not only a commonsense policy but also as a way to forestall more extreme Democratic measures in Congress. These diplomatic talks would eventually culminate in the Angell Treaty of 1880.

Yet, these moves weren't enough for those Democrats who wanted the full termination of Chinese immigration to America. Cartoons by George Frederick Keller in the *San Francisco Wasp* frequently portrayed the Chinese as diseased invaders. An 1880 cartoon titled "Devastation" portrays the Chinese as ravenous hogs, animals frequently associated with filth and contagion. Likewise, another drawing the next year known as "A Statue for Our Harbor" shows a Chinese Statue of Liberty. At its base are filth and rats, while several beams of light shine on San Francisco with such labels as *disease* and *poverty*. In fact, as late as 1881, as the Chinese Exclusion Act was being debated, newspapers once again sought to connect the Chinese to cholera.[58] Nor were these views only held by Democrats on the West Coast but also spread throughout the nation. Dr. Joseph Jones, who headed the Louisiana Board of Health, warned against the "filthy ... unprincipled, vicious, and leprous hordes of Asia," blaming them for the reintroduction of leprosy into the state in the 1880s. In his view, this was caused by "their practice of taking water in their mouths and spitting it out on the clothes they iron is more than ever disgusting when considered in connection with the possible transmission of disease by this means."[59]

Heavily pushed by the Democratic Party of the West Coast, this view of the Chinese as importers of vice and viruses led to the passage of the

Chinese Exclusion Act in 1882. Though initially vetoed by President Arthur, it was passed once more and eventually signed into law. Legal Chinese immigration was largely ended into the United States until the passage of the Magnuson Act in 1943 and the Immigration and Nationality Act of 1965.

Despite the ending of large-scale Chinese migration to the country, those that resided on the West Coast remained a political target for decades. Perhaps not surprisingly, disease remained the catalyst for many of the moves against them. During the fifth cholera pandemic, which blanketed the planet in the 1880s and 1890s, residents of California once more assumed that it would arrive on the shores thanks to the Chinese. On August 29, 1892, Li Yung Yen, the Chinese Consul-General in San Francisco, issued a proclamation ordering all Chinese residents in the state to clean up their homes and neighborhoods in order to prevent the arrival of cholera in America. As the San Francisco–based *Morning Call* writes, "The word 'cholera' blanches the yellow cheeks of the pagans and makes them show the whites of their almond eyes."[60] Dr. J.W. Keeney, the leader of the San Francisco health office, quickly moved to launch inspections of Chinatown. However, this move was largely opposed by the Republican mayor, George Sanderson. A public dispute soon erupted between the two men, which showcased the opposing political views of the Chinese at the time. Keeney's focus seemed to be squarely set on the Chinese neighborhoods of the city, with him publicly announcing, "There is no need for anyone to fear the cholera in this city."[61]

Many in the general public shared Keeney's view at the time. The editorial board of the San Francisco–based the *Morning Call* opined white citizens frequently pointed out public health nuisances to the health board for rectification. "But a startling difference obtains among the Mongolians. Who ever heard of a complaint of a nuisance having been filed by a Chinaman?"[62]

Yet, Chinese residents seem to have quickly responded to the call of their foreign consul and moved to clean up their sections of the city. Interestingly, this merely provoked more anti–Chinese sentiment from the usual sectors. Their quick move to accept foreign commands was contrasted with their supposed refusal to adopt local ordinances. "The Chinese pay little heed to the local government, but when a hint comes to them from a representative of the Peking Government they are all eyes and ears."[63]

Much diminished fears of Chinese-spread contagion emerged on the more Republican East Coast. While local citizens followed with interest newspaper stories that detailed the hunt for a Chinese immigrant who was sought to be stricken within the city, it was largely portrayed as an isolated incident.⁶⁴ At the same time, a Connecticut periodical pointed out that the Chinese rarely actually get the disease due to their habit of boiling water for tea.⁶⁵

But the most notable of these political attacks against the Chinese occurred in 1900 when an ancient nemesis finally reached American shores. As early as 1892, newspapers began reporting the presence of a mystery pestilence in China. As the Chinese largely attempted to employ only traditional methods to drive away the illness, including the firing off of guns, it spread through the area.⁶⁶ The disease continued to rage unabated in both Hong Kong and Canton and was soon recognized to be bubonic plague. A mass exodus of Chinese residents was reported, the "labor market is paralyzed," and deaths reached 100 per day by early June.⁶⁷ Reacting swiftly, Mayor Levi Ellert of San Francisco announced a quarantine of ships coming from Yokohama in 1894 and ordered the use of chlorine gas to delouse Chinese passengers but none of any other nationality.

Yet, much as with the cholera scare of 50 years before, the disease was seen as a "disease of filth, and it is little likely to invade any ordinarily clean American city."⁶⁸ Newspapers were quick to highlight how the thousands of deaths a month in Hong Kong were only of Chinese, with no Westerners falling ill.⁶⁹ Though rats had recently been speculated to be the vectoring agent of bubonic plague, it was thought that the Chinese were actually acquiring the illness from consuming these rodents.⁷⁰ In fact, the plague was seen as a good opportunity to further restrict the slow migration of Chinese into California. As one San Francisco paper explained in 1894, "The Chinese plague is a bad thing for China, and it would be worse for the United States. But if it assists us in keeping Chinamen out of the country for a little while it may afford some ... rest and permit us to wrestle with our emigrant evils."⁷¹ A Democratic congressman from California, Anthony Caminetti, soon proposed a national quarantine to forestall just such a tragedy.

Over the summer of 1898, newspapers again carried stories of an outbreak of the plague in Hong Kong. Yet, apart from morbid curiosity, little attention was paid to the possibility that the disease would cross the ocean. Then, on October 28, newspapers reported that the French ship *Duchess Anne* had arrived in San Francisco flying the yellow flag of quarantine. Public health officials sailed out to the bark only to discover that the captain and a sailor had both died of the bubonic plague while transiting the Pacific.

Though officials placed the ship in extended quarantine, subsequent deaths in Chinatown began the spread of rumors that the disease had entered the city.⁷² Newspapers began to question official accounts of the situation and spurred on panic. "Extraordinary efforts are being made to suppress information regarding the appearance of a disease supposed to be the dreaded bubonic plague in Chinatown, but the public is gradually learning the facts."[73] Police were stationed around Chinatown to "warn whites that they had better keep out" while the situation was both investigated and presumably allowed to run its course among the Chinese.[74]

Local papers, especially the *San Francisco Call* were quick to refute these stories as little more than yellow journalism. City health officials were confident by the end of November that no cases of the plague had actually occurred in the city's Chinatown. While no major eastern paper subsequently retracted its story, the entire plague scare largely subsided by December of 1898.

Only a few months later, in 1899, the ship *Nippon Maru* from Yokohama approached California and reported two cases of the disease on board. Authorities reacted quickly and quarantined the vessel at Angel Island. A thorough search of the boat found eleven Chinese stowaways aboard. Shortly afterward, two Japanese managed to jump ship, probably fearing that they would catch the plague and die. Their bodies were soon after found in San Francisco Bay and an autopsy afterward revealed signs of the plague.[75] The Chinese and Japanese passengers were evacuated to Angel Island and held in confinement until their health could be guaranteed. A territorial battle broke out between the health officials of San Francisco and Washington, D.C., with the former insisting that the ship remain in quarantine and once again be fumigated, while the latter announced it clear of all illness.

Yet the move did little to calm fears. A story soon spread that two Japanese crewmembers had jumped ship rather than stay in quarantine. They drowned in the process, and their bodies were eventually recovered and taken for autopsies after a cursory examination showed plague marks on their corpses.[76] Subsequent studies showed that both men had in fact been infected, causing the quarantine to be continued even longer. The situation was further complicated by the fact that ships full of men returning from military duty in the Philippines were expected to dock soon in San Francisco as well. Luckily, the precautions put in place by health officials worked, and by July the *Maru* was allowed to dock once no further cases of the plague emerged. Papers were once again quick to criticize the fear-mongering of some elements.

A few months later, *The Scranton Tribune* ran an astrological article asserting general predictions for the coming year. "As Saturn, the cause of all great troubles and mighty evils is now in the home of Sagittarius ... watch out for epidemics ... plagues of flies, bugs, and water epidemics."[77] The coming month would deliver much of what this prediction promised.

VIII. "The Wretched Refuse"

After several more months of fear, the plague arrived in Hawaii around the turn of 1900. On December 12, 1899, newspapers in Hawaii reported the first two deaths from bubonic plague on American territory. Both men were Chinese bookkeepers who worked at stores in Honolulu. Hawaiian authorities moved quickly to contain the disease, as more cases were being reported. Inspections were performed of quarantined areas, refuse was burnt, a hospital ship was sought out, and those traveling between the islands were to be medically examined. For his part, Sanford Ballard Dole, the first president of the Republic of Hawaii, sought to remind citizens that "plague is a child of filth … there is no danger to those whose houses, persons, and food are cleanly."[78]

Weeks of quarantine followed as reports of additional cases and deaths slowly emerged. Though the exact origin of the illness was still debated, anger and focus were once again turned toward the Chinese. "Many believe that if the plague were present in Honolulu the inhabitants of Chinatown would be carried off by the hundreds, on account of the filthy conditions of the district."[79] Health officials targeted the garbage, refuse, and homes of these individuals in their efforts to prevent a wider spread of the contagion.

At the same time, the fire department of the city was used to burn down various Chinese buildings once they were shown to have harbored plague victims. Over the first few weeks of January, over 40 buildings were incinerated on orders of the local government. The chief of the San Jose, California, fire department, who was vacationing in Hawaii at the time, expressed his support for the process during an interview with a local newspaper. "I have profited in no small measure by the work of the Honolulu Fire Department in burning the condemned and infected buildings."[80] Yet, this "benign" practice was to change dramatically only a few days later.

On January 20, 1900, the Honolulu Fire Department began a blaze to reduce infected structures in Chinatown on Nuuanu between Beretania and Kukui. Yet, after two hours of a controlled burn, the winds shifted direction and the fire began to spread. The steeple of the Kaumakapili church caught fire, as did several buildings beyond it. Soon, a great conflagration had developed, which engulfed most of Chinatown in flames. Worse yet, as the population of the neighborhood was still under quarantine, escaping citizens found themselves colliding with soldiers at the checkpoints. "Mobs charged the guards along River street in an effort to get out of danger."[81] Rather than let them through, more soldiers and volunteers were called out to hold the line. "Citizens were armed with ax and pick handles and went immediately to the assistance of the guard. But for these reinforcements the crazed Asiatics would have overrun Honolulu's plague-free territory like a pestilence ... even women stood shoulder to shoulder with the men."[82] Fear of the epidemiological danger posed by the Chinese outweighed humanitarian need and basic decency. Eventually though, authorities moved to remove the Chinese citizens in an orderly fashion so as not to have a scattering of them around Honolulu.

By the time the smoke had settled, 38 acres of Honolulu covering some 11 blocks had been reduced to rubble and ash, and thousands of Chinese residents were left homeless. Yet, hopes abounded among many that this accident would spell an end to the epidemic. As one mainland paper claimed, "The bubonic plague is now believed to be under control." The reduction of Chinatown was thought to have surely destroyed the pathogens that lurked there.[83]

Whether due to the purging effect of the fire or the quarantine procedures of the health office, the plague slowly began to retreat on the island. By March 31, 1900, health officials in Honolulu officially declared the epidemic to be over. All told there were 70 confirmed cases and 61 deaths, though almost certainly many of both categories were simply not reported. The plague, though certainly sensational, caused little serious loss of life in the islands. A far bigger fear was its potential impact should it reach the mainland.

With the frequent transit of passenger and sugar ships between San Francisco and Honolulu, it was thus only a matter of time before the bacteria hit the mainland. This terror came to fruition on March 7, 1900, when the body of a deceased Chinese laborer, Wong Chut King, was discovered to have the plague during an autopsy. Chinatown was almost immediately put under a strict quarantine with passengers on street-cars even being forced to confine themselves inside trolleys as they skirted the area. The region was soon after disinfected: the houses were washed with sulfur dioxide and mercury bichloride, while carbolic acid was dumped into the sewers. The latter move probably only helped to spread the disease further as it drove subterranean rats out into the streets.

At the same time, many in San Francisco actually attempted their best to cover up any evidence of an outbreak, weighing the economic impact of disease in their city to be worse than any fear of the Chinese. Surgeon General W.K. Van Reypen was quick to assure the public that "the climatic conditions of the United States preclude the possibility of the plague ever getting within this country. It is a disease of the Orient, and seldom, if ever, attacks Europeans."[84] Likewise, only the day after the initial quarantine was ordered, the *San Francisco Call* opined, "These diseases ... prove to be largely racial," and called for restraint against overzealousness.[85] It was soon even suggested that the entire incident was merely a ploy by the famously nativist Democratic Mayor James D. Phelan to enrich himself

VIII. "The Wretched Refuse"

and his supporters.[86] Republican governor Henry Gage likewise sought to ignore the issue for economic reasons.

After three days of quarantine and complaints from both the Chinese and local businessmen, the quarantine was lifted. The anti-quarantine *San Francisco Call* applauded the action in its usual xenophobic way. "Notwithstanding the evils of the presence of the Chinese here, which no one questions, their right to be here is settled by the treaty."[87] Yet less than 24 hours later, three test animals injected with discharge from the glands of the deceased Chinese resident died. Once again, the pendulum of public opinion swung toward quarantine and house-to-house disinfection. The Chinese resisted the move, with many fleeing and sneaking into the American section of the city. Families even hid bodies in their homes to avoid having their relatives dissected in autopsies.

More bodies were soon discovered and though the governor of the state refused to act out of fear of losing trade, other states did. A number of states cut off intercourse with California while several countries in Central and South America quarantined ships arriving from San Francisco. A massive cleanup of 1,200 homes in 1901 and the election of a more proactive governor in 1903 helped to finally eradicate the pestilence by 1904. In the end there were 126 reported cases of the illness of which 122 died.

Though East Asian immigration and travel certainly did import the bubonic plague to America, its actual effect was minuscule compared to previous, legendary outbreaks of the illness. Yet this did not stop some nativist elements from using the outbreak to push for not only tighter restrictions on the Chinese but a complete ban on all Asian immigration as well. The creation of the Japanese Exclusion League in 1905 and the subsequent segregation of Japanese and Korean students in public schools in the Bay area developed in part due to these plague fears. Jack London took this anti–Asian concept to a startling conclusion when he published his short story "The Unparalleled Invasion." Commenting on the rapidly expanding population of China, London's story recommended employing disease offensively to wipe out the population of East Asia. Despite traditionally positive Sino-American relations, the arrival of disease along with Chinese immigrants served to strain even this close bond, further alienating the ethnicity and limiting the country's ability to modernize through access to foreign capital and education.

A similar story unfolded two decades later in Los Angeles. Unlike San Francisco, which had a large Asian minority population, LA had a sizeable Mexican population. Yet, both were treated as outsiders by the California population. Therefore, in late September of 1924, when a suspected case of pneumonic plague broke out in the Macy Street District, public anger turned against Mexican residents. On September 28, 1924, Jesus

Lajun was diagnosed with a venereal disease. Over the next few weeks, Jesus, his daughter, and the nurse that cared for them all fell ill and died from a disease that quickly spread to hundreds of others as well. It would take a month for the health department to correctly identify the culprit as the plague. Los Angeles quickly placed armed police officers around the Mexican districts of the city, ordering homes to either be cleaned or face destruction. At the same time, local newspapers refused to cover the true nature of the epidemic, referring to it as pneumonia instead. USPHS surgeon Benjamin Brown even sent coded messages to the surgeon general so as not to spread alarm.[88] As for national newspapers, reports only began to surface in November, by which time the outbreak had largely run its course.

The targeting of the Irish and Chinese as importers of disease were not occurrences that were peculiar to the 19th century. Throughout the 20th century, disease was often used by politicians to target immigration to the country. Yet, that is not to say that the two factors were not connected. Pandemic disease especially tended to be of foreign origin, and those arriving in the country were often suffering from malnutrition and illness. During the 2021 border crisis, millions of individuals pushed across the southern border of the country at the height of a global pandemic. Republicans were quick to point out the hypocrisy of requiring mask and vaccine mandates for American workers, while little to no testing or treatment was done on the migrants. Florida governor Ron DeSantis took aimed at President Biden's lax border enforcement, connecting it to spreading cases of the 2019 coronavirus.

> He's imported more virus from around the world by having a wide open southern border. You have hundreds of thousands of people pouring across every month. And it's not just from Mexico. In fact, it's rarely from Mexico. You have over a hundred different countries where people are pouring through. Not only are they letting them through, they're then farming them out all across our communities across this country. Putting them on planes, putting them on buses, do you think they're worried about COVID for that? Of course not. So he's facilitating ... who knows what new variants are out there? But I can tell you whatever variants are around the world, they're coming across that southern border. And so he's not shutting down the virus, he's helping to facilitate it in our country.[89]

While the connection between immigrants and disease has been well established, some have historically preferred to use it as a political cudgel to attack immigration rather than the illness itself. Conversely, others have willfully and blindly ignored the connection in the hopes of gaining political power from these newly arrived people. Pestilence and politics are always intertwined.

Chapter IX

Rashes and Reforms

Disease wasn't simply used as political fodder to attack presidents and other public figures but also began to be employed to target institutions and public problems as well. Oftentimes this criticism was legitimately placed if their failures to prevent or treat disease led to the deaths of Americans, while other times it was pure political theater. At the same time, for those who were actually pushing to reform or improve society, it became a useful catalyst to garner either fear or disgust from the public. Where divine command or economic advantage failed to sway voters, nosophobia succeeded. The disease of the 19th century helped to begin the social, political, and economic modernization of the country.

The Missing Act of Burr the Musical

One of the earliest examples of this involved the consummate example of politics at the time, Aaron Burr. Early New York City received most of its water from either private wells or Collect Pond, a large body of water near Pearl Street in lower Manhattan. Yet, a century of human habitation had largely turned Collect Pond into a miasmic swamp. Under the epidemiological thinking of the time, it was a commonly held belief that polluted sources of water were breeding grounds for disease, thus making its existence a concern to the neighborhood and city officials. Years later, following the filling in of the notorious body of water, Dr. John Bard recounted, "Every summer, the inhabitants of the houses on the north side of it ... were subject to malignant intermittent, and several ... yearly died. Since the draining of that place, these houses are become as healthy as any in the neighborhood."[1]

While some resorted to buying water imported from Brooklyn, others turned to the city government for a solution. As early as 1796, the city of New York requested proposals for providing fresh drinking water to residents, yet in the end, little action was taken. The *Commercial Advertiser* of

New York City carried an article in 1797 detailing a petition by Dr. David Ramsey of South Carolina written to the state government to ensure clean drinking water in Charleston to counter the threat of yellow fever.[2] The next year, a similar proposal was made in New York City by Dr. Joseph Browne. The Westchester physician urged the creation of a private, stockholder company, which would pipe in clean water from the Bronx River to the residents of lower Manhattan. His proposal coincided with an outbreak of yellow fever that year, which no doubt influenced the members of the city council to finally act.

Though ultimately favored by the city council, the idea was amended to replace a private company with city control, funded by new state loans and taxes. As this required official approval by the state of New York, the discussion moved up the river to Albany. At that time, the head of the assembly was Aaron Burr, who also happened to be the brother-in-law of Browne. Burr seized upon the moment to push for the private company option, with his own financial and political interests in mind. His ultimate aim was to use the proposed water company as a financial conduit to establish a massive bank that would rival Alexander Hamilton's in the city. Burr had hopes of placing himself at the head of politics in New York but would need a large war chest to do so.

Burr utilized bribery, the interception of communications, threats, promises, the exclusion of delegates from meetings, and whatever underhanded political means he could in order to help push the legislation through the Assembly. Part of this involved a 10-day trip to Manhattan to once more convince the city council of the benefits of a private company. Portraying the entire undertaking as a public health endeavor, he even managed to enlist the support of his rival, Hamilton, who worked hard to persuade the mayor and council. Once assent was given, Burr used legislative tricks to push it through both the Senate and Assembly without a formal vote, and on April 2, 1799, the Manhattan Company became a reality.

The new company was allowed to transport water from outside of the city back to lower Manhattan. To accomplish this, it was granted vast leeway, including not being responsible for repairing any streets that it damaged while installing pipes and, more radically, it was allowed to invest its profits as it saw fit. This last measure allowed Burr to invest 95 percent of the initial $2 million raised through the sale of stock in the construction of the Bank of the Manhattan Company (Chase Manhattan), with only $100,000 going to the water project. Due in part to this, practically no effort was made to transport new water into the city. Instead, Burr's company merely sank more wells into the already polluted region of Collect Pond.

The Manhattan Water Company proved to be an epidemiological

IX. Rashes and Reforms 93

disaster for New York City. Not only did it not provide the necessary amount of clean drinking water to the city that it had been contracted to, the water it did provide was most likely significantly contaminated. Likewise, it failed to aid other problems that the city was facing including sanitation and fire management. During a yellow fever outbreak in 1803, the company was forced to suspend service for weeks to undertake much needed repair, worsening the already deadly conditions. Lawsuits and complaints followed and proved to be one of the many catalysts for the duel between the now Vice President Aaron Burr and Alexander Hamilton in 1804.

Though Burr had already been removed from the company in 1802 due to outstanding debts, it continued to serve as the primary water supplier to lower Manhattan for the next three decades. Even after most of Collect Pond had been filled in, the homes constructed there began to sink into the ground due to the continued presence of groundwater. With upper-class families and businesses refusing to settle in the region, it quickly became a slum for recent immigrants and those on the lower rungs of society. The Five Points, as it became known, would witness some of the worst riots and the highest incidents of cholera death during the antebellum period. "Every day's experience gives us assurance of the safety of the temperate and prudent, who are in circumstances of comfort.... The disease is now, more than before rioting in the haunts of infamy and pollution.... The broken-down constitutions of these miserable creatures, perish almost instantly on the attack."[3] A few years later, a new prison was constructed in the area as well. Known locally as The Tombs, this Egyptian revival structure became notorious for the conditions of its lower level due to the remnants of the Collect Pond. None other than Charles Dickens visited in years later and recorded his observations.

> What! do you thrust your common offenders against the police discipline of the town, into such holes as these? Do men and women, against whom no crime is proved, lie here all night in perfect darkness, surrounded by the noisome vapours which encircle that flagging lamp you light us with, and breathing this filthy and offensive stench! Why, such indecent and disgusting dungeons as these cells, would bring disgrace upon the most despotic empire in the world! Look at them, man—you, who see them every night, and keep the keys. Do you see what they are? Do you know how drains are made below the streets, and wherein these human sewers differ, except in being always stagnant?[4]

The problem of providing drinking water to Manhattan from outside the city was finally addressed in the 1830s. The cholera pandemic as well as the Great Fire of 1835, finally convinced the public and the city council of the need to address the issue. Democratic Mayor Cornelius Lawrence approved the creation of the Croton Aqueduct, which, when completed in 1842, brought millions of gallons of water a day from the Croton River into receiving tanks in Manhattan. Though the project helped to provide clean drinking water to thousands of families, it inadvertently led to other epidemiological problems, as the now-unused Collect Pond led to a rise in the water table in lower Manhattan, further flooding homes and leading to depressed property values and the growth of slums.

Other cities in the region slowly followed the actions of New York City. Philadelphia began to pump 3.9 million gallons of water into the city daily beginning in 1823 through a public works project of a similar nature to Manhattan's. This was likewise in response to the yellow fever epidemics that routinely visited the metropolis. Boston and Baltimore chose to largely use private companies to complete the task during the antebellum period. For the vast majority of other cities and towns, however, private wells remained the standard for many decades.

Miasmic thinking likewise led to the development of sewer systems around the same time. The *New York Herald* reported in 1859 "the soil at this day is nothing better than a sponge, from which poisonous exudations are emitted in the hot season, causing intermittent fevers and other local diseases."[5] The same cholera epidemics that pushed the construction of the Croton Aqueduct likewise led New York City to begin construction of a proper sewer system in 1849. Interestingly, despite their previous support for improved sanitation to confront disease in the city, the local Democrats blasted the Whigs for the excessive costs of the project as well as their handling of cholera in Manhattan. "If a waste of money ... entitles the whig party to a continuance of power, then indeed the present authorities have a just claim to re-election."[6] Clearly this chastisement had more to do with politics than with actual science.

Disease became a frequent method by which reform was pushed in the 19th century. Dorothea Dix, who famously campaigned to improve asylums and prisons, utilized information about the outbreak of illness at these institutions. In her 1845 report on the general state of prisons in the country, she singled out Sing Sing for the "great amount and severity of autumnal sickness," which she linked to the "use of bad water ... and the want of suitable clothing."[7] Her 1847 memorial on the state of prisons in Illinois and 1852 work on insane asylums in Maryland made similar claims.[8]

Metropolitan Board of Health

The epidemiological lessons of the Civil War led many cities to create or reform their own boards of health during the1860s and 1870s. During the 1860s, as the population of New York City continued to swell with increased immigration, attention began to be paid to the living conditions in the expanding tenement houses there. In one famous case, Dr. Stephen Smith investigated a tenement building that was responsible for the vast majority of disease cases visiting his hospital. Despite his best efforts, he quickly realized that little action could be taken as no laws or codes were in place that required action by the landlord. In the end, Smith worked with the editor of the *New York Evening Post*, William Cullen Bryant, to threaten the landlord with a public shaming campaign in order to produce the desired result.[9]

Smith joined with the influential Citizens Association, which aimed at reforming various social and political aspects of life in New York, to push forward a health bill. Knowing the resistance of the Tweed-controlled Democratic Party, the bill was brought to the state legislature instead.[10] Despite these political maneuvers, the statewide Democrats and several lukewarm Republicans combined to defeat the measure over the winter of 1864. This vote became a major component of the electoral campaigns that ensued the next year. A letter to the editor of the *New York Evening Post* mentioned holding those Republicans who voted against it and "must have been influenced by some improper motive" to task.[11] The voters of New York responded, and that year a wave of Republicans were swept into office, with a large number being members of the Radical wing who were focused on reform.

Part of this impetus for this was the reemergence of cholera in New York City. The Civil War was barely over; troops were returning from the battlefield, warships from their patrols, and a steamer named the *Atalanta* was drifting slowly and menacingly into New York Harbor. The ship had departed Le Havre, France, loaded with 525 passengers in steerage and wouldn't arrive in New York until October of 1865. Reports of illness and death onboard the ship reached Manhattan before the vessel. In all, it was reported that there had erupted 60 cases of cholera aboard the *Atalanta* with 16 deaths. Taking a proactive stance, the city of New York brought the hospital ship *Florence Nightingale* downriver from Brooklyn to serve as a quarantine station for the infected. Thirty-six more would develop the illness while on the hospital ship with four more deaths by November 10.

At the same time, the experience of the previous cholera pandemics, as well as the work of Dr. Snow, had revealed to many that poverty and intemperate living may not be the only vectors for the illness. On November 23, Dr. Walter J. Hadden wrote to the mayor and council of Jersey City emphasizing that though the disease may begin by striking the poor, it was blind as to class and would spread to all segments of society.

> Now this dreaded pestilence of cholera hangs over us, and we know where it will strike first; first among our poor, on account of ill ventilation of the places in which they reside, where the walls reek with organic accumulations, the air poisoned from the exhalations of so many human beings herded together, whose systems are weakened by the inhalations of foul air, eating of bad food, and the vices and diseases they have engendered. It will carry off the enfeebled, the dissolute and miserable. Yet it will visit the houses of the rich as well. It will strike inscrutable blows among the healthy, as well as the diseased, and once established, will create sad havoc among all classes.[12]

Other medical commentators joined moral crusaders to push for action to clean up the streets and slums of the New York City area.

> Now Sir, all of us who are at work among the poor practically, know that are plenty of such dens of crime, and "nests of fever" ... Here we know that thieves, and vagrants, and prostitutes are bred and educated. When next Spring or Summer, the pestilence suddenly breaks out in the city, its first grim appearance will be in these "lodging houses," and in these it will revel. From these centers it will radiate all over the city and the Union. Quarantine will not be of the slightest use, when such fertile receptacles for the seed of the disease are here all prepared.... Such hideous dens must be broken up....[13]

Thus, in February of 1866 the New York Senate voted 26 to 3 to pass the legislation through, with one Democratic paper lamenting, "Oh public necessity, what crimes are committed in thy name."[14] Democrats and Whigs overwhelming voted against it, seeking to place its success or failure purely on the shoulders of Republicans. Its passage in the Assembly afterward, though by a closer margin of 74 to 28, was still overwhelming. The *New York Times* opined that it "washed its hands of responsibility," as the Republicans "preferred a party machine to a health board."[15] Despite the politics of the passage, the Metropolitan Health Act of 1866 created the first modern board of health in the country.

Democrats utilized both the bill itself and its passage to not only attack the Republican Party but push for amending the state's constitution. "The Health Bill is a measure of usurpation and wrong, and it may fail in the end ... it will weaken the party that originates it. Like all projects to invigorate the Republican organization in the city, the democratic majority will be augmented by its passage."[16]

The politically controversial law was quickly put to the test as April of 1866 saw the re-emergence of cholera in New York City. The fourth cholera pandemic circled the globe in the 1860s and 1870s, sickening and killing millions. Now, with its arrival in Manhattan, Governor Reuben Fenton issued a state of emergency, granting exceptional powers to the newly appointed board of health. Among these was the ability to enforce existing statutes concerning sanitation as well as liquor excise laws. The latter was due to the still standard belief of many that intemperate living was the cause of disease or at least made one more susceptible to it.

The New York City Board of Health moved quickly to address the numerous problems in the city's response to cholera. Between March and November of 1866, some 31,077 orders emerged from its office and addressed issues of sanitation, property management, housing, the regulation of bars and eateries, and numerous other topics. Included in these were 4,000 yard-cleaning orders and 770 cistern cleanups. So vigorous was its action, that the *New York World* accused it of "terrorism," arguing that its actions would counterproductively "frighten the community into depression of nervous force and consequent disease."[17] The Democratic-leaning *Brooklyn Daily Eagle* criticized the Board of Health for refusing to pay the standard rate for advertising its new health codes in its paper. The Board instead had apparently sought preferential treatment due to its benefit to the public, as the paper was the largest circulator in the city.[18]

Despite these political battles, New York City was able to weather the cholera pandemic much better than other parts of the country. In total, some 500 fatalities were reported in the city of 1.2 million people, while Brooklyn reported between 800 and 900 deaths, Philadelphia 834, Cincinnati 1,200, St. Louis 3,500, and New Orleans 1,350. Cincinnati unfortunately waited until almost 90,000 were stricken before organizing a board of health to fight the disease, thus losing almost 0.6 percent of its population. St. Louis's casualty figures represented an astonishing 1.5 percent of its population, while New Orleans' was helped spread by a race riot that broke out in July of 1866 and was quelled by infected soldiers. Boats then completed the spread of the disease across the already devastated South, with 510 dying in Vicksburg between August and September alone (which represented almost 6 percent of the population), and another 500 falling victim in San Antonio. Total deaths for the nation are estimated to be anywhere from 10,000 to 40,000. Yet, New York City had proven that, despite its filth, reticent population, and large immigrant base, defeat of disease was possible. Charles Rosenberg perhaps best characterizes the success of the Board of Health. "There is no date more important than 1866, no event more significant than the organization of the Metropolitan Board of Health. For the first time, an American community had successfully organized itself to conquer an epidemic."[19]

A Splendid and Sickly Little War

Cuba had been in a state of rebellion against the government in Madrid since 1895. Over the next three years, battles on the island were accompanied by the Spanish use of reconcentration camps and the outbreak of disease to kill hundreds of thousands. Yellow journalists in the United States were quick to use the notion of illness to both paint the Spanish as brutal conquerors as well as to produce fear in Americans of refugees spreading sickness here. The *New York Sun*, one of the most notorious of papers pushing for war, began to shift from its relatively neutral and accurate portrayal of the presence and impact of disease on the island in early 1897. Instead, it began to push the notion that disease was purely the fault of the Spanish. Throughout 1896, both *The Sun* and other papers noted that smallpox was endemic to the eastern end of Cuba. Now, the former paper informed its readers that "the smallpox was introduced here by the 200,000 soldiers from Spain," because "the Spanish common people are not cleanly in their habits."[20] Yet even worse, because of the unprecedented outbreaks on the island, "Cuba is now a focus of disease, and became a scourge of danger, perhaps to the world." The island was "a far greater danger to the United States than the much-feared bubonic plague of India."[21] The implication to readers was clear, America needed to act to prevent a pestilential catastrophe both off our coast and in our cities.

Though the road to the conflict of 1898 was heavily debated and an official act recognizing that a state of war existed between the U.S. and Spain ultimately only passed the Senate by a vote of 42–35, once war was declared, the feeling in the country turned more favorable toward its undertaking. This was no doubt added by the rapid string of victories visited upon the Army and Navy both in the Philippines and the Caribbean.

As President McKinley was himself quite reluctant to go to war, partisan political anger was instead directed at others in his administration. Most notable among these targets was Secretary of War Russell Alger. The former governor of Michigan quickly became a leading proponent of recognizing Cuba and involving the country in securing its freedom.[22] This stance led him into conflict with many who were opposed to imperialism. At the same time, as secretary of war, he became a natural target during the war for any errors that occurred.

As early as January of 1898, newspapers were not only reporting on an episode of sickness that Alger suffered through but used it to attack him as well. *The Anaconda Standard* commented, "Alger's disease is only typhoid, not Klondike fever, to which he has been so recklessly exposing himself."[23] Once war had broken out, Alger became the most frequent target for those who wished to critique the administration. As early as June 8, only a few days after the arrival of the U.S. Flying Squadron in Cuba, the *Salt Lake Herald* was already labeling Alger as "incompetent."[24] While some of these attacks were general, several began to specifically focus on certain aspects of the campaign.

IX. Rashes and Reforms

In early June, Governor Hazen Pingree of Michigan publicly criticized both the quality of food and clothing being provided to American soldiers.[25] Though Alger defended the quality and quantity of meat being provided to the men in the field, the accusation would reemerge frequently over the next few months. In mid-July of the next year, the *Lexington Gazette* would even refer to the "Alger meat" being supplied to soldiers in Cuba.[26] Events began to escalate even more quickly, as reports surfaced that men were being sickened by rotten meat at the unfortunately named Camp Alger near Falls Church, Virginia.[27] While the sick list increased daily, the cause of the epidemic was eventually discovered to have been typhus. Despite this, most newspapers continued to blame Alger for the fiasco.

Within weeks, a similar situation erupted at Camp Merritt in San Francisco. Disease so ravaged the encampment that newspapers soon rechristened it the "Camp of Death."[28] Once more, Alger became the target for those wishing to find someone to blame for these massive casualties from disease. An article on August 4 proclaimed, "Alger's course is condemned on every hand."[29] Additional newspapers ran stories over the next month detailing the "general incompetency" of the secretary in dealing with these and other issues.[30] Attacks soon started to come from even other administration officials, particularly outgoing Secretary of State John Sherman. The latter had strongly opposed involvement in the conflict and now held the pro-war Alger responsible for the suffering and death of American soldiers and sailors in the Caribbean.[31]

Yet, perhaps the most damning of indictments came from Teddy Roosevelt. As the American army wasted away in front of Santiago, some general officers petitioned Maj. General Shafter to allow their units to return stateside while negotiations took place. Once their request was denied, the group asked Roosevelt, the only commander present who was not regular Army, to draft a circular letter detailing the current situation. Known as the Round-Robin Letter, it was soon leaked to the press back in America and created a sensation among the public that was unaware that the vast majority of deaths taking place in the war were from bacteria and not bullets. The V Corps was quickly brought back to quarantine camps in Long Island, Roosevelt rose to fame as a man of "moral courage," and Alger was further chastened.[32]

With the war winding down to a successful conclusion, the American public was jubilant with the outcome of the brief but splendid campaign. Despite this, calls were issued for a thorough investigation and analysis of the preparation for war. While many of the issues to be addressed by the proposed committee were frequent criticisms of the conflict, such as supplies, equipment, health, and transportation, it was largely meant to serve as a means by which to improve the military for future conflicts. President McKinley consented to the idea and by the end of September had organized the 12-man Dodge Commission presided over by General G.M. Dodge.

Over the next few months, witnesses, experts, and reports were paraded past the committee as they sought both problems and solutions. Despite this, its transactions were relatively mundane, not surprising considering the general success of the conflict. Then, on December 21, 1898, General Nelson Miles delivered bombshell testimony before the commission. While discussing the general failure of the supply system to Puerto Rico and Cuba, Miles began to discuss the quality of meat arriving on the front lines. Amidst his testimony, he referred to the food given to the men as "embalmed beef."[33] The line resonated with both senators and the public and quickly derailed the otherwise predictable outcome of the hearings. General Miles went still further, announcing that he was carrying out his own investigation into the meat scandal, something that "would show that those in high authority agreed to making an experiment that endangered the health and lives of thousands of soldiers."[34] His testimony included the following evidence presented from other commanders in the field.

> -The beef seemed to be of inferior quality and was anything but palatable. Quite a number of men could not and did not eat it.
> -The meat was utterly unfit as an article of diet for either sick or well. It had no nutriment in it, and turned the stomachs of men who tried to eat it.
> -The meat produced disordered stomachs, was not nutritious, soon became putrid, and in many of the cans was found in course of putrefaction when opened.
> -The meat issued presented such a repulsive appearance that the men turned from it in disgust. "Nasty" is the only term that will fitly describe its appearance. Its use produced diarrhea and dysentery…
> -The meat was a miserable apology for food in a hot climate, a slimy-looking mass of beef scraps, unpalatable to the taste, and repulsive to the sight. Competition for the contracts placed the prices so low that only tailings and scraps were used for canning….[35]

The story became a sensation, with many blaming the embalmed beef for the high death rates by disease suffered by the men on the islands. Almost 90 percent of the deaths during the brief, but highly successful, war came about due to disease rather than bullets or bombs. While this had always been a truism of conflicts dating back to ancient times, it was largely ignored in popular histories due to its connections with personal intemperance as well as failures in supply and sanitation. Now, the public was actively acknowledging this fact and politicians quickly scrambled to make political hay out of the situation.

IX. Rashes and Reforms

A bitter feud developed between Miles and Brigadier General Charles P. Eagan. The latter had been responsible for the maintaining food supplies from the U.S. to the Caribbean during the war and took personal umbrage to Miles' statements. Eagan personally appeared before the Commission in January of 1899 to call Miles "several different kinds of a liar."[36] The feud between the two became personal and bitter, leading to threats of court martials. Ultimately, however, it was Eagan who was court-martialed, with his trial becoming a national sensation. The trial unfolded quickly and he was suspended from active duty until his retirement in December of 1900.

Ultimately, however, the Wade Board, which was formed to specifically investigate the accusations of General Miles, found his claims to be exaggerated. In its May report, the commission found the meat to be "generally good."[37] While many flocked to Miles defense, seeing a cabal of government and industry associated interference, others saw a different political connection.

At least as early as March of 1899, while the various war commissions were drawing to a close, talk began to circulate that General Miles was being considered for the presidency in 1900.[38] Though assumed by many to be a Republican, he appears to have been largely apolitical, and his military experience and role as a critic of the current administration would make him a potential alternative to the controversial William Jennings Bryan. Yet, not all in the party were so eager, with the *New York Sun* running an article in early March: "The Democratic Party will not run the momentous campaign of 1900 on the grub issue."[39] Other newspapers stated that the McKinley administration was largely sidelining him as much as possible during the latter stages of the "embalmed beef" investigation in order to prevent him emerging as a potential political threat.[40]

In fact, some even saw Miles' testimony and one-man crusade as purely political theater. The *Kansas City Journal* even went so far as to blast the General's "yellow journal friends and yellow war record," suggesting that he choose Emiliano Aguinaldo, the Filipino rebel leader, as his running mate.[41] Moves were made to discredit the entire "embalmed beef" episode on these grounds.

Talk of Miles' campaign increased as the year progressed, with he himself formally stating his willingness to run in April of 1900.[42] Overall, he was seen as favored by the gold Democrats and lent some military weight to the party. Yet, Bryan had a stranglehold on the party machinery and most in the party preferred an anti-imperialism/pro-silver message for that year. For his part, the latter campaigned extensively and rarely mentioned either Miles or Adm. Dewey by name.[43] In the end, William Jennings Bryan won the nomination with little resistance and Miles went on to aggressively campaign for him. The general returned in 1904 to seek the nomination a second time, with newspapers billing it as a grudge match between him and his old rival Roosevelt. Yet, once again, he didn't progress far into the campaign season.

The issue of diseased meat reemerged a few years later thanks to Upton Sinclair. A renowned socialist writer, he published an exposé, *The Jungle*, on the meat industry in Chicago. Interestingly, his original intent was to show the horrible treatment of immigrant labor by monopolistic industries in the country.[44] The work was originally run in serial format by the *Appeal to Reason* in 1905, a socialist newspaper out of Kansas. After much effort by his part, he was able to enlist a national publisher and the work was released to a much wider audience in February of 1906.

Sinclair's famous quip of "I aimed for the public's heart and by accident hit it in the stomach" was extremely accurate. While the focus of his work was the hardships faced by immigrants, the vast majority of readers instead reacted viscerally to his depictions of the meat-making process. Amidst the references to the terrible conditions of both what went into the product as well as the process by which it was done, Sinclair resurrected the claim of embalmed beef. "It was stuff such as this that made the 'embalmed beef' that had killed several times as many United States soldiers as all the bullets of the Spaniards; only the army beef, besides, was not fresh canned, it was old stuff that had been lying for years in the cellars."[45]

One person who was cautious about the exposé was President Teddy Roosevelt. The Republican president, despite his generally progressive agenda, was doubtful of Sinclair due to his socialist leanings.[46] In fact, only the previous year, the author had made national news for organizing a national group to push the study of socialism at the collegiate level.[47] Therefore, in order to investigate the veracity of the claims, Roosevelt dispatched investigators to Chicago. The subsequent Neill-Reynolds Report verified much of what had been written and not surprisingly was seized upon by General Miles.[48] When called in front of Congress, Charles P. Neill recounted that not only was filthy meat and general debris swept up into the meat-packing vats but also "the expectoration of tuberculosis and other diseased workers."[49]

Sinclair's book, the report of Neill and Reynold, and the complaints of the public eventually resulted in the Meat Inspection Act. Signed into law on June 30, 1906, by President Roosevelt, it was a revolutionary act that did much to improve the quality of meat in the nation. Around the same time, the issue of quack medicine helped produce the Pure Food and Drug Act, which expanded the concept of government inspection to cover various consumed products.

Disease helped to push many of the reforms that emerged during the

19th century in America. While cost normally derailed many of these proposals, once the element of contagion was brought up, citizens and politicians were more willing to act. Yet, even here, politics played an important role limiting success. Interestingly, much of the urban improvement of the late 19th century was pushed by the Sanitary Movement, a scientific philosophy that rejected the germ theory of disease and instead relied upon traditional notions of miasma. Many of the Republican governors, boards of health, and Congressmen of the northeast, especially post–Civil War Radical Republicans, proved open to these ideas as they seemed to present more opportunity for involvement and improvement then did the ideas of Doctors Snow or Reed. Even though the scientific basis of their ideas were ultimately misguided, they managed to produce some of the great systems of civilization that would define modern American cities.

Chapter X

The Pox of Progressivism: Vaccinations

The reliance upon divine intervention to prevent or cure disease slowly shifted toward looking to the medical community as Western civilization progressed. Now, with the onset of the 20th century, this reliance was shifted further toward government. While medicine was still seen as the cure for illness, its prevention, its mitigation, and the organization of the medical resources needed to confront it were all seen as falling within the bailiwick of government. Pestilence was a source of power for politicians; germs required governments to control them. Nowhere was this connection stronger than within the Progressive movement in 20th-century America.

In his 1941 work, *Escape from Freedom,* Erich Fromm differentiates between Negative and Positive Liberty. The former had characterized the American political experience since the founding of the country. By definition, it represented the "freedom from instinctual determination of his actions."[1] What this looked like in reality was the creation of a government whose sole purpose was to protect the citizen from the loss of their rights or their property. Government existed to make sure nothing was taken away from the person; in this, it was a negative form of liberty.

As the 19th century wore on, however, there emerged a push in some circles for what became known as Positive Liberty. This was the concept that people should be able to fully articulate their wishes and desires but acknowledged that societal, political, and economic constraints existed in the way. To some, therefore, government became a vehicle by which to push the improvement of man and society. With the acknowledgment of disease as perhaps the greatest danger to citizens, it became one of the first areas to be tackled by progressive governments.

The dangers of Positive Liberty lie in two facets. The first is the ever-growing need to feed more power to the government in order to provide equality of outcome. This invariably comes from stripping away the rights

X. The Pox of Progressivism: Vaccinations

and freedoms of the population. The second occurs with the associated preference for science over ethics. Growing out of mid–19th-century Positivism, it argued for a focus on data-driven solutions to problems in society. This normally leads to the concept of a government by experts, who would direct people for their own best interests. The danger comes from both a reliance on science in a way that transforms it into unquestionable dogma, as well as a tendency to drift toward utilitarianism. These various trends led to a political approach to disease in the early 20th century that often produced more harm than good.

The start of this trend can be seen in the emergence of the vaccine movement in America in the late 19th century. As discussed previously, the history of vaccination begins early in the American experience. The efforts of Mather and Boylston not only saved countless lives in Boston but also began the very public debate over the practice. Variolation was certainly not without its hazards. A staunch proponent of the procedure, Benjamin Franklin published a work on the practice by Dr. William Heberden in 1759. In his foreword to the lengthy pamphlet, Franklin detailed both the history of the practice in America, as well as the reasons for opposition to it. He particularly chose to focus on a recent outbreak of the disease in Boston in 1753–1754. Interestingly, he noted that as the disease erupted, many rushed to be variolated, creating an environment in which "the numbers inoculated in every neighbourhood spread the infection likewise more speedily among those who did not chuse Inoculation; so that in a few months, the distemper went thro' the town, and was extinct."[2] Though this certainly served to produce herd immunity faster, it also fueled speculation among residents that the inoculation had made the situation worse.

In his foreword, Franklin notes that some residents accused doctors of covering up the number of deaths caused by the practice, while at the same time claimed that town officials were exaggerating the reported number of the unvaccinated who died. The accusations eventually led local town officials to develop a process for collecting accurate information to inform the public. Magistrates would record and report all deaths under oath while accompanied by public observers who represented both the pro- and anti-vaccination camps.

Interestingly, while the gathered data shows that survival rates for those vaccinated was far superior to those who acquired the disease naturally, with only around 1.5 percent dying as opposed to almost 10 percent, this was still seen as higher than acceptable by many. Proponents of the practice chided parents for sending their young or unfit children in for variolation, or else blamed doctors for rushing and not following up with their patients, while opponents of the practice blasted the roughly 30 total deaths that did occur following variolation as medically unnecessary.

For his part, Benjamin Franklin identified three main reasons for the opposition to the practice. These included "scruples of consciousness" over its moral lawfulness, the strength of family opinion, and the often-excessive cost of the practice. The last of these tended to confine the procedure to the wealthier classes, creating a socioeconomic divide that was likewise reflected in the politics. To help combat the first two concerns, Franklin recommended that doctors experienced with the procedure provide more pamphlets and information to the public, as politicians were too ignorant of the science to assuage the people.

Yet, public misgivings over variolation were certainly not unfounded. With little to no regulation in the medical community and an improper understanding of the science, doctors occasionally produced disastrous episodes. In 1767, Dr. John Smith began to practice variolation in Yorktown, Virginia, only to produce a local epidemic of smallpox when he failed to monitor the location and status of his patients. The decision by Dr. John Dalgleish the next year to likewise provide the remedy in Norfolk led to a local riot. An "anti-vaccine mob" attempted to disrupt his practice twice, in both 1768 and 1769, ransacking homes and assaulting patients. This was in part caused by anti-vaccination feelings but also targeted the home of the wealthy, Loyalist Dr. Archibald Campbell where the operation took place.[3] Once again, a clear political divide existed between those who favored and opposed the practice, which reflected larger issues at the time.

Many of the initial states subsequently passed laws to either forbid or heavily restrict the practice of variolation. Wealthy families, such as the Washingtons, Jeffersons, and Adamses, continued to pursue the practice, giving further proof of the, at least, economic divide that separated the two sides. Boston remained at the forefront of the practice despite a general ban there as well. Following the eruption of an epidemic in 1764, town leaders suspended the law to allow for a variolation campaign. The one notable exception to this were the vaccination efforts of General Washington during the Revolution. As mentioned previously, Washington's own pro-vaccination views when combined with a public fear of the disease's use by the British in a biological attack allowed for the public health campaign to move ahead.

As the 19th century dawned, the discovery by Edward Jenner of what would become the smallpox vaccine provided for a safer method by which to protect the public against the deadly illness. Thomas Jefferson, an ardent supporter of both science and vaccination, became an eager proponent of Jenner's work. During his presidency he frequently corresponded with the British doctors and others to discuss and push the practice. While the federal government had little power in this area at the time, he used his pen and voice to support the procedure. For example, in 1802, he encouraged the visiting Shawnee chief, Black Hoof, to be inoculated along with some of his warriors in Washington.[4]

Nearly a decade later, Congress moved to provide at least limited government support for the practice. In 1813, Congress, heavily led by the Democrat-Republicans and supported by President Madison, passed the "Act to Encourage Vaccination." It established a National Vaccine Agency under Dr. James Smith of Baltimore. Furthermore, it legislated that the U.S. Postal Service would be required to transport vaccine material for free if it weighed under 5 oz. Combined with orders for all military personnel to receive the vaccine, this was largely the extent of what the federal government could do to encourage the practice.[5]

However, this effort did not last long, with Congress allowing the agency to dissolve in 1822. The push for this was led by Congressman Hutchins G. Burton (DR) of North Carolina. While noting that he felt the original legislation was passed with "the purest principles of benevolence," it has nonetheless led to "one of the greatest calamities which has for several years befallen that part of the country in which I reside."[6] An outbreak of the disease had occurred in North Carolina in early 1822, which many locals blamed on the practitioners of the Vaccine Agency, as vaccine material had been accidentally mailed to an unsuspecting physician. Over the next few months, Burton's political rhetoric only intensified, accusing the federal government of turning a blind eye while citizens were "slaughtered by hundreds with indifference."[7] Burton was supported by several other Northern and Southern congressmen, including Dr. William Eustis of Massachusetts, while opposition mostly came from Northern members of the House, including Dr. Lewis Condict of New Jersey and several who would eventually join the National Republican and Whig parties. A lengthy debate ensued in Congress in late April, with Burton expressing the support of President Monroe for the dissolution of the Agency. Eventually, Congress voted to end its mandate, with the House approving the measure by a vote of 102 to 57.[8]

The vaccine movement reverted to the state level during the Jacksonian Era that followed, but it saw little appetite for a push even on that scale. Even Massachusetts, the birthplace of both variolation and vaccination in the country, began to disregard the process in the 1830s. In 1838, a delegation of the Massachusetts Medical Society appeared before the Whig dominated state assembly to ask for a repeal of the smallpox laws of 1792 and 1797. These had mandated the strict isolation and observation of smallpox cases, whether naturally caused or inoculated. The medical community, which had been hesitant to support Jenner's methods initially, now argued that isolation was both costly and intrusive of a patient's liberty. The political establishment sided with the experts and repealed the laws.

What followed was a predictable explosion of the disease, with over 26 times as many deaths occurring from 1838 to 1855 as had happened from 1812 to 1837.[9] This led, not surprisingly, to a much more Draconian policy in 1855. The Know Nothing sweep into the state legislature and governor's office that year produced one of the most aggressive reform campaigns of the 19th century. Hundreds of bills were passed in 1855 alone, including a revolutionary vaccine mandate signed by Governor Henry Gardner. It called for the mandatory vaccination of all manufacturing companies, alms houses, school personnel, lunatic hospitals, prisons, and any other organization wholly or partially supported by the state. Most notably, it called for the mandatory vaccination of all children attending public schools as well. Additionally, local boards of health were given the power to vaccinate entire towns if needed. With no religious, moral, or medical exemptions allowed, the Know Nothing bill stood as a sweeping and revolutionary piece of legislation. Yet, with no statewide board of health in place to enforce the measure until 1869, it's debatable how widespread or effective it was. In fact, death records show an average smallpox fatality rate of 150 per year continuing from 1855 to 1873.

Vaccination efforts did not seriously improve in Boston until the outbreak of another epidemic in 1872. The 1,040 deaths experienced by the city did more to drive people to the doctor than did any number of Know Nothing mandates. A similar story unfolded in New York City in 1869. Following an outbreak of the disease the year before, the city's board of health began to investigate vaccination levels, ultimately discovering that less than half of all school children in Manhattan were inoculated against smallpox. Dr. Harris of the New York State Board of Health took an aggressive stance against the disease, undertaking door-to-door vaccination campaigns on blocks where positive cases were found. By 1870, the city government was recommending that all citizens be inoculated against the disease. Therefore, it was perhaps not surprising that in 1873, New York City moved to require vaccination for all children entering public schools, followed up by a mandate for all janitors as well in 1875.[10]

Public debate dominated New York City Board of Education meetings for the next several years. The public was quick to point out the logical fallacy in mass vaccination. "If vaccination is a protection against smallpox, those who are vaccinated can have nothing to fear from those who are not, and the policy ... is absurd."[11] This argument cut at the logical basis for a vaccine mandate and served to expose the paternalistic thinking and desire for power that were beginning to drive state action and progressivism.

This became more outwardly revealed during the very public journalistic debate that ensued between the Democratic Party–aligned *Brooklyn*

Daily Eagle and its competitor, the *Union*. In a November 1875 article, the *Union* proclaimed, "If parents willfully neglect to take precautions against contagious disease [it is] the right of 'decent people' to take the case into their own hands ... to supply the remedy."[12] Public health was a public concern, which the people could contract to the government. The editors of the *Daily Eagle* in turn argued that this was not only undemocratic but a fallacy, suggesting that it makes as much sense as "because it is admitted that sobriety is desirable we must forsooth force men by statute to abstain from drink ... the degradation of some newspapers is admitted, therefore we should abolish liberty of the press and pass gag laws."[13] In a similar vein to debates over vaccine mandates in the modern day, the *Daily Eagle* argued: "We desire to affirm our belief that everybody should vaccinate ... but we object to force." It wasn't the science that was causing debate but whether a free people should be ruled by it.

Over the next decade, a number of groups arose that were against the forced mandating of vaccinations. Probably the first of these was the Anti-Vaccination Society of America, which was organized around 1879. Inspired by the actions of William Tebb, a British businessman and social reformer who had established a similar organization in the United Kingdom, it was organized by those opposed to vaccination as well as those who saw mandatory inoculation as an affront to personal liberty. While the two groups had similar concerns, their opponents would often paint the latter wing as being anti-vaccine as well in an effort to discredit them. As the famed abolitionist and minister Moncure Conway pointed out in an 1879 letter regarding the similar situation in London, "There is steadily arising in this country a rebellion against compulsory vaccination ... by prosecutions and punishments of some respectable and intelligent families, the authorities have been the means of constituting an Anti-Vaccination Society."[14] The Society would go on to publish newspapers, compose a hymn, and held conferences during which medical professionals railed against the effectiveness of vaccination.[15] Similar societies were set up over the next several years, including the New England Anti-Compulsory Vaccination League (1882), the Anti-Vaccine League of New York City (1885), and the Anti-Vaccine League of America (1908). Many times, these were composed largely of medical professionals, some of whom rejected the germ theory of Pasteur and instead supported the views of Antoine Béchamp and others. Progressive politicians and their newspaper mouthpieces railed frequently against these groups, with the *New York Times* recommending in 1885 that since "neither ignorance now imbecility can justify any person in establishing himself as a distributing center of pestilence ... the sanitary authorities should not forbear, when occasion arises, to subject every member of the Anti-Vaccination League to compulsory vaccination."[16]

Contemporaneously, more and more states moved to mandate smallpox vaccination. By 1899, Maryland, Arkansas, Georgia, Iowa, Mississippi, and the Choctaw Nation had all followed suit. As these pieces of legislation came at a time of improving sanitation and declining rates of infection, they naturally provoked further opposition from those opposed to vaccinations or germ theory, as well as those who saw themselves as liberty-minded individuals. Unfortunately, the push for mass immunization also increased the risk of accidental contamination or death.

Disaster finally struck in 1901 in Camden, New Jersey, when nine children, who had been recently vaccinated against smallpox, died of tetanus. An outbreak of the disease in early October, which killed an eight-year-old girl, her father, and seven of her siblings, had compelled the Camden Board of Education to announce it would enforce an 1887 law that mandated the vaccination of schoolchildren. By the end of the month, nearly 5,000 young people had undergone the process in what would normally be seen as a very successful campaign. Yet, over the next few weeks, nine young people died of tetanus, all but one of whom had been vaccinated by H.K. Mulford, the main distributor for Camden. During a contemporaneous vaccine push in Philadelphia, in which more material from Mulford was used, an additional three people perished from tetanus.

A public outcry ensued, one which was quickly seized upon by those opposed to vaccinations or mandates. The president of Camden's Board of Health, Dr. H.H. Davis, stated on November 15, "Vaccinated persons will be in danger until a heavy rainfall ... none of them have been caused by vaccines, but by the tetanus germs in the filth of the air," an odd use of miasma theory to defend the vaccines developed under the germ theory.[17] This began a standard trope that the process of vaccination was safe, but the patients themselves were causing their subsequent illness due to their ignorance and filthy living styles. Under pressure from parents, the Board of Education ultimately brought in Dr. Albert Barnes to help investigate the matter. Interestingly, he worked as a chemist for Henry K. Mulford at the time, which would clearly result in a less than unbiased account. Barnes claimed, "The patients' arms after vaccination were neglected by the parents ... [they] had been exposed to infection from every possible source." On November 30, 1901, the Board of Education finally released its findings, claiming that the source of the infection was a period of "dry weather."[18] Despite these claims, subsequent outbreaks and investigations would prove years later that Mulford's batches were most likely contaminated, yet the desire to push vaccination by various interest groups clearly outweighed the interests of the public.

Newspapers continued to fight over the need for mandatory vaccination, with many citing the "smallpox scare" then ensuing not only in the

United States but also around the world. "Never in the history of Christendom has there been such a scare of the disease known as small-pox ... every citizen of this country should get vaccinated and if he does not do so of his own free will then the law should compel him to do so. Go and get vaccinated."[19] The extremes of the way in which fear gripped many can be seen in an anecdote carried by the *Waterbury Democrat* in November of 1902. The author relates how a train conductor, while collecting tickets, saw a passenger holding a dog that had a red ribbon wrapped around one of his legs. At the time, this was a traditional symbol of vaccination. When questioned, the female passenger responded, "Yes, he's just been vaccinated. The smallpox scare may come again this winter, so I've had him seen in good time."[20] The *New York Times* referred to opponents of the practice as a "familiar species of crank," with "absurdly fallacious" arguments.[21] At the same time, other periodicals pushed against the craze. The Republican-leaning *Washington Herald* published numerous articles and opinion pieces from doctors citing the inefficiency of vaccinations or the illegality of mandates.[22]

For its part, the federal government used the scare as well as the incidents of contaminated vaccines to push the Biologics Control Act of 1902. Coming four years before the famed Food and Drug Act, it allowed for the oversight of all vaccines and antitoxins being produced in the country and mandated labeling requirements.

The response from the public, as mandates increased, was the launching of several notable lawsuits. Some of these attempted to argue against the science of vaccination or else claimed that the potential harm outweighed the benefit. One of the earliest was the case of *Blue v. Beach* in Indiana in 1900. Launched by the general secretary of the Anti-Vaccination Society of America, it ultimately failed before the state's supreme court. Additional cases proliferated in the 1890s and early 1900s across the country, with all failing to make their point.

Some also pursued religious arguments, banking on the First Amendment to protect them from mandates. Interestingly, religion seems to have played little role in the vaccine debate since the era of Cotton Mather, though this may have simply been due to the lack of mandates and enforcements rather than a lack of doctrinal opinion. The onset of compulsory mandates at this time coincided with the rise of a new religious sect, the Church of Christ, Scientist, founded by Mary Baker Eddy. The philosophy of Christian Science viewed disease as a mental error to be corrected by prayer rather than a physical one to be addressed by medicine. While the religion did not expressively forbid the use of medical treatment, it saw it as useless when compared to the power of faith. When questioned on the topic of vaccination, Eddy herself responded, "Rather than quarrel over being vaccinated, I recommend that, if the law demand an individual to submit to this process, he obey the law; and then appeal to the gospel to save him from any bad results."[23] Despite this, it did not stop many practitioners, including her own son George Glover, from launching lawsuits.

Finally, in 1905, one of the numerous anti-mandate cases reached the Supreme Court. Known as *Jacobson v. Massachusetts*, it was brought by a pastor from Cambridge who was fined in 1902 when he refused to obey the mandate enforced by the city during a smallpox scare that year. Jacobson argued both against the medical necessity of the vaccine as well as professing that the Massachusetts statute violated the Fourteenth Amendment. In a 7–2 decision, the Supreme Court rejected his appeal. The Harlan Court reaffirmed the notion of "police powers" for the state but did establish restraints upon it. For a statute or mandate to be constitutional, it would need to satisfy the areas of necessity, reasonable means, proportionality, and harm avoidance. The Jacobson case would become the standard case used by future courts concerning the power of government with regards to public health, being cited 69 times in the next century.[24] At the time, the *New York Times* gleefully reported, "The contention that compulsory vaccination is an infraction of personal liberty and an unconstitutional interference with the right of the individual to have the smallpox if he wants it, and to communicate it to others, has been ended [by the U.S. Supreme Court].... [This] should end the useful life of the societies of cranks."[25]

This recognition of the expanded police powers of the state with regards to health is best represented by the aggressive actions of the New York City public school system in 1906 that led to the infamous Adenoid Riots. As the school year was coming to a close, Principal A.E. Simpson of PS 110 moved to provide not only mandated vaccinations to students but also brought in doctors to perform adenoid surgeries as well on a group of "defective" students. The latter was a common practice at the time and was thought to reduce the risk of serious infections for children. Simpson later claimed that letters were sent home to parents and permission obtained for the procedure. The school's motive was to save parents the trouble of having to take their own children uptown to Bellevue Hospital.

The procedures were carried out quickly and without fanfare but, as the students returned home to tell their parents about men with razor blades cutting their throats, rumors quickly began to spread. The Lower East Side was filled with tenements that housed recent Eastern European and Jewish immigrants. Only two weeks earlier, a pogrom in Bialystok in Russia had seen the murder of 80 Polish Jews and, for many, these tales from their children produced terror and anger. On June 27, 1906, mobs of parents descended upon nearly a dozen schools in the area to rescue their children.

X. The Pox of Progressivism: Vaccinations

The *Evening World* reported, "Police reserves from 6 stations were called to handle the hysterical women," but they could do little to stop the mob from trying to force their way into the schools. A riot soon ensued, as bricks were thrown at windows, a teacher was assaulted, and men attempted to tear apart the doors. "Scores of mothers and fathers of children in the schools were actually insane."[26] A fire drill was eventually called to evacuate the children to their parents in order to prove they were not being harmed. Speculation was rampant at the time that the rumors were spurred by local, unscrupulous physicians, known as "snips," who specialized in the procedure and were angry that the Board of Health was depriving them of business.

Further court cases followed, all of which were based upon some notion of a constitutional right to avoid mandated vaccinations. Included among these were *Zucht v. King* (1922), *Prince v. Mass.* (1944), and *Maricopa County Health Department v. Harman* (1987). Yet, the power of state and local governments with relation to their ability to force inoculation upon a citizen was only finally successfully challenged in 1966. At the height of the civil rights movement in America, Assemblyman Alexander Chananau of New York was proposing a new and stricter polio vaccine mandate for school children. In response to protests from some religious groups as well as the Board of Health, a clause was put in place that allowed for religious exemption from the practice. New York became the first such state to do so, a move quickly followed by most others. By 1980, all states in the country had pushed through mandatory vaccines for schoolchildren. Yet, religious exemptions still existed for certain communities, most notably among Hasidic Jews, some devout Muslims, and Christian Scientists, while conscientious objectors also made up a certain percentage.

A combination of forces began to converge in the 1990s and early 2000s in America to create a minor measles epidemic. Vaccine hesitancy among the above-mentioned religious groups increased following the rise in Jewish and Muslim immigration in the 1990s. At the same time, an earth-shattering study was released by the journal *The Lancet* in 1998, which hypothesized a connection between the MMR vaccine and autism. Authored by Dr. Andrew Wakefield and 12 of his associates, it drew tenuous connections between increasing rates of autism and increasing rates of vaccination. Though caustic scientific debate ensued, Wakefield's idea was quickly picked up by notable celebrities, including Robert DeNiro and Jenny McCarthy, by Robert F. Kennedy, Jr., who published on it extensively, as well as by many in the general public. Though the research of Wakefield was eventually discredited, many in the public were not so easily swayed.

By the early 2000s, vaccination rates at several schools in California,

New York, and other states were far below what was needed for herd immunity. Most notably, the Waldorf schools of the Bay Area in California reported rates as low as 22 percent.[27] While these tended to be left-leaning institutions and clear geographic clusters of vaccine hesitancy were observed in more liberal enclaves, studies at the time also found some vaccine hesitancy among conservatives as well.[28] Outbreaks of measles began to creep upward as the second decade of the 2000s progressed, with 220 cases reported in 2011 and 687 in 2014.

An outbreak in December of 2014 at Disneyland in California quickly spread across several other states as well as Mexico and Central America in 2015. Not only did this epidemic become a political talking point in the discussion of illegal immigration during the 2016 election cycle, but it also resulted in California becoming the first state to eliminate the religious exemption clause from its vaccination mandates. This move was followed a few years later by Maine and New York as well, while West Virginia and Mississippi never allowed such a claim.

Nor were laws mandating vaccines only developed for schoolchildren. Concerns over the transference of diseases from animals to humans, as well as its impact on the agricultural economy, led to numerous laws requiring the inoculation and testing of certain animals. Yet, in many cases, this produced resistance in a similar way to human mandates. One of the more notable examples was the Iowa Cow War of 1931. Daniel Webster Turner, a progressive Republican governor of Iowa, began to enforce a 1929 law that required the testing of cattle for tuberculosis. Funded by a property tax hike, it was opposed by many farmers for both economic and practical reasons. Rumors abounded that the practice either produced sudden abortions in the cattle, lowered the quality and quantity of milk that was produced, or else was unreliable.[29]

In a repeat of the Whiskey Rebellion of 1794, farmers of Cedar County, Iowa, rose up in 1931 to oppose the law's implementation. The movement began with a march by thousands on the capital at Des Moines. Yet, as no legislative help was forthcoming, they soon moved to obstruct the veterinarians and tax collectors who were sent to carry out the law. In September of that year, two doctors accompanied by dozens of officers were accosted by hundreds of angry farmers. Turner responded decisively, dispatching 2,000 national guardsmen the next day. As one newspaper reported, "People learned that martial law will mean the cessation of all civil law ... they were told that it amounts to a dictatorship of the county."[30] Protests were rapidly suppressed and prevented, key members of the Farmers Protective Association were arrested by the military, and the testing campaign was finished. States were prepared to use force to ensure health mandates.

X. The Pox of Progressivism: Vaccinations

Vaccination has been a politicized topic in America since it was first practiced in the early 18th century. It has intersected debates over religious freedom, constitutional rights, bodily autonomy, immigration laws, and the power of the state. The battle of vaccines has reflected the progressive belief in the growing power of the paternalistic state. Many of these notions would reach a boiling point in 2021 as vaccine mandates to confront the novel coronavirus began to be enforced on both the state and federal level. The notions of negative liberty and utilitarianism, which accompanied the process in the late 19th century, were thoroughly embraced by the Progressives and the Democratic Party throughout much of the 20th century and beyond.

Chapter XI

The Pox of Progressivism: Culling the Herd

The Constitution was enacted less to define the government than to limit it. From the beginnings of the country, the fight over federalism and the proper division of powers between state and national governments has been paralleled by the battle over the size and role of government on either level. Progressivism, which began on the local and state level in the 19th century, slowly began to push for stronger federal government with the dawning of the 20th. It couched these efforts in terms of combating what it saw as the problems of modernity. Yet, as can be expected, philosophical debates between the parties arose over the scope and methods of this expansion. Some of the most spectacular episodes of growing political power, especially those with terrifying results, occurred as a means by which to tackle disease.

Forced Health Care

As previously observed, the power of state governments to tackle disease, vis-à-vis vaccine mandates and quarantine rules, had steadily grown as the 19th century progressed. For its part, the federal government remained largely absent from these state level issues, save for the mandatory vaccination of soldiers during wartime. The first moves to change this occurred during the Hayes administration when two separate entities were created to help stem the spread of disease into and throughout the country.

The first of these national level organizations was the Marine Hospital Service. In 1798, the Congress approved the creation of hospitals in major port cities to service the crews of ships. These would be funded through the leveling of a 1 percent tax on the income of all sailors. In June of 1870, following an investigation that showed the complete disorganization in the hospital system, the various buildings were organized under a federalized Marine Hospital Service operating out of the Treasury Department. Introduced by Senator Zachariah Chandler (R–MI), it was rapidly moved through Congress and signed into law by President Grant. Slightly later, the Democrat-led 46th Congress of the United States (1879–1881) pushed a bill through the House proposed by William Felton (D–GA) that granted the MHS the power to organize quarantines of vessels arriving in American ports.

Increased impetus for the act emerged in the early summer of 1878 as a massive yellow fever epidemic emerged in the Mississippi River Valley. Tens of thousands of deaths later, the Marine Hospital Service organized a commission under Colonel T.S. Hardee to address any deficiencies in the handling of the outbreak. Not surprisingly, the Hardee Commission eventually returned a report that blamed the city government of New Orleans for failing to properly contain and advertise the presence of the disease. Its inaction allowed the contagion to spread the length and breadth of the river, killing over 20,000 and costing millions in lost business. The recommendations of the Committee were for the creation of a national system of quarantine to handle future outbreaks.[1]

For those who favored a centralization of power, the tragedy of the yellow fever epidemic of 1878 provided just such a catalyst. At the same time, for still others, it made practical, public health sense to organize efforts on a national level to prevent the arrival of contagions that would in the end cross state lines with little effort. Fear of a repeat of what occurred during the summer of 1878 resulted in the drafting of legislation in 1879 that created a National Board of Health with powers to effect internal quarantines. Support for such a radical move came from a variety of sources, including pro-business Republicans, a concerned Southern public, and Radical Republicans. Yet, even from the beginning, concerns existed among conservatives over this expansive addition to federal authority. In May of 1879, the Senate moved to place various limitations on the original House bill, seeking to use the NBH to merely supplement state actions.[2] A conference was subsequently organized between the leaders of the NBH and various Southern industries and interests to find a more moderate approach to the strategy of internal quarantines. As one Southern Democratic newspaper opined, "The subject of inland quarantine ... is one which may be either a blessing or a curse to the people, and hence demands extreme care and deliberation in its management."[3]

The return of yellow fever during the summer of 1879 led to the quick enforcement of local quarantines. Some states, such as Tennessee, announced that they would work in conjunction with the NBH to staunch the spread of the illness.[4] Yet, very quickly it was realized that the outbreak was far less severe than the previous one and, at the same time, the actions of the federal agency were soon seen as both overzealous and ineffective. Quarantines failed to stop the spread of the disease, as its vectoring agent was unknown at the time, but they did severely damage local industry. Democratic newspapers in the South quickly turned against the Board, using its failures to tarnish the Hayes administration. "It was the duty of Mr. Hayes to appoint as members of the board ... such physicians as are experts in sanitary science and familiar with pestilence ... it is very plain that the board as at present organized is a costly humbug."[5] New Orleans, one of the largest port cities in the nation, vociferously protested against the quarantines by both the federal government and other states, calling them "unjust ... as her officers declare there is not a case of yellow fever in the city."[6] By the early fall, lawsuits were even being prepared in various states, with one Florida politician referring to quarantine as "a relic of ignorance and barbarism."[7]

In December of 1880, a quarantine convention was held to discuss the issues raised by both the frequent yellow fever outbreaks as well as the dispute over federalism and public health measures. In the end, regional committees were organized to study the issue and present the findings to Congress. Yet, the fate of the National Board of Health was ultimately decided not by constitutional concerns but by bureaucratic infighting. In 1883, as cholera once more threatened the Western Hemisphere, a Democratic Congress moved to strip funding from the NBH. The move was largely orchestrated by Surgeon General John Hamilton, who favored the use of the Marine Health Service as an effective tool of national quarantine. Many Republican papers, including the *New York Post*, argued against the move, stating that the creation of the NBH was based upon "sound public sentiment and demand for sanitary protection."[8] Yet, the interests of the Marine Health Service for power, anger among Southern Democrats, business concerns of some Republicans, and conservative opposition, all united to kill the agency.[9]

Though the growth of federal authority in the management of public health was temporarily slowed by conservative forces in the 1880s, state authority continued to grow exponentially. In 1894, the Brooklyn Board of Health was in the midst of pushing mandatory vaccination for smallpox on residents of the city. Two expressmen, John H. Smith and Thomas Cummings, protested the move and refused to receive the shot. In response, the Board of Health had them forcibly quarantined inside their stable by the city's police department. Both men sued for their freedom, and Justice William Gaynor of the Brooklyn Supreme Court, a well-known libertarian, issued a ruling in their favor, arguing that "if the commissioner had the power to imprison an individual for refusing to submit to vaccination I see no reason why he could not also imprison one for refusing to swallow some dose."[10] In his subsequent decision, Justice Gaynor declared, "Arbitrary power is abhorrent to our system of government ... if the legislature desired to make vaccination compulsory, it would have so enacted."[11] Yet, Dr. Zachary Taylor Emery, the top health official for the city, continued to undertake aggressive and extralegal measures to ensure vaccinations and quarantines. Overnight raids by police-backed doctors swept through Italian neighborhoods, often leading to violence.[12] Though Emery claimed victory in quelling an epidemic, legal battles and costly lawsuits subsequently plagued Brooklyn for years.

A few years later, the state of Texas likewise took aggressive action against its citizens in order to combat pestilence. An outbreak of smallpox in late 1898 in the city of Laredo began to alarm state health officials. By January, over 10 percent of the town was reported as having been infected, finally prompting Health Commissioner L.T. Blunt to act. A strict quarantine was enforced, homes were fumigated, and vaccines were strongly encouraged. As March dawned, these regulations became stricter, with officials blaming the large Mexican population of the city for non-compliance.

Blunt himself arrived in Laredo on March 16 and soon after summoned a contingent of Texas Rangers to enforce his health decrees. Protests and riots soon followed, especially among the Mexican population. On March 20, 1899, while searching the house of Agapito Herrera, a gun battle ensued between the Rangers and Herrera's men. Following the latter's death, a large, angry crowd gathered, leading to yet another riot that saw one person killed and eight wounded. The next day, the governor sent in the 10th U.S. Cavalry, stationed at Fort McIntosh, to restore order. Though two dozen additional men were arrested, order was largely restored to the town. The quarantine would continue until May 1, at which point the collapsing infection rates allowed for it to be lifted.

Yet, these and other forceful confrontations were only the tip of the progressive spear of public health power. The evolving notion of public health and "the public good" slowly embraced the concept of utilitarianism, pushing personal rights and notions of fundamental liberties to the back. One of the most famous examples of this concerns the infamous Typhoid Mary.

Mary Mallon was born in Ireland around 1869, immigrating to America in 1884. Like most young Irish women of her time, she found work as a domestic. In Mary's case, this involved cooking for wealthy families in New York City. Yet, Mary was unique in that she was an asymptomatic carrier of *Salmonella typhi*, better known as typhoid. This bacterial illness was one of the largest causes of casualties during the Civil War and at the time had no known cure.

In 1906, Mary was engaged in cooking for the family of the wealthy Manhattan banker Charles Henry Warren at their summer home in Oyster Bay. That summer, typhoid sickness suddenly erupted among the well-to-do family, sickening most of its members. The outbreak threatened to cause a scandal and ruin business in the affluent summer resort town. In response, the property owner contacted various medical experts, eventually calling in Dr. George Soper. Upon his arrival, the doctor investigated all possible sources and vectors of the illness but could not find a reasonable cause for it. The only odd clue was that the family's cook had vanished three weeks after the outbreak began.

Soper eventually tracked down Mary Mallon and began to piece together a history of employment in various cities that coupled with local outbreaks of typhoid. His attempts to interview her or obtain samples of her urine and feces all proved to be fruitless. "Indignant and peremptory denials met our appeals. We were unable to make any headway. Mary's position was like that of the lawyer who, on being told by the judge that the facts were all against his client, said that he proposed to deny the facts. Mary denied that she was a carrier."[13] At the same time, she continued to work as a domestic in various households, eventually helping to cause an outbreak in 1907 that infected over 3,000 in New York City.

Finally, Soper convinced the city to act. Mary was forcibly seized by the authorities and tested for the bacteria. "The implication was plain. The cook was virtually a living culture tube in which the germs of typhoid multiplied and from which they escaped in the movements from her bowels. When at toilet her hands became soiled, perhaps unconsciously and invisibly so. When she prepared a meal, the germs were washed and rubbed from her fingers into the food."[14] When the results came back that showed her to be a carrier of the illness, she was detained at Riverside Hospital on North Brother Island.

In an interview with Dr. Bensel, the sanitary superintendent of the health department, the *New York Tribune* questioned whether or not the Mallon case could serve as a tool for disease management in the future. To the reporter's shock, Bensel strongly cautioned against it. Professing that "New York has many walking pesthouses," the doctor pushed the idea that the sheer number of the infected and the cost associated with finding and confining them all would prove to be an impossibility.[15] Shockingly, no mention was made as to the legal or ethical concerns in the practice. Instead, the diseases were seen as dangerous terrorists. "They are a greater menace to any community than bomb throwers and Black Hand artists."[16]

While imprisoned, Mary was experimented on with various treatments and doctors offered to perform an exploratory surgery to remove part of her liver, though she "balked" at the notion. Instead, she remained in confinement, cooking and cleaning for the facility, and was even offered a marriage proposal by a Michigan farmer living in an isolated region.[17] Finally, after three years of confinement and numerous lawsuits, including a $50,000 suit for wrongful imprisonment, the hospital agreed to release her under the promise that she not seek work as a domestic.

For the next five years, Mary disappeared. Living under assumed names, she continued to work as a cook, spreading sickness and death wherever she went. Finally, in 1915, she was once more arrested. As Soper himself opined in a 1919 article on the subject:

> Mary's status after her second arrest has been totally different from that which she possessed after her first. This is true both as to the legal aspects and public sympathy. Whatever rights she once possessed as the innocent victim of an infected condition, precisely like that of hundreds of others who were free, were now lost. She was now a woman who could not claim innocence. She was known willfully and deliberately to have taken desperate chances with human life, and this against the specific instructions of the Health Department. She had been treated fairly; she had been given her liberty and was out on parole. She had abused her privilege; she had broken her parole. She was a dangerous character and must be treated accordingly.[18]

This time she was confined to Riverside for the remainder of her life, dying in a weakened mental state in 1938 as a "medical prisoner."[19]

Typhoid Mary's case, and those of many others at the time, became an inspiration for further such seizures of the sick in the name of public health. Another famous example was the case of John Early, a Spanish-American War veteran who was forcibly quarantined numerous times by both state and federal governments from 1908 to 1938. Medical experts fought both each other and the government over whether Early had leprosy and if it was contagious. Early himself made a dramatic appearance at the Willard Hotel in Washington, then housing Vice President Marshall and numerous senators, in 1914, and actively petitioned Congress to enact legislation to humanely help other lepers in the nation. As he himself wrote:

> To demonstrate how easy it is for a leper to mingle in cities, I planned my present trip six months ago. I knew that it is only when a great truth is sent home to the hearts of the people that attention is paid to it. I knew that if I mingled among the well-to-do and the rich and exposed them to contagion that they would arise out of selfprotection and further my plan of a national home. That is why I chose the Pullman car, why I slept at the best hotels, ate in the best restaurants. No one cares what happens to the poor. If I had kept to the slums in my travels, the agitation would have been little. I had no desire to hurt anyone. I do not believe that the present stage of my disease is contagious. I had the money to travel as I did. I saved my wages and my pension for months to do so, and I hope the lesson has struck home.[20]

The State and STDs

The American entrance into World War I exposed certain economic, technological, and infrastructural weaknesses of the military. Despite Charles Evans Hughes' campaign for "preparedness" in 1916, Wilson's victory meant that less preparations were taken before our declaration of war in April of 1917. One of the startling revelations that emerged afterward was the number of draftees who had to be rejected for physical or epidemiological reasons. Some 8 percent of regular army soldiers and 40 percent of draftees reported some form of venereal disease.[21] Among these were those young men who were found to be stricken with syphilis during their initial medical evaluation, a number that amounted to 13 percent.

States moved to address these issues early in the conflict, relying on the connections of disease and military strength to push extreme legislation. In Washington state, the city of Pullman appealed to Congress directly, arguing that in order to protect its citizens who were being sent off to fight, as well as those back home upon their return, "the Chamber of Commerce of Pullman hereby petitions Congress to pass a law giving military authorities full power and making it their duty to eliminate prostitution within 10 miles of an army camp or navy yard."[22]

Congress moved to seize upon this reality and these requests to further assault the traditional target of prostitution. The result was the Chamberlain-Kahn Act of 1918, which was passed as part of the military appropriations bill that year. Interestingly, despite claims that this was in response to military concerns, it was enacted in November of that year, shortly after the Armistice. George Chamberlain (D–OR) and Julius Kahn (R–CA) were well-known western proponents of both the war and military strength and saw the long-term value of a healthier population.[23] The surgeon general, Rupert Blue, stated at the time that venereal disease was "a national menace ... a plague that, far more easily communicable than leprosy, has to be stamped out of the nation."[24]

This legislation gave power to the armed forces to indefinitely detain individuals who were deemed dangerous to the military. Over 20,000 women would be arrested and quarantined over the course of the war in various states. They were forcibly held, examined, and imprisoned, some for up to a year.[25] In the end, many who did not suffer from venereal disease would acquire it due to the forced examinations. Yet, despite the loss of civil rights, proponents argued that the efforts of the government were largely successful. Prostitution was pushed further toward extinction and the nation as a whole would suffer no recorded casualties from these diseases during the war. In fact, 96 percent of the 48,167 cases of venereal disease that were treated by the military were contracted by the men before they joined the Army.[26]

Syphilis had grown to replace smallpox and cholera as the dread of society. Since at least the late 15th century, the disease had ravaged the population of Europe. Initially thought to be confined to soldiers, sailors, and sex workers, it was used as a moralizing agent by many and helped in part to influence the Protestant Reformation. But it was to be the hereditary nature of the disease, the passing of the "sins of the father" onto the family, as well as the manner through which it was originally acquired, that would make it such a loathsome contagion. With the expansion of the state's policing power with regards to disease, governments moved to take drastic steps to end the plague in the early 20th century.

Paul Ehrlich's discovery of Salvarsan as a cure for syphilis in 1909 provided an even greater impetus for tackling the disease. Apart from the moral stigma associated with it, progressives felt that nothing stood in the way of eradicating the illness with proper help from the government. Considered rampant from 1900 to 1920, some contemporary writers argued that 10–15 percent of the general population was infected.[27]

Many questioned whether to treat the illness at all. Some feared it would lead to increased immoral activity, with such a deadly consequence no longer being a deterrent to vice.[28] Many also wondered whether doctor-patient confidentiality should be cast aside in the better interests of the community at large. The American Medical Association went so far as to update its code of ethics in 1912, adding in two addendums to deal with infectious disease.

> 1. There are occasions, however, when a physician must determine whether or not his duty to society requires him to take definite action to protect a healthy individual from becoming infected because the physician has knowledge, obtained through the confidences entrusted to him as a physician, of a communicable disease to which the healthy individual is about to be exposed. In such a case, the physician should act as he would desire another to act toward one of his own family under like circumstances. Before he determines his course, the physician should know the civil law of his commonwealth concerning privileged communications.
>
> 2. At all times, it is the duty of the physician to notify the properly constituted public health authorities of every case of communicable disease under his care, in accordance with the laws, rules, and regulations of the health authorities of the locality in which the patient is.

As always, state governments took the lead in attempting to control syphilis. By 1916, nine states had passed laws that included the illness as grounds for banning a marriage. In 1935, Connecticut took this a step further, requiring blood tests for all those seeking to be married in the state. At the same time, "a marriage license issued in 1935 or any previous year will be invalid after January 1, 1936."[29] This broad expansion of government power and invasion of medical privacy initially cast a chilling pall over applications for marriage. In Connecticut alone, the first six months of its presence saw a 50 percent drop in marriages within the state, followed by steeper declines in subsequent months.[30] It soon became apparent that many couples merely crossed state lines or married in secret to avoid the new law.[31]

The Roosevelt administration soon attempted to create similar mandates on the national level, in its ever-increasing efforts at acquiring more power. In 1936, Surgeon General Thomas Parran proposed a comprehensive plan to tackle syphilis. It initially consisted of four components: (1) widespread testing to uncover cases, (2) examination of all persons who came in contact with an infected individual, (3) blood tests before marriage and birth, and (4) increased education on the disease.[32] The result of these plans was the much pared down National Venereal Disease Control Act of 1938, also known as the La Follette-Bulwinkle Act. Rather than pushing for federal control of the problem, Congress moved to merely fund state efforts, appropriating $15,000,000 for the undertaking. Part of this was due to the aggressive actions already being undertaken by the various states. Within only three years of Connecticut's marriage law being enacted, 25 other states had already followed suit. Likewise, New York pioneered the Twomey-Newell Bill in 1938, which mandated blood tests for pregnant women.

Many states would go on to adopt even more stringent provisions, completely outlawing the marriage of those with any STDs. The idea was heavily pushed by the United States Public Health Services in the 1910s and 1920s and was eventually adopted by several states.[33] Included among these were Nebraska, Wyoming, Delaware, Oklahoma, and South Carolina. Though these were eventually repealed in the latter half of the 20th century, some remained on the books as obscure laws only to be discovered by accident years later. Interestingly, some even proposed that diseased people be encouraged to marry other stricken people and forced to use birth control in order to create dead ends for illness.[34]

Yet, many opposed these moves on economic, libertarian, or scientific grounds. The cost of providing the tests to those who couldn't afford them was immense, as was the loss of revenue for states who enacted the requirement and saw their young couples cross state lines. Likewise, the law failed to capture those who engaged in common-law marriages. Thirdly, it was argued by many that the vast majority of those who were afflicted by the disease tended not to marry and thus would not be discovered. Others pointed to the possibility of false positives or of the test itself spreading unwanted infection. Finally, in the case of New York's mandatory testing law for expecting mothers, some worried that it would reduce pregnancies or lead women to avoid doctors and thus neglect prenatal care.[35] It was seen by many that these moves were "a product or outcome of sensationalism and high-powered propaganda in which sensational promises and panaceas are substituted for a serious-minded weighing of the problems involved."[36]

Despite these substantial objections, the laws remained in force for decades. Beginning in the 1980s, states finally moved slowly to abolish the practice. This was due to both the reality that very few cases were being discovered as well as concerns over privacy rights. Montana became the last state to abolish the practice in 2019, ending nearly 80 years of forced blood testing for syphilis in the nation. Likewise, legislation was proposed around the same time to finally eliminate the ban on marriage in Nebraska for those suffering from venereal diseases.

Eugenics

The concerns over syphilis in children went far beyond a simple public health issue and instead represented the growing practice of eugenics. The latter was primarily concerned with affecting reproductive practices through the science of heredity. As such, it focused on preventing unwanted life, creating fitter life, creating more life, and ending undesirable life. At its core, eugenics was built around the concept of placing a value on human life, particularly its value to the nation. It emerged from a combination of science, nationalism, atheism, and progressivism.

While some have historically viewed the origins of eugenics in the West as stretching back to the infanticide practices of Sparta and Rome, these tended to revolve around poor scientific understanding or concerns over resources more than a concept of purity. The roots of the modern concept can more precisely be traced back to the era of the publication of Darwin's *Origin of the Species* in 1859. The notions of natural selection, unnatural selection, and heredity were soon seized upon by some and applied to humans as well. As one of its founders opined, "The creed of eugenics is founded upon the idea of evolution."[37]

Perhaps the most famous early proponent of this was Francis Galton, a relative of Darwin. His 1869 work *Hereditary Genius* proposed that intelligence was largely an inherited trait. Darwin followed up with his own work on the subject, *The Descent of Man*, in 1871, that likewise touched on the issue of inherited traits in humans. Galton and his subsequent followers began to argue that just as humans had for thousands of years selectively bred plants and animals to promote certain traits, the same should take place with people. As one historian opined, "If Darwin wrote of 'man and nature' as they were.... Galton wrote of 'man and nature' as they might be, even as they should be."[38]

Eugenics saw clear ethnic distinctions in how disease spread. With the demise of miasma theory, notions of cleanliness and filth being the divide between those who would avoid contagion and those who would fall prey now gave way to ethnic or "racial differentiation in immunity."[39]

Galton's ideology was influenced by Malthusian fears of limited resources, Protestant notions of perfectionism, and the post–French Revolution notions of nationalism. Eugenicists felt that not only was the improvement of the population necessary due to these factors, it was also now possible thanks to a better understanding of science. All that was needed was for governments to assert their power more aggressively over the population.

In the United States, the American Eugenics Society was formed in 1921 and sponsored newspapers, books, plays, classes, and even musicals in an effort to spread its message. As previously discussed, the various marriage laws seeking to identify and treat, or outright ban, those suffering from venereal diseases from marrying were often portrayed as eugenic in nature.[40] As one newspaper commentator opined in 1921:

> But as our civilization advances we are beginning to see that marriage is really a matter in which the state has a great deal of interest. It is the duty of society to transmit a better and a stronger race to the next generation ... hence we have a movement for a study of eugenics with the object of eradicating disease and of securing the insuring healthy and vigorous offspring.[41]

Some supporters of eugenics wished to go beyond simply the policing of marriage, advocating for even more invasive action by the government to benefit the population. As famed clean living movement supporter John Harvey Kellogg once said, "A new and glorified human race which sometime, far down in the future, will have so mastered the forces of nature that disease and degeneracy will have been eliminated."[42]

A popular scientific literary genre around the turn of the 20th century involved the study and publication of family histories. Far from simply just experiments in genealogical curiosity, these were meant as anthropological studies of the moral and biological degradation of isolated families. Perhaps the first of these to gain national notoriety was Richard Dugdale's 1877 *The Jukes: A Study in Crime, Pauperism, Disease, and Heredity*. Others quickly followed over the next few decades, all purporting to show the genetic descent of disease, criminal behavior, and low intelligence among families. Due to the theorized, purely hereditary nature of these conditions, no amount of education or reform was thought to be capable of correcting the problem. Instead, many eugenicists began to favor a more aggressive approach.

The role of the government in embracing eugenics to counter disease took a far more disturbing turn in the latter half of the 1920s. Kellogg and others at the time favored an aggressive policy of forcibly sterilizing those who were deemed mentally or physically unfit. The first reference to the notion in the 19th century can perhaps be traced to Dr. Gideon Lincecum, a Texan physician who proposed a sterilization law in Wisconsin in 1849. Yet, it would take another 56 years before a state legislature finally passed just such a bill. Pennsylvania moved in March of 1905 to legalize the forced sterilization of those perceived to be mentally or physically unfit due to hereditary conditions. Republican governor Samuel Pennypacker quickly vetoed the piece of legislation, arguing:

> It is plain that the safest and most effective method of preventing procreation would be to cut the heads off the inmates, and such authority is given by the bill to this staff of scientific experts.... Scientists like all men whose experiences have been limited to one pursuit ... sometimes need to be restrained. Men of high scientific attainments are prone ... to lose sight of broad principles outside of their domain.... To permit such an operation would be to inflict cruelty upon a helpless class ... which the state has undertaken to protect.[43]

Instead, it would take until 1907 for the first state to fully pass a sterilization law. This occurred in Indiana, with much of the proposed text being provided by the Eugenics Society. Eighteen other states soon followed, including Oregon where the law was sponsored by Bethenia Owens-Adair. The latter was not only one of the first officially licensed female doctors in the state but had been a strong proponent of strict blood tests for marriage as well.

Yet, some doubted the constitutionality of such a law, with both conservatives and Catholics staunchly opposed to it. New Jersey's attempt at passing just such an act was eventually ruled unconstitutional by the state's supreme court in 1913, with the justices stating that it denied people equal protection under the law. In 1924, the Commonwealth of Virginia passed its own statute allowing for the forced sterilization of individuals who were deemed defective in some way, as it benefited "the health of the patient and the welfare of society." Almost immediately, Albert Sidney Priddy, the superintendent of the Virginia State Colony for Epileptics and Feebleminded, moved to find a patient to use as a legal test case.

The person chosen was Carrie Buck, an 18-year-old girl and patient of the hospital. Carrie's mother, Emma Buck, was well known in Charlottesville for alleged prostitution, immorality, drug use, and feeblemindedness and would end up as a patient in the colony as well. Carrie herself had been adopted and raised by a middle-class family that approached the public welfare office in 1924 in an attempt to have her institutionalized. The primary motive seems to have been an unexpected pregnancy, either caused by Carrie's own "immorality" or else rape. She was declared to be feebleminded and epileptic and sent off to the Virginia State Colony.[44] Priddy took a strong interest in Buck upon her arrival and quickly moved to embark on the process for sterilization.

The legal battle over the sterilization law would eventually end up in the U.S. Supreme Court, a move heralded by the eugenics movement and progressives who sought to make it the law of the land. The pro-sterilization argument utilized elements of eugenic thought, economics, progressivism, and disease management to present its case. Harry H. Laughlin, the superintendent of the Eugenics Record Office, whose ideas had been used to help craft the law, wrote a deposition in which he pointed out both the hereditary mental illness of the family as well as the alleged syphilis of the mother.[45]

A week-and-a-half after the trial opened, the judges returned an 8–1 decision in favor of allowing the state to sterilize Carrie Buck. The decision of Chief Justice Oliver Wendell Holmes is often well known for his famous phrase "three generations of imbeciles are enough." Yet, his legal reasoning for this went beyond simply the notions of hereditary traits and eugenics, and instead leaned heavily on the medical policing powers of the state. "The principle that sustains compulsory vaccination is broad enough to cover cutting the Fallopian tubes." Holmes cited *Jacobson v. Massachusetts* as the ground for which to allow for the mandatory sterilization of individuals. In fact, this was the only prior case cited in his ruling.

> We have seen more than once that the public welfare may call upon the best citizens for their lives. It would be strange if it could not call upon those who already sap the strength of the State for these lesser sacrifices, often not felt to be such by those concerned, in order to prevent our being swamped with incompetence. It is better for all the world, if instead of waiting to execute degenerate offspring for crime, or to let them starve for their imbecility, society can prevent those who are manifestly unfit from continuing their kind.[46]

The lone dissenter was Justice Pierce Butler, a staunch Catholic conservative.

After the ruling, over a dozen additional states enacted similar laws, and many other countries followed suit as well. Mental and physical diseases had become enough of a concern of the state to allow for them to ensure these weaknesses would not damage the genetic strength of the nation. As one contemporary newspaper wrote, "We may look forward to the day when those elements in society which are most dangerous ... will not be allowed to reproduce their kind."⁴⁷ The same periodical went on to acknowledge that while "there are some who profess to fear that the spread of compulsory sterilization laws may bring about a reign of doctors with power to unsex not only the unfit but also their personal enemies, certain classes of society, the poor ... and even troublesome minor races ... it is highly improbable."⁴⁸

Birth Control Movement

Around the same time, a push was made by other progressives to limit the births of "undesirables" in other ways. The chief architect of this was Margaret Sanger, a well-known eugenicist who sought to use birth control and sterilization to limit the spread of disease and what she felt to be inferior people. Over the course of several books, numerous articles, and pamphlets, Sanger propounded a view for increased access to birth control and contraceptives for women that hinged heavily on notions of disease, in sharp contrast to the more socioeconomic arguments of later proponents of birth control and abortion. Sanger's thinking can be divided into three main components: (1) a fear of Malthusian catastrophe, (2) the goal of preventing pregnancy-related or -worsened diseases, and (3) eugenically controlling diseases and infirmities.

In keeping with many others at the time, Sanger subscribed to the idea that the human population would always naturally increase to unsustainable amounts, at which points war, disease, or famine would be required to dramatically reduce it.⁴⁹ Thus, overpopulation was seen as the root cause of "pauperism, ignorance, crime, and disease."⁵⁰ Much of her 1922 publication, *The Pivot of Civilization*, was devoted to this idea. In part, Sanger argues, it was man's successful confrontation of pestilence in the 19th century, which was not followed by a concerted reduction in birth rates, that has produced overpopulation. Our success over disease would be our undoing.

Margaret Sanger spent much of her writing detailing the impact that pregnancy could have on a woman's body and health. At the time she began pushing for birth control, she claimed that childbirth was the second leading cause of death among women, just narrowly being nudged out by consumption.⁵¹ At the same time, women who were already suffering from tuberculosis, diabetes, or any of a number of other conditions could see their health potentially worsened by the ordeal. In addition, she claimed that pregnancy could lead to biological or physiological issues in women, ones that would be completely avoided with birth control. Finally, Sanger and others argued that if a woman simply refrained from sex, then her husband would stray outside of marriage, leading to a rise in venereal diseases.[52]

The final philosophical underpinning of Sanger's thought was influenced by her belief in eugenics. In 1916, she gave an address in Chicago titled "The Child's Right Not to Be Born," which leaned heavily on the notions of only producing perfect children. While religious leaders had long considered disease to be the "dispensation of God," Sanger argued that science and knowledge of the role of hereditary illness could now change that.[53] Diseased parents, such as those with consumption or syphilis, and ones with congenital deformities or mental illnesses, would undoubtedly produce diseased children.[54] Humanity had long waged "war against insects, germs, and bacteria" in order to defeat illness and now could do the same through preventing births.[55] Fighting against contraceptives was, in the words of Dr. Max Hirsch, "like a person who would fight contagious diseases and forbid disinfectants."[56]

To Sanger and the American Birth Control League, which she helped to found in 1921, the goal was to not only prevent the illness-caused death of millions of women but to create the perfect American race as well. She aimed to "put into women's hands knowledge that will save her from giving birth to any more babies destined to certain poverty, misery, and perhaps to disease and death."[57]

The political debate over the legality and morality of birth control would continue for decades. Many on both sides would likewise resort to the topic of disease to help push their viewpoint. Some proponents leaned on the idea that pestilence was a far greater threat to society to acquire support from certain Protestant and Jewish sects.[58] Despite this, the Catholic Church remained staunchly opposed to the idea. In fact, many in the latter religion expressed concerns that the use of contraceptives could lead women to likewise avoid marriage or seek additional sex partners, leading to an explosion in venereal diseases. Many continued to push Malthusian fears of overpopulation leading to the outbreak of pandemics, while others claimed that disease and birth control were the cause of population fluctuations, including that which helped to bring down the Roman Empire.[59] Interestingly, during debate in the Connecticut state legislature as to whether to allow birth control, expert witness Dr. George Keefe claimed that birth control itself actually led to disease, and "pregnancy ... has a salutary effect on some diseases."[60]

Acceptance of birth control began to slowly spread through the United States, often propelled forward by notions of disease. By 1926, 15 cities were offering courses on contraception to "diseased mothers."[61] These programs only expanded during the era of the New Deal and the 1960s. The legal debate was effectively settled in 1965, when *Griswold v.*

Connecticut struck down that state's restriction on the sale of contraceptives to married couples as a violation of the right to privacy. This was followed by a similar ruling in favor of unmarried individuals in 1973 in *Eisenstadt v. Baird*. Finally, both cases would go on to substantially influence the Court's ruling in *Roe v. Wade* that legalized abortion as well. Planned Parenthood, which had fought to ensure legalized infanticide, had succeeded Sanger's original American Birth Control League in 1942 and had been pushing for abortion as a method since 1955. Ironically, Sanger herself had always argued that access to birth control would help to eliminate abortion, an act which she saw as unwarranted and vile.

Medical Experimentation

The push by progressivism to grant more power to the government in order to fix the problems of society, which invariably led to the dehumanization of the very members of that society, reached perhaps its darkest extent in the medical experimentation of the middle half of the 20th century.

Medical experimentation has existed for centuries but seems to have been rather rare until the beginnings of the modern era. During the latter half of the 19th century various doctors and scientists practiced surgical or biological experimentation on unsuspecting patients. Oftentimes these were prisoners, minorities, or orphans. Yet, these were often small studies, performed by individual researchers of their own volition, and many, such as the work of Dr. Roberts Bartholomew, were heavily criticized by the American Medical Association.

The Public Health Service began to embark on its own medical experimentation in 1914. A variety of occurrences including crop failures and economic hardship had unleashed an epidemic of pellagra across the South in the early 20th century. With the disease being responsible for the death of more people in the region each year than tuberculosis, fears of the illness spreading to the North prompted the U.S. government to dispatch Dr. Joseph Goldberger to the region in 1914. The latter had previous experience investigating outbreaks of illness in both the U.S. and Mexico and had in fact contracted both yellow fever and typhus during these travels.[62]

Dr. Goldberger spent months studying the disease and the conditions that could have caused it in the Deep South. As part of this, he employed a series of volunteer prison inmates who were given the diet of an average poor Southerner in exchange for an official pardon from the state. Within months, the volunteers had contracted the disease, exhibiting all the classical symptoms. Despite his efforts, Goldberger was harassed and derided by critics, both those who religiously clung to the new infectious model of disease and those who saw his results as drawing connections between poverty and disease. Despite this, the public nature of his experiment and the fact that the prisoners volunteered for it, at least avoided recrimination for its undertaking.

Yet, the experiments of the Public Health Service took a decidedly darker path in the 1930s. Around that time, the Julius Rosenwald Fund worked with various state and federal agencies to investigate and treat syphilitics across the nation. In the first few years of 1930, they partnered with the USPHS to undertake a larger scale study and treatment of the disease among a group of blacks in Alabama. After examining the region, the Public Health Service settled on Macon County, which was argued to have a 30 percent-plus incidence rate of the disease. Yet, despite receiving assistance and support from the Tuskegee Institute, the study was unable to gain local funding and thus eventually lost the matching funds offered by the Rosenwald Fund. Yet, rather than curtail the project, the directors of the USPHS moved to turn the study into one that did not involve treatment and that instead merely observed the impact of syphilis on untreated individuals.

Racialist ideas at the time held that syphilis was prominent among blacks and that likewise they were not known for seeking treatment. "The stoicism of these men as a group; they still regard hospitals and medicines with suspicion and prefer an occasional dose of time-honored herbs or tonics to modern drugs."[63] The study would eventually track 600 subjects over the next 40 years, offering them free treatment, free medical exams, and even funeral expenses in order to gain their trust. Yet, despite promises of treatment for their "bad blood," only placebos or minuscule doses of medicine were provided to them.

As the years progressed, the government went to extreme lengths to ensure that their subjects were not treated for syphilis. Local doctors and health offices were told to refrain from providing medication and, in the 1940s when many of the men went for medical exams before their local draft board, the USPHS exerted its influence to have them removed from the army. Even once penicillin was found to be an easy and effective treatment for the disease in 1947, the USPHS denied it to the men of the Tuskegee Experiment. This occurred despite the same department's efforts to set up rapid treatment centers across the nation. The actions of the USPHS now directly violated federal law, as Congress had passed the Henderson Act in 1943, which mandated the public funding of treatment for those with syphilis and tuberculosis.

The experiments continued into the 1960s, by which point many began to internally admit that the initial suppositions of the Public Health

XI. The Pox of Progressivism: Culling the Herd 133

Service were wrong. Far fewer men had the disease in the county than originally predicted. Likewise, despite the beliefs and best efforts of the investigators, some 30 percent of participants managed to obtain penicillin by 1952.[64] It would take the exposé of whistleblower Peter Buxtun in 1972 to finally bring the study to national attention and to an ignominious conclusion.

Congress quickly moved to pass legislation in 1974 that outlined new requirements for human experimentation in the form of the National Research Act, but the damage was already done. News of the Tuskegee Experiment eroded the already thin trust of many blacks in the government and medical fields. The average life expectancy of that group dropped by 1.4 years immediately after the 1972 revelations, a drop which has been attributed by some to a distrust of seeking medical treatment.[65] This trend would impact both the AIDS crisis of the 1980s as well as vaccination efforts during the 2019 pandemic.

Yet, Tuskegee was not the only instance of vast government overreach in the study and treatment of disease in the Cold War period. Concerns over disease and its impact on the military pushed the USPHS to participate in a number of extreme experiments during the 1940s–1960s. Several of these continued to use prisoners as test subjects, some knowingly and others against their will. The former is best represented by the syphilis experiments at Terre Haute Prison in 1943 and the Stateville Penitentiary Malaria Study in 1944. While prisoners did volunteer, there were still several ethical issues raised at the time. In fact, Nazi defendants at Nuremburg would reference these undertakings in their own defense. Following these trials, the American government sought to continue venereal disease testing abroad to avoid local scrutiny. From 1946 to 1948, the USPHS used both infected prostitutes as well as the direct administration of bacterial and viral agents to transmit various diseases to prisoners in Guatemala. Likewise, the Willowbrook State School on Staten Island in New York utilized intellectually disabled children for horrific studies in the transmission of hepatitis during the 1950s to 1970s.

By the 1950s, the discovery of penicillin as a cure for most STDs led to a decline in this type of research. But fears of syphilis were quickly replaced by concerns of biological weapon usage by the Soviets. In order to better understand and prepare for these threats, the American government moved to undertake experimental research. Yet, the impact of disease is always felt when it hits a sizeable population, thus any study would have to be done on large groups of people.

During the 1950s and 1960s, the American government undertook a series of biological experiments that involved the releasing of pathogens in various cities across the country. Some of the more famous of these included Operation Sea Spray in San Francisco in 1950, Operation LAC off of South Carolina in 1952, and Project 112 during the 1960s. The last of these involved the release of biological agents in the New York City subway and at National Airport in Washington, D.C. These tests employed generally harmless bacteria in order to simulate biological attacks, yet despite this, several cases of illness and at least one death have been attributed to them.[66] These experiments were accompanied by Operation Whitecoat, a 20-year project that saw enlisted men, army volunteers, and conscientious objectors subjected to medical experimentation to test investigative techniques and treatments. Two of the principal diseases tested on the men in an effort to prepare for biological warfare were Tularemia and Q-Fever. Though informed consent was certainly practiced based upon the lessons of Nuremberg, there still remained many elements of the experiments that would violate ethical considerations today.[67]

Revelations of these practices during the 1970s did much to end the use of human subjects in medical experimentation. By the 2000s, as evidenced by Operation Dark Winter, investigation into biological warfare had become more of a tabletop exercise designed to fine-tune government responses. Yet, the U.S. government did not completely abandon its investigations into disease research, with the new public scrutiny doing much to drive them into more dangerous directions.

The late 20th century saw the rise of gain of function research in virology. Though the term did not gain widespread circulation among the public before 2012, as early as 2001 studies began to be published on the process. Scientists, often with government funding and encouragement, experimented on altering and strengthening bacteria and viruses in order to make them more deadly and/or transmissible. The given purpose was to learn how to treat advanced microbial mutations and threats.

One of the first recorded instances occurred in 2001, when scientists in Australia accidentally developed a far more lethal strain of mousepox.[68] The next year, a group of scientists in New York chemically created the extinct virus polio, while in 2005 another group from the CDC resurrected the exact strain of H1N1 that was responsible for the 1918 Spanish Flu Pandemic. The federal government soon took an interest in these practices and by the time of the Obama administration was using the NIH to fund grants for almost two dozen such projects.

Yet, many in the scientific community began to question the ethics and dangers of these experiments. In 2011, the U.S. government reacted to an experiment that aerosolized the H5N1 virus by having the National Science Advisory Board for Biosecurity suppress the studies' reports. Though they were subsequently allowed to be published the next year, it did lead to the drafting of new guidelines by HHS for funding such research. Matters

XI. The Pox of Progressivism: Culling the Herd 135

worsened in 2014 when various episodes of poor security at CDC labs surfaced. The misplacement of smallpox cultures, the contamination of samples, and the potential exposure of employees to anthrax led to complaints by both scientists and politicians. Over 200 scientists signed the Cambridge Working Group declaration, calling for a halt to epidemiological experiments "until there has been a quantitative, objective and credible assessment of the risks, potential benefits, and opportunities for risk mitigation, as well as comparison against safer experimental approaches."[69]

In response, President Obama announced a pause in 2014 on all funding for gain of function research that involved influenza, MERS-CoV, and SARS-CoV. "Following recent biosafety incidents at Federal research facilities, the U.S. Government has taken a number of steps to promote and enhance the Nation's biosafety and biosecurity, including immediate and longer-term measures to review activities specifically related to the storage and handling of infectious agents."[70] This was meant to coincide with a full study to be undertaken by the government on ways to improve safety.

Yet, in the meantime, Dr. Anthony Fauci, the head of the National Institute of Allergy and Infectious Diseases, undertook to outsource gain of function research to China. Hundreds of thousands of dollars flowed into the Wuhan Institute of Virology specifically where experiments were undertaken on SARS-CoV strains. Though the White House lifted the moratorium in December of 2017, the NIAID continued to utilize the institute in Wuhan, renewing its funding grant in 2019. Only with the subsequent outbreak of a pandemic in the city and rumors of its origins within those labs did the Trump administration pull all funding in early 2020.

During the ensuing litany of investigations that characterized Congress' response to the pandemic of 2019, Senator Rand Paul personally sought answers from Dr. Fauci about U.S. funding of gain of function research in China. After numerous denials from the head of the NIAID, the NIH finally admitted to the practice in October of 2021.[71] In response, several Republican senators pushed for the passage of the Viral Gain of Function Research Moratorium Act that would once again put a halt to the practice.

> More than a year and half after the initial outbreak of COVID-19 in Wuhan, serious questions remain regarding the origins of this deadly virus and its possible connection to federally-funded gain of function research in China. The American people deserve to know the truth, and until a full and transparent investigation is guaranteed and real oversight is imposed on this risky line of research, no taxpayer dollars should be squandered by unelected bureaucrats operating in the dark.[72]

The history of 20th-century progressivism and disease is one of faulty science, poor decisions, a stripping away of liberty, eugenics, and death. While science, individual decisions regarding health, and private industry have revolutionized public health in the nation, politicians have often simply used it for perverse ends.

CHAPTER XII

Disease and the Democratic Process

Many factors, beyond simply political ideology, go into the process of electing people to office. Appearance, rhetorical skill and style, advertising, money, and a host of other variables certainly play roles in varying degrees in the decision of the voter. Yet, one of the more interesting and historically underappreciated ones has been the role of personal health and illness. Likewise, once in office, the specter of sickness can be damaging to an official's hold on power, and this concern has therefore driven officeholders to extreme ends to cover up these instances.

Election of 1812

Perhaps the first instance of illness becoming a political issue in terms of a presidential campaign occurred in 1812. That year saw War Hawks and Southern Republicans pushing for war with the United Kingdom over its policy of impressment and its active assistance of Native American attacks on the United States. James Madison was running for re-election and hoping to use the vote as a national referendum on the conflict. Yet, not all members of his own party supported the push toward war. Many began to rally around his Northern vice president, George Clinton, with the Baltimore *Whig* suggesting in March of 1811 that he would make a better leader than Madison.[1] Some felt his background to be better suited to the perspective war than that of Madison, while Northern interests hoped that his ties to New York would lead him to prevent a war entirely.

While there was no active campaigning done by office seekers at the time, supporters and detractors frequently spoke about both Madison and Clinton. Yet, at the age of 72, Clinton seemed to many to be too old and perhaps infirm to hold office. Clinton himself expressed concern about the issue in a letter to President Jefferson in 1804, writing about his "old Age and ill health."[2] In August of 1811, Thomas Jefferson wrote to Benjamin Rush detailing his own declining health as a mirror for Clinton's health.

> It is wonderful to me that old men should not be sensible that their minds keep pace with their bodies in the progress of decay. Our old revolutionary friend, Clinton, for example, who was a hero, but never a man of mind, is wonderfully jealous on this head. He tells eternally the stories of his younger days, to prove his memory. As if memory and reason were the same faculty. Nothing betrays imbecility so much as the being insensible of it. Had not a conviction of the danger to which an unlimited occupation of the Executive chair would expose the republican constitution of our government made it conscientiously a duty to retire when I did, the fear of becoming a dotard and of being insensible of it, would of itself have resisted all solicitations to remain.[3]

First Lady Dolley Madison spoke of these concerns in a letter in March of 1812 at the height of the presidential election season, writing, "The Vice-President lies dangerously ill."[4] The fears of Madison and others would come to fruition a few weeks later as Clinton died from a massive heart attack. Though Federalists and some anti-war Republicans rallied around his nephew, DeWitt Clinton, Madison managed to secure his reelection and, with it, war with England. Though Clinton's ill health was not used as a political tool on a wide scale, it represents the start of a trend. The health of a candidate could and should perhaps become the concern of the voting public.

Election of 1824

The politicization of a candidate's health continued with the 1824 election cycle. While the nomination and election of William Crawford, the current secretary of the Treasury to President Monroe, seemed assured, the sudden collapse of his health threw the election into chaos. He appears to have developed erysipelas around that time, better known as St. Anthony's Fire.[5] Typically caused by streptococcus bacteria, the condition left him covered in a large, red rash. Suddenly in the fall of 1823, Crawford suffered a paralytic episode that left him blind, deaf, and dumb.[6] Some have connected the onset of this to the lobelia and other medicines being used to treat him at the time. Confined to his bed for eight weeks, Crawford's closest associates did their best to restrict the flow of information regarding his condition. His absence was largely written off as a bout of some minor ailment. Writing to James Madison in October of 1823, President Monroe queried, "How is Mr. Crawford—and when do you think that he will be able to move? His family, were recovering their health, when I left the city."[7] John Q. Adams likewise simply lumped Crawford into a larger list of politicians and notables who were seasonally ill at the time.

XII. Disease and the Democratic Process

> There has been a very sickly time here these two Months; though not much mortality among persons of your acquaintance.... Mr Crawford continues ill at Mr Senator Barbour's in Virginia—Mrs Crawford who has just recovered from illness herself, went yesterday accompanied by Dr. Sim, to join her Husband. He is convalescent, but has been so ill, and recovers so slowly that he will probably not be here for several weeks.[8]

Yet as the months wore on, those in the political sphere began to take note of the health of the designated successor. Crawford's absence from the official nomination caucus held in Congress in February of 1824 spoke volumes. An attempt by the candidate to travel to Monticello and gain Jefferson's blessing shortly afterward was derailed by a second illness that only further led people to question his electability.[9]

Following these episodes, states and local party organizations soon moved to nominate rival candidates. In February of 1824, Massachusetts nominated John Quincy Adams to be president and soon after Pennsylvania chose General Andrew Jackson. A relapse of Crawford's condition in the late spring and early summer merely worsened his political chances. Writing to Crawford in April, Thomas Jefferson noted, "I enquire always with anxiety of the state of your health, and am concerned to learn that your convalescence is more slow than I had wished and hoped."[10] A four way contest thus developed between Crawford, Adams, Clay, and Jackson.

Interestingly, while many ignored Crawford's illness, periodicals and commentators seized upon the health scares of Clay. Reports surfaced in both late 1822 and 1823 that the senator was dead or dying.[11] Suffering from a "bilious fever," Clay was confined to his bed in Ohio where he had traveled to for business. Treatments with mercury seemed to have only worsened his conditions, and at least one newspaper, the *National Intelligencer*, reported his demise.[12] Due to the lack of communication across the states, residents and friends in Louisville believed the worst. Writing in February of 1823, Henry Shaw sarcastically related how "you was sick—I mourned over it—you died I wept for you—you regained your health, I rejoiced & thanked my God for your deliverance."[13] While his condition improved enough to allow for his return to both Kentucky and the nation's capital, his health remained rather frail overall throughout 1823.

Crawford seems to have actually recovered much of his faculties by the fall of 1824, and many of his more ardent supporters were still reasonably confident of victory in the election. Thomas Jefferson himself noted, "There is nothing publicly interesting. That question will surely lie between Crawford and Adams; and whether it will go into Congress is still uncertain."[14] Yet, in the end, Crawford finished a distant third in terms of electoral votes and fourth in popular totals. His victories in Virginia and his home state of Georgia, as well as several electoral votes in New York and Maryland, were enough to edge out Henry Clay but fell far behind Adams and Jackson.

Due to the lack of a clear winner, the 12th Amendment was invoked and the vote was thrown into the House of Representatives. The contest that followed was largely between Adams and Jackson, with Crawford siphoning off votes in the South from the latter. Clay and Adams then famously orchestrated what became termed the "Corrupt Bargain," pushing enough votes in the West toward Adams to secure his ascension to the presidency. The bitterness that resulted between Adams and Jackson tore the political tranquility of the nation apart and gave birth to the Second Party System. Political parties were reborn in America thanks in part to chaos that resulted from the health woes of Crawford and led to the subsequent political duels between Jackson and Clay that would culminate in the election of 1832.

Election of 1832

The wide scale and public politicization of a candidate's health would further emerge on the scene during the election of 1832. Occurring at the height of the cholera pandemic, disease was already being used as a political issue by both parties. Yet, the huge amounts of public animosity toward both candidates, Henry Clay and Andrew Jackson, likewise resulted in their own personal lives becoming partisan topics.

More than almost any other president, Jackson's health issues defined both his life and his first term in office.[15] Plagued by malaria, a virulent kidney disorder, a bullet-caused lung abscess, and decades of self-inflicted lead poisoning, General Jackson was far from a healthy man.[16] From 1824 to 1828, Andrew Jackson lost all of his teeth in rapid succession, a classic symptom of prolonged mercury poisoning. Meanwhile, he often complained of intestinal issues, paranoia, and violent mood swings, all of which could have easily arisen from a kidney disorder, probably produced by over two dozen years of lead poisoning.[17]

The 62-year-old president's letters at the time are full of references to his ill health. One of the first, penned only a few weeks after his inauguration, stated candidly, "My labours have been great, my health is not good," while another written to his brother-in-law John Donelson shared the former's now apparently well-established opinion, "My time cannot be long here on earth."[18] In fact, by September of 1829 President Jackson was already discussing his plans for a quiet retirement to the Hermitage.[19]

By the fall, he unexpectedly cancelled his remaining obligations for the year and set out for Rip Raps, an artificial island adjoining Ft. Calhoun

XII. Disease and the Democratic Process 141

where he had a modest hut built that bore the sobriquet of the Summer White House.[20] The president would continue to use Rip Raps throughout his time in office, often deciding momentous policy decisions while there, such as the removal of government funds from the Second Bank of the United States.[21] The National Republican press quickly latched onto both Jackson's relocation from the house of the people to a hardened military fortress, as well as to rumors of his declining health.[22] At the height of the Maysville Road debate in 1830, Jackson became very sick due to his kidney dysfunction. Secretary of State Van Buren was not only forced to help the ailing Jackson up the White House stairs but actually became the leader of the famous veto movement.[23] With the demise of William Crawford's political career in 1824 due to illness, Jackson's various health issues were of legitimate concern to voters in 1832.

Compared to Jackson, Henry Clay was a frailer looking but much healthier individual. Yet that is not to say he escaped impact by disease at various points in his life. It was largely thanks to the illness of the famed Revolutionary George Wythe that a young Henry Clay was able to begin his legal and political career. Likewise, his yearly, arduous journey from Kentucky to the national capital often resulted in the sickness of his family. During the harsh winter of 1816 his entire family was struck down with sickness. As he himself recorded, "Mrs. Clay & all my children, except my two sons, are with me. Unfortunately the youngest of them (Laura) took the whooping cough on the journey, and we are at this moment despairing of the recovery of the youngest Laura."[24] She died a week later and was buried in Congressional Cemetery. The heat and swamps of the capital were well known for contributing to an unhealthy environment there, with seasonal fevers being blamed for various sicknesses and the deaths of officials and their family members. Each year, Clay was not alone in having to carefully weigh the decision of whether to risk either the pestilential terrors of the capital or the illnesses of travel.

Clay's personal experiences with the travails of interstate travel in the early Jeffersonian Era certainly had an effect on his views of infrastructure. Though he did not personally connect the issues of health and transportation in his letters, they did make frequent references to the conditions of the roads connecting Kentucky to the capital, commenting on the tremendously negative effects that weather had on travel.[25] In 1817, he wrote to William Thornton, "Still I should think that, until the Country is more cultivated, occasional instances of Ague & fever & intermittens will occur in the months of August & September."[26] Clearly though, the death of several of his children while en route to Washington would have personalized the terrible reality of transportation in the country. During his time in the House, he constantly pushed for the expansion of roads to the West, lambasting Congress for failing to stretch the Cumberland Road beyond Wheeling, so "that we might have a way to reach the Capitol of our country ... in the advancement of the national prosperity."[27]

Henry Clay and the Whigs quickly seized upon Jackson's perceived lackluster response to the cholera pandemic, combining it with the president's dissolution of the U.S. Bank to produce a formidable platform.[28] In Congress, Clay introduced a resolution two weeks after Jackson's letter, requesting the president to set aside a day of fasting and prayer in order to implore God to "avert from our country the Asiatic scourge which is now traversing and devastating other countries."[29] The Democrat Senate approved the measure the next day by a vote of 30 to 13, with almost half of the president's party breaking ranks to support the bill. The overwhelmingly Democratic House, though, voted to table the measure in July. Clay must have expected the bill to go no further than the Senate but continued his verbal assault regardless. The next day, he addressed the Senate, pointing out that the resolution was "recommendatory" rather than "obligatory," further tarnishing Jackson in public opinion. Though a well-known agnostic, Clay even went so far as to point out that while, "I am a member of no religious sect.... I have ... a profound respect for Christianity ... its usages, and its observances."[30]

Jackson's decision, however, was not as universally condemned by Christians as Clay had hoped it would be. Both Baptists, who were dominant in Southern, Democratic areas, as well as Catholics, supported the president's affirmation of a separation between church and state.[31] Far from simply expressing his own irreligious beliefs, the president may have actually been adroitly appealing to the beliefs of his main constituents, Southerners and Irish urban dwellers.

Upper-class Whigs were not left untouched by the scourge either. William H. Maynard, a state senator from New York, was organizing a trip to Ohio in June of 1832 when he was stricken with the illness. Maynard was an influential member of the Anti-Masonic Party and was hoping to travel to the state to cement an alliance between the two main anti–Jacksonian parties. Unfortunately, his death reduced these prospects. Stronger support from the Anti-Masonic Party would have allowed Clay and his party to win New Jersey, Vermont, and possibly Ohio as well.[32] As Clay himself lamented in a later October letter to James Brown, "The Ohio Election has gone against us ... owing, as it is said, to the want of arranging a proper concert between the Anti Masons and N. Republicans."[33]

As the election grew closer, some newspapers even began to report the death from cholera of Henry Clay himself. With Jackson's well-known use of the media at the time, this was reminiscent of a similar attack by Adams on Jefferson in 1800. Clay had to take the unprecedented step of informing his friends that he was in fact very much alive. "You may probably hear that I caught the pestilence, and have been long since dead and buried. You are authorized to contradict, most positively, such a report if you should hear it."[34] Clay himself utilized the disease as a foil for his attacks on the terrors of Jacksonian Democracy. "Jacksonism! It is worse than the Cholera, because it has been more universal, and will be more durable. The Cholera performs its terrible office, and its victims are consigned to the grave, leaving their survivors uncontaminated. But Jacksonism has poisoned the whole Community, the living as well as the dead."[35]

In the end, despite legitimate concerns over Jackson's physical and mental health, the 65-year-old president was reelected to office. His victory showed his continued popularity among the "common man" and a lack of appreciation for health concerns in politics.

Election of 1944

Concerns over illness would keep several additional presidents from seeking re-election, most notably Chester A. Arthur in 1884 and Woodrow Wilson in 1920. Though rumors and speculation about their health ran rampant in newspapers, they themselves largely decided against seeking reelection for a number of reasons, and the topic therefore did not become a major campaign issue. The next time that illness did become a topic of political debate was in 1944.

Historians are now more aware of the immense health problems facing Franklin D. Roosevelt since at least his second term in office. Yet, even after almost a century, mystery and obfuscation still cloud much of this speculation. Regardless, it had become clear to even most citizens by 1944 that the health of the country's wartime president was declining. Following his return from the Tehran Conference in December of 1943, he was reported to be suffering from influenza.[36] The shah of Persia would even write to Roosevelt a few months later, expressing his concern:

> I was distressed to hear, by your letter of February 10th, that you had been laid up for some time with an attack of the "flu" and hope you are now enjoying the best of health and strength. You will need all your accustomed vigour and energy to bring to final accomplishment the colossal and unprecedented efforts your country is making, under your brilliant leadership, for the early termination of the war and the establishment of a just and lasting peace.[37]

Despite this, it is unknown exactly what Roosevelt was suffering from at the time. Yet, as pointed out by the shah's letter, what was clear to Democrats and many others was the perceived indispensability of Roosevelt to bring the war to a successful close.

With the approach of FDR's sixty-second birthday only a few weeks later, pro-administration newspapers went out of their way to proclaim the health of the president. The *Ypsilanti Daily Press* reported that Roosevelt was "in excellent health" and quoted his personal physician who opined that he was "in the finest general health of any man of his years he had known."[38] Yet, only a few months later, the same paper reported, "The question of President Roosevelt's health today was causing considerable concern."[39] The article went on to state that it was now an open rumor in the capital that Roosevelt would not run for a fourth term.

Nor was this purely American speculation but seems to have become common knowledge and a common concern among the various allied nations. The *Detroit Evening Times* published a shocking exposé in April of 1944 that the British Ministry of Information was providing propaganda pamphlets to American soldiers not only promoting the idea of a fourth term for Roosevelt but also assuring them of his pristine health.[40] For its part, the White House spent much of 1944 issuing statements from Vice Admiral Ross T. McIntire, the president's personal physician, about his robust constitution.

Yet, this did little to tamp down rampant speculation from even members of his own party that he wouldn't run. In April of 1944, Democratic Senator Burton K. Wheeler of Montana opined that not only could his party not win the 1944 election, but "I am certain that Mr. Roosevelt does not want the nomination," due to his health issues.[41] While Wheeler was making this speculation, Roosevelt himself was on a three-week vacation in the South seeking to improve his health and rid himself of his alleged influenza and bronchitis.

Roosevelt's health also led to increased political speculation over a possible successor. His current vice president, Henry Wallace, represented the extreme left wing of the party and was quite unpopular with large segments of the population. The *Western News*, out of Montana, summarized the view of many by calling Wallace an "unbalanced dreamer," going on to say that it would be a "catastrophe for the nation if Roosevelt should pass away ... and Henry Wallace should step into the presidential office."[42] These considerations continued right up to the Democratic convention held in mid–July that year. Rumors ran rampant among convention delegates that pro–Wallace members had pushed the president, "much against his wishes, to seek another term, with Wallace as his running mate, and then to resign ... a few months after the election."[43] Yet, ultimately, the political fears over Roosevelt's declining health and what it would mean for the party pushed delegates to reject Wallace and replace him with the more conservative Senator Harry Truman of Missouri.[44]

With the onset of the campaign season between Roosevelt and Thomas

Dewey in the late summer, questions of the president's health became a frequent target for Republicans. Democrats derided these attacks. "There is one thing which ought to be taboo in this campaign ... the gossip about the physical characteristics of the two nominees for the presidency."[45] Robert E. Hannegan, chairman of the Democratic National Committee, went so far as to accuse Republicans of undertaking a "whispering campaign" about the health and illnesses of President Roosevelt.[46] Though the Republicans for their part denied these allegations, the very raising of them merely brought the issue more into the public eye. Meanwhile, the White House physician continued to release glowing reports about the president's health.

Dewey's campaign certainly did seize upon the issue, focusing on convincing voters that who they were really electing was Truman. As one newspaper ad asked, "Do you want to take the chance that Harry Truman may be President if Mr. Roosevelt's health fails, as it very likely may?"[47] Political pundits at the time speculated that this issue was pushing the election in Dewey's favor.[48]

In order to put an end to this speculation, the Democrats sent Roosevelt on a two-week tour of numerous states in the northeast and Midwest. Often traveling in an open car through fierce wind and rainy conditions, he delivered speeches to millions. Yet, as these were generally considered to be safe districts for him, the tour seemed to be more of a promotion of his health than his policies.

Despite the apparent health concerns of many, Roosevelt ended up being elected to a fourth term by his usual wide margin, tallying 432 electoral votes to Dewey's 99. Yet, with only 53 percent of the popular vote in his favor, it was his closest election yet. Just under six months later, President Roosevelt passed away, a victim of the numerous health issues that had plagued him for years.

Election of 1956

A little over a decade later, similar attacks and concerns would appear during the reelection of Dwight D. Eisenhower. Despite his openness about his health issues, in sharp contrast to the Roosevelt White House, the public was no less concerned about his capability to continue for another four years in office. Democrats launched a "Nervous About Nixon" campaign, much as Republicans had raised concerns about Wallace and Truman years before. Ike himself did little to help things, frequently speaking about his health issues and even suggesting that he might not run again. Within party ranks, vicious fights broke out over whether or not to retain Nixon should Ike's health actually fail.[49]

Numerous commercials and televised speeches were utilized to limit the strain of actual campaigning on Eisenhower. Predictably enough, this simply increased concerns among the public that the sitting president was too infirm to campaign, let alone govern the nation. Democrats seized upon this fear, running a short commercial which asked Americans whether they were "Nervous about Nixon? President Nixon?" Adlai Stevenson himself announced that he would not publicly make the health of the president an issue during the campaign, though his statement simply brought the topic more attention.[50]

The Republicans responded to these health concerns by finally pushing Ike out into the field. As he always did, the president responded strongly, giving speeches and meeting people. As younger brother Milton Eisenhower succinctly put it, "It doesn't matter what you say"; Eisenhower simply had to appear healthy and in command.[51] All of this campaigning had a deleterious effect on Ike's health. Over the course of a little more than a month, he developed a persistent cough, heart palpitations, abdominal pain, dizziness, and diarrhea. None of this, though, could prevent his unparalleled popularity from securing forty-one states and 57 percent of the popular vote, two more states than in 1952. Yet, the potential ramifications of weakening the sitting president in an attempt to court votes could have had enormous consequences at such a volatile time during the Cold War.

Election of 1960

The personal health of the candidates again became a political issue during the election of 1960. During the first contest between two men from the Greatest Generation, the illnesses of both relatively young politicians became objects of concern for the public. Initial questions first arose among Democrats themselves, as supporters of Lyndon Baines Johnson attempted to portray John F. Kennedy as a diseased and sickly man at the height of the national convention.

While Johnson stayed above the fray, his supporters began to speak to newspaper reporters about Kennedy's health. Chief among these were John Connally, the future governor of Texas, and India Edwards, one of the most powerful women in the DNC. Both informed donors and the media that Kennedy was suffering from Addison's disease, a generally fatal ailment. India opined, "If it were not for cortisone, Kennedy probably wouldn't be alive."[52] Coming only 16 years after the re-election and subsequent death of Roosevelt and following Ike's own health scares, the issue resonated with voters. The young senator from Massachusetts was quickly

XII. Disease and the Democratic Process 147

defended by his supporters and family. Not only did Robert Kennedy deny the allegations, a doctor's report showing JFK's excellent health was produced, and Johnson's own heart disease was raised in response. To counter these damning claims, the Kennedy campaign put out a letter from its medical team stating that JFK did not suffer from Addison's caused by tuberculosis. This was, in effect, true, as his Addison's was caused by either steroid abuse or his APS II, but it was clearly a sly manipulation of his medical history. Nixon's camp quickly released its own glowing medical report, showing that the young Republican was far healthier than both Democratic contenders.[53]

Kennedy's competition with Richard Nixon during the election that year saw his health brought to the fore once more. The Democratic candidate was kept in action by a competent support team that included medical help as well. An aide followed Kennedy around with a black bag filled with various medications. For obvious reasons, the existence of this valet was kept secret from almost everyone. While campaigning in Connecticut only forty-eight hours before the election, Kennedy's people lost his medical bag, causing fear and chaos among his staff. The candidate himself called up Governor Abraham Ribicoff to say, "There's a medical bag floating around and it can't get in anybody's hands ...You have to find that bag ... it would be murder."[54] Nixon was no less willing to use Kennedy's illnesses against him than Johnson had been. In episodes eerily foreshadowing the Watergate break-in, the offices of two of JFK's doctors were ransacked in the fall of 1960, including that of future White House physician Janet Travell. Luckily for the Democratic candidate, his records were filed under a pseudonym. Shortly before the election, Representative Walter Judd of Minnesota, who had given the keynote speech at the Republican National Convention, challenged Kennedy to reveal the true depth of his ailments. Thanks to his subterfuge, JFK was able to portray himself as an energetic healthy campaigner and for the most part was able to dodge this inquisition. In fact, this was one of the reasons that the Kennedy campaign leaned upon his youth so much, despite the potential handicaps of being portrayed as inexperienced.

Yet, interestingly, Nixon's health would become the greater centerpiece in the final showdown between both men. The election of 1960 was perhaps most famous for the inclusion of televised debates between the two men. In this medium, the relaxed, tanned, and confident Kennedy proved to be more appealing to voters. Nixon—who had just undergone knee surgery for a serious staphylococcal infection, had recently been ill, had experienced significant weight loss associated with both events, and had only just emerged from a fourteen-state tour that had seen him once more injure his leg—seemed to appear as a sickly individual.[55] Interestingly,

Kennedy's tan appearance had less to do with his careful cosmetic preparation for the debate and more to do with a visible side effect of his Addison's disease. Regardless, it became a commonly accepted political truism that those who saw the debate held JFK to be the winner due to Nixon's appearance, while those who listened to it on the radio chose Nixon based upon his commanding answers.[56] Youth, vigor, and attractiveness would go on to define Camelot and become a trope for almost all subsequent Democratic candidates for the next half century.

Elections of 1972 and 1988

The postwar era saw a rise in mental health awareness and treatment in America. At the same time, this increased occurrence of both saw it enter into the political field as a legitimate concern of voters. While many candidates have had their mental state questioned by both opposition leaders and the media, most notably Andrew Jackson, Barry Goldwater, Richard Nixon, and Donald Trump, the first case of a diagnosable condition arose during the election of 1972.

George McGovern of South Dakota managed to bypass much more moderate and popular choices due to a variety of issues and events and eventually became the choice of Democrats to run against Richard Nixon in 1972. Yet, quite apart from his own extreme stance on many issues, his biggest liability seemed to be his choice of vice president. Much as the presidential nomination process had been chaotic, so too was that for the choice of running mate. Out of the seventy-nine names that had been thrown into the mix, Senator Thomas Eagleton of Missouri emerged as the consolation choice.

Republican opposition research quickly investigated the past of both men. On July 19, 1972, Sam Krupnick, a Nixon supporter from Missouri, wrote to the president's secretary to share that Eagleton was alleged to have spent time in the Malcolm Bliss Mental Hospital in St. Louis, Missouri. Though Krupnick offered "acute alcoholism" as a potential cause, the truth was actually far more damning to the McGovern campaign.[57]

Senator Eagleton had checked himself into a mental hospital for depression in the 1960s three times. Beyond that, on two of these occasions he had undergone electroconvulsive shock therapy. The McGovern team was taken by surprise when these accusations began to surface. Eagleton had never been its first choice and had not been fully vetted prior to the convention's vote. Scrambling to perform damage control, Eagleton confronted the issue head-on. In an address two weeks later he told the public, "On three occasions in my life, I have voluntarily gone into hospitals as result of nervous exhaustion and fatigue."[58]

Though McGovern announced that he backed his running mate 1,000 percent, concerns soon began to surface. As his campaign manager and future presidential candidate Gary Hart of Colorado said, "This was the height of the Cold War. The key here wasn't how do we feel about mental illness or therapy or anything like that. The key was—finger on the button." Though a poll at the time showed 77 percent of Americans did not care too much about the issue, McGovern soon decided to drop his running mate as a candidate. Only eighteen days after his selection, Eagleton was off the ticket. In the end, though this certainly helped to damage McGovern as a viable candidate, it probably was only one contributing factor to his already flawed and failed campaign.

A similar issue emerged during the 1988 fight between Vice President George H. Bush and Governor Michael Dukakis. While President Reagan had been viciously hounded by claims among Democrats that he had fallen into dementia during the second half of his presidency, he turned the tables and issued a similar claim against Dukakis in 1988. In August of that year, only a few months before the general election, when asked for a comment about the Massachusetts governor, President Reagan responded that he "did not want to pick on an invalid."[59] This came upon the heels of months-old rumors that Dukakis had been previously treated for clinical depression and that his wife had been suffering from an STD.

Though Dukakis at first moved slowly on releasing medical records, the Democratic campaign soon changed course and quickly began to flood the media with forms, reports, and testimonials. Though the issue did not destroy his campaign, Dukakis later admitted that it added yet another element of doubt and suspicion to an already tottering run for the presidency.[60] His poll numbers had already been collapsing and continued to do so until November, when he lost to Bush 426 to 111.

Elections of 1992, 1996, and 2008

Old age itself has become a target for politics in recent years. While the notion of an "elder statesman" was once revered in the republic, as the Democratic Party moved toward choosing younger and younger candidates since the 1950s, it gave way to the idea of youthful vigor and connecting with "modern voters." With the exception of Lyndon Johnson, all Democratic candidates between 1952 and 2016 were younger than their Republican rivals.[61]

Kennedy was perhaps the first to actively run on this concept, with commercials embracing him as someone who was "old enough to know, but young enough to do," despite only being four years younger than

Nixon. Men such as Eisenhower and Reagan were portrayed as doddering old fools, unhealthy in both mind and body. These attacks would pick up steam in the late 20th century and early 21st, as the age gap between Democratic and Republican candidates widened significantly.

During the 1992 campaign between President George H.W. Bush and William Jefferson Clinton, the Democratic governor from Arkansas was 22 years younger than his rival, representing an entirely new generation in politics. While an emphasis on this was to be expected, Bush didn't help matters by falling ill during a meeting with the Japanese. On January 9, 1992, after having spent the morning playing a strenuous tennis game against the emperor and crown prince of Japan, the sixty-seven-year-old president attended a dinner at Prime Minister Miyazawa's home. During the banquet, Bush suddenly began to vomit and then fainted, all of which was caught on camera. The embarrassing incident was quickly disseminated to every major television network around the world, producing both weeks of jokes as well as true concerns about the health of the elderly leader, especially when compared to the youth and vigor of Governor Bill Clinton.

The administration reported that the president was suffering from a mild case of influenza. With his own aged presidency coming so closely upon the heels of Reagan's, questions soon began to be raised. The *New York Times* couched its coverage with references to Bush's age, writing:

> Mr. Fitzwater said today that the President, who is 67 years old, required no medication beyond an anti-nausea drug, but that Mr. Bush still experienced "some weakness" and that as a result, his morning schedule had been canceled. He said the President had a good night's sleep and would resume his schedule this afternoon. "The doctors are certain that there is no other illness or any other problems related to this, that it's a simple case of the flu." he said. "The President is human; he gets sick."[62]

Though only one of several missteps by the Bush campaign, it did little to help his falling poll numbers. He was soundly defeated in his bid for reelection by Clinton later that year.

Four years later, Democrats undertook similar attacks against Senator Bob Dole. The seventy-three-year-old war hero was even older than Bush and appeared even more frail due to his wartime injuries. The Clinton campaign relied upon such obviously loaded terms as "old policies," "dysfunctional," and "worn-out rhetoric" to raise questions in the minds of voters.[63] Dole did little to help his cause while on the campaign trail, famously falling off of a stage during an event and mentioning the long-defunct Brooklyn Dodgers in a speech. Once more, the younger and more popular Clinton secured victory.

XII. Disease and the Democratic Process

This trope would be repeated a third time in 2008, when once more two men of different generations ran for the White House. In this case, the 47-year-old Barack Obama took on the 72-year-old John McCain. As early as June of 2008, CNN ran a segment asking, "Is Sen. John McCain too old to be president?"[64] The Obama team recycled many of the same charges that had been thrown against Dole a decade before, stressing the age of his ideas as well as the confused nature of the candidate.

The release of John McCain's health records became a talking points issue during the campaign, with many speculating that the Republican candidate had something to hide. The majority of this concern resolved around his bout with melanoma in 2000. Various newspapers began requesting access to the documents as early as March 2008, well before the actual convention of either party was held.[65] To help head off further speculation, McCain released all of his records in May of that year. To his credit, the candidate had previously released 1,500 pages of medical information in 1999, during his first run for the presidency, perhaps the greatest trove of political health documents ever to be given to the American public.

Not surprisingly, while professing concerns about McCain's advanced age, few media outlets turned as much negative attention to Obama's extreme youth. Though the Democrats released their candidate's health records shortly after Republicans did, it was merely a short, undated summary by a physician. In addition, the letter glossed over the candidate's smoking habit and contained a bizarre reference to his "good intake of roughage and fluids."

McCain's advanced age weighed upon the thoughts of many voters and was one of the prime factors in his decision to adopt a much younger running mate. His thoroughness in releasing more than 1,500 pages of medical information perhaps merely magnified the issue in the public's eyes. In the end, though the election was not decided by age or health concerns, these stories perhaps distracted some voters from the true issues.

Election of 2016

The election of 2016 saw two candidates, one 70 and one 69, engage in a bitter campaign that politicized the health and illnesses of each other. Though slightly younger than some previous candidates and seemingly healthy, the media and pundits seized upon the slightest specter of mental or physical illness.

Donald Trump certainly received the most scrutiny of the two, with his age, weight, general health, and mental well-being attacked furiously for months on end. Even claims about his height and the size of his hands became fodder for liberal media analysts. The two most frequent accusations, though, concerned his weight and his psychological health. Media outlets would often point out that the Republican candidate was clinically obese, using this to question his overall health.[66] Yet, while Trump was certainly one of the largest presidents, his weight was in fact equal to Teddy Roosevelt's, a man famous for his health and aggressively active lifestyle, and only 14 pounds heavier than Bill Clinton, a man lauded for his youth and vigor despite serious cardiovascular issues. With the liberal focus on confronting "weight bias" and embracing body positivity occurring at the same time as these attacks on Trump, many saw it as the height of hypocrisy.[67]

Likewise, many jumped at the opportunity to examine candidate Trump's mental health, arguing that he suffered from any number of psychoses and was therefore unfit for office. Once again, these attacks were not unique. In 1964, *Fact* magazine published an article titled "The Unconscious of a Conservative: A Special Issue on the Mind of Barry Goldwater." It contained opinions from an alleged 1,189 psychologists and psychiatrists stating that the Republican candidate was unfit to serve as president. The backlash from the public was intense, and the APA soon updated its Principles of Medical Ethics to include the following provision on public diagnosis, "It is unethical for a psychiatrist to offer a professional opinion unless he or she has conducted an examination and has been granted proper authorization for such a statement." Better known as the Goldwater Rule, it became the accepted standard among psychologists for the next half century.

Yet, beginning in 2016, many members of the profession violated the rule by once more expressing their professional opinion on a candidate. Dozens of articles were written and numerous interviews given on television and online, all pointing to various alleged psychoses of the Republican candidate. One of the more prolific on this front was Dr. Bandy X. Lee of Yale Medical School. Not only did she write several articles purporting to identify mental abnormalities in Trump, but she also helped to organize and participate in a call to the House Judiciary Committee in 2019 suggesting that they consider his "dangerous" mental state during the impeachment investigation as well.[68] These accusations by Lee and others merely increased as his presidency went on.

For his part, Donald Trump frequently bragged about his health, especially when compared to previous holders of the office and candidates. In December of 2015, his personal physician, Dr. Harold Bornstein, issued a one-page written report in which he stated, "If elected, Mr. Trump, I can state unequivocally, will be the healthiest individual ever elected to the

XII. Disease and the Democratic Process 153

presidency."[69] Democrats and various media outlets alternatively mocked or questioned the report, demanding a more thorough accounting of his health. Months of refusals by Trump followed until early September of 2016, when he presented a recent physical to Dr. Mehmet Oz during an appearance on the latter's show. Yet, this did little to tamp down speculation, with physicians continuing to offer opinions on his potential or theoretical health concerns for months.[70]

Yet, all of this stood in sharp contrast to the largely passive coverage of Hillary Clinton's health. Only the very few conservative media outlets that existed attempted to address the health issues of the Democratic nominee. Speculations about her health stretched back to at least 2012, when the then secretary of state suffered an apparent fall at home, which resulted in an alleged concussion. Her spokespeople claimed that Clinton was suffering from the flu at the time and had collapsed in her house due to dehydration. As she had been scheduled to appear before a Congressional investigative committee over her role in the Benghazi attack and now moved to cancel her participation, Republicans quickly labeled her illness "Benghazi Flu."[71] Over the next month she was likewise hospitalized for what was claimed to be a blood clot related to her concussion and began to appear for the next two months in very thick glasses. After Dr. Drew Pinsky speculated on his show about possible brain damage related to the incident, his program was cancelled by HLN.[72]

Throughout much of 2016, while making frequent campaign stops, Clinton also suffered from numerous coughing fits that were quickly seized on by conservative pundits. The left-leaning *Atlantic* went on to publish a lengthy piece referring to concerns over the coughing as right-wing propaganda.[73] Liberal media outlets only began to mention the incidents in September of 2016, months after they had started. Republicans also began to circulate pictures of Clinton needing assistance walking up flights of stairs, seeking to establish still further proof of her ill-health.

The most serious incident occurred in early September of 2016, when video emerged of a barely upright Clinton being carried into a van by handlers as others moved to shield the scene from cameras. The campaign would later claim that she "overheated" while attending the 9/11 memorial and had to be assisted into her transportation.[74] Yet, many doubted this as temperatures at that time were only in the high 70s. Subsequent reports blamed the incident on pneumonia, with doctors stating it may last into late October.[75] Many saw this as a convenient attempt to forestall speculation about any subsequent incidents before the election.

In the end, it is difficult to say if concerns over the health of either candidate impacted voting trends. Both likewise seem to have passed the next four years without major medical issues. Regardless, presidential health had now become a well-publicized and speculated-upon topic during elections.

Women's Suffrage Sickness

The visual appeal of a candidate, their perceived healthiness and vigor, were long thought to be of importance to women voters. While research on this fact is divided, what is generally agreed upon is that female voters have historically focused more energy and effort on public health issues then men have.[76] In fact, issues of disease helped to launch the women's suffrage movement in the first place and nearly derailed it as well.

Thought the question of whether to allow women to vote stretches back to colonial times, it gained increased momentum after the Civil War. Though the sparse population of the western states, when combined with the pro-suffrage polices of the Republican Party and the racist attitudes of the Democratic Party, led to women's voting occurring in those states first, the idea soon began to gain steam across the country. Interestingly, women on both sides of the argument used the ideas of a woman's traditional role in the home to push their views. For suffragists, the notion that empowering women with the right to vote would lead to healthier, cleaner, and disease-free households was a common tactic. A broadside created by the New York State Woman Suffrage Association at the start of the 20th century pointed this out.

> She can care for her own plumbing and refuse, BUT if the plumbing in the rest of the house is unsanitary, if garbage accumulates and the halls and stairs are left dirty, she cannot protect her children from the sickness and infection resulting.
> She can open her windows to give her children the air that we are told is so necessary, BUT if the air is laden with infection, with tuberculosis and other contagious diseases, she cannot protect her children from this danger.
> A woman can open windows to give her children fresh air, but they will get sick if the air is filled with disease.
> Alone, she cannot make these things right. Who or what can?
> The city can do it—the city government that is elected by the people to take care of the interests of the people.
> And who decides what the city government shall do?
> Do the women elect them? NO, the men do.
> So it is the men and not the women who are really responsible for the
> Unclean Houses
> Bad Plumbing
> Unwholesome Food
> Danger of Fire

XII. Disease and the Democratic Process

Risk of Tuberculosis and Other Diseases
In fact, MEN are responsible for the conditions under which the children live, but we hold WOMEN responsible for the results of those conditions.[77]

Much as with every other group in American history, disease was used as a metaphor both for and against the suffragists. In 1911, during the campaign in California to extend voting rights to women, the chair of the Democratic Party called the entire notion of women's suffrage "a disease."[78] At the same time, the suffragists themselves relied heavily on recounting the conditions that their members faced in prison whenever they were locked up for illegal actions. Frequently, these stories focused on diseases they acquired there as a way to garner sympathy. Virginia Bovee signed a sworn affidavit in 1917 stating:

> The prisoners with diseases are not always isolated, by any means. In the colored dormitory there are now two women in advanced stages of consumption. Women suffering from syphilis, who have open sores, are put in the hospital. But those whose sores are temporarily healed are put in the same dormitory with the others. There have been several such in my dormitory.[79]

The movement began to gain further momentum during World War I when, for various reasons, Republicans and many Democrats began to favor a national move to expand voting rights. A vote on a new amendment to the Constitution was held on September 30, 1918, falling only two votes short of what was needed to pass. Though disappointed, most supporters felt that active campaigning by them would help to influence the upcoming midterm election and allow for a subsequent revote. Unfortunately, this was the moment that the Spanish flu struck America.

The massive pandemic, which killed over 650,000 Americans, sent home hundreds of Congressmen, shut down the country, and put an end to all campaigning. A supporter of the amendment in Louisiana opined, "Everything conspires against women's suffrage. Now it is the influenza."[80] Carrie Chapman Catt, who fell ill herself, spoke pessimistically about the future:

> These are sad times for the whole world, grown unexpectedly sadder by the sudden and sweeping epidemic of influenza. This new affliction is bringing sorrow into many suffrage homes and is presenting a serious new obstacle in our Referendum campaigns and in the Congressional and Senatorial campaigns. We must therefore be prepared for failure.[81]

Yet, despite the near cessation of political activity by men in the country, pro-voting women and their allies undertook a concentrated letter writing and pamphlet dispersal campaign aimed at key voting districts. In the end, Republicans were able to gain 24 seats in the House and 6 in the Senate, enough to pass through the legislation that would become the 19th Amendment in June of 1919.

Chapter XIII

Immigration and Illness in the 20th Century

As previously discussed, disease was often an invader, a foreign entity not only with regard to the human body but the body politic as well. Even before its mechanism of spread was properly and scientifically understood, the connection between pestilence and the movement of people was well known. The long and well-documented history of the use of quarantines to attempt to stave off the spread of epidemics provides proof of this. With immigration being so closely associated with the history of America, its role in the spread of disease became further ammunition for those who wished to politicize the practice. While some of this concern was well founded as disease certainly did often accompany immigrants, at other points it was grossly exaggerated for political ends. Political debate over the arrival of the Germans in the 18th century, as well as the Irish and Chinese in the 19th, and their connections to disease were continued in the 20th with regards to Italians, Jews, and Hispanics, as well as many others.

Though the arrival of Germans into Pennsylvania in the 18th century and the mass immigration of Irish in the Black Forties had led to concerns over the importation of disease, only the movement of Chinese into the country produced significant legislation. Yet, this was to change with the growth of "new immigration" in the late 19th century. Recycling many of the old disease-related tropes lobbed against the Irish, combined with the preference for legislative solutions to these concerns, some in the American government moved to politicize and restrict the latest arrivals to the country.

The new immigration of the late 19th century saw a shift in the origins of those coming to America from northern and western Europe to southern and eastern areas of the continent. Italians, Poles, Russians, and Jews began to make up large segments of those landing at Ellis Island or other port facilities. Many of these were driven by economic opportunity or political unrest. In the case of the Jews, violent pogroms were underway

XIII. Immigration and Illness in the 20th Century

in many areas east of the Oder River. Much as with the earlier arrival of the Irish, economic fears and religious biases led to resistance by some to this new wave of migrants.

This was in some ways fueled by the growing push by progressives to federalize more and more functions that had previously been within the bailiwick of states. Immigrants, who could easily travel over state lines upon their arrival and whose actions and the diseases they could potentially import could impact the general American populations, were soon seen as something to be regulated by Congress. Though preceded by such pieces of legislation as the Page Act of 1875, this thinking was finally enshrined in the Supreme Court decisions of *Henderson v. Mayor of City of New York* (1875) and *Chy Lung v. Freeman* (1876). Congress moved to further examine the issue, with the Committee on Foreign Affairs reporting back in 1879 that a limit on immigration was desirable as a way to curtail the influx of disease into America.[1]

The first general resulting piece of legislation was to be the Immigration Act of 1891. For the first time in American history, immigrants could be prevented from entering due to a number of undesirable characteristics, including disease. All ships arriving in the country were to have their passengers undergo a medical examination, with those who failed being either hospitalized or deported depending upon their condition. The legislation was generally favored by both parties, with *The Evening World* of New York opining, "America is not the sink for foreign refuse to be washed into. We are free enough to demand that only material from which free men can be made shall be suffered on our shores."[2] Ellis Island was opened in New York harbor at this time to help document and medically regulate arrivals.

Newspapers began to report on the number of immigrants coming into the country, as well as those detained due to disease. Invariably, Italians became the predominate group to be singled out in print.[3] Likewise, despite the successes of identifying and preventing sick individuals from entering the country, disease continued to be a political tool by which many pushed for still harsher restrictions on Italians and others. A Minnesota newspaper at the same time ran an article on an outbreak of "Italian itch" in Pennsylvania.[4] Though it is unclear what the malady actually was, the arrival of Italians was blamed for it. A Texas journalist reported shortly afterward that taking notes or coins from Italians were the surest ways to acquire the infection, a thinly veiled attempt to economically isolate the new arrivals.[5] An outbreak of typhus in 1892 in New York was likewise blamed on the Italian and Russian community.[6]

These charges and attacks continued over the next two decades, undoubtedly helping to push the next act that further restricted immigration. Passed in 1907, this law expanded upon the medical exclusion of immigrants, by not only detailing specific conditions that would make them inadmissible but also making their family members or traveling companions subject to detention or deportation as well. Shortly after this, speaking at a meeting of the Men's Club of New Haven, Connecticut, in 1907, the county health officer praised not only the efforts of city leaders but also the "excellent immigration laws of the country," for keeping the country free from "great disease epidemics."[7]

Yet, these increasingly restrictive laws were still not good enough for those who wanted either a full cordon sanitaire around the country or else who simply opposed immigration of certain groups. The Associated Press published a piece in December of 1907 titled "Diseased Immigrants Are Menace to New York."[8] It reported that despite current laws and the best efforts of officials, the number of pestilential immigrants arriving daily was simply overwhelming. Over the next decade, newspapers continued to report on local outbreaks, invariably blaming Italians or Slavs for the sicknesses.

The question of immigration, invariably wrapped up with the issue of disease, would go on to become one of the main topics during the election of 1920. Known as the Solemn Referendum, the battle between Warren G. Harding and James M. Cox was to be a trial by the electorate of over two decades of Progressivism. Though both men favored maintaining the current restriction on Asian immigration, a vote for Harding was seen as approval of a more restrictive system for those crossing the Atlantic as well.

In 1921, the notions of eugenics, public health, and immigration collided to produce the Emergency Quota Act of that year. As the new year dawned, and a new Congress and president prepared to take their places, newspapers ran articles asking for a careful consideration of the impact of immigration on the health and genetics of the nation. The House Committee on Immigration subsequently released a report warning of a flood of Jewish immigrants, most of whom were "wasted by disease."[9] At the same time, the Commissioner General of Immigration, Anthony Caminetti, issued his findings on the current situation in Europe. Caminetti, a staunch proponent of limiting immigration, had been dispatched to the Continent by Wilson shortly after the election. Upon his return in January of 1921, he warned of an "influx of typhus infected aliens unless prompt measures are taken to keep out the diseased who are preparing to sail for this country in the spring."[10] Though many argued that the existing laws and measures of quarantine available at the time were more than adequate to address this impending disaster, others weren't as sure.

Opposition to the bills being proposed in Congress quickly grew, aimed at exposing many of the falsehoods of Caminetti and others. Jewish groups especially were organized, as they appear to have been one of the primary targets of public concern. Employees at Ellis Island began to speak out about the terrible conditions there, arguing that it was "disease-ridden, a plague hatchery and a dangerous menace." Dr. Royal S. Copeland went on to claim "Immigrants gather more germs at Ellis Island than they bring in."[11]

The main proponent in Congress of decisive action was Representative Albert Johnson, a Republican from Washington State. A long-time subscriber of eugenics, the congressman had frequently spoken out in favor of halting immigration, especially now that typhus threatened our borders. Surgeon General Hugh Cumming, another Wilson holdover, spoke in front of Congress in February of 1921, providing further evidence of the dangerous situation. Johnson himself began to push for the immediate establishment of delousing stations to tackle immigrants afflicted with "disease bearing vermin."[12] A jurisdictional tug of war erupted between the federal government and the state of New York, as the former attempted to seize control over quarantine facilities at Ellis Island. Throughout February, newspapers carried stories of Ellis Island being overwhelmed by both the number of immigrants coming in as well as the eruption of illnesses there.[13] As one newspaper blared across its headline that spring, "The typhus germ cannot be Americanized."[14]

Yet, interestingly, the inauguration of the Harding White House saw a collapse in general media coverage of the issue. The expected spring offensive by typhus never materialized. The existing quarantine facilities and practices of New York and other port cities seem to have prevented the epidemic from materializing. Despite this, Johnson and others continued to push for a restriction on immigration, though not the total one that was suggested back around January.

The resulting piece of legislation would become known as the Emergency Quota Act of 1921. Passed overwhelmingly by Congress in May, it was signed into law by President Harding on May 19, 1921. The act called for a reduction in immigration to a level of 3 percent of the number who emigrated from a particular country in 1910. Meant as a compromise measure between complete suspension of immigration for a year and no action whatsoever, the legislation was specifically designed to stay in effect only until June of 1922. In 1924, an even more restrictive and long-term law was overwhelmingly passed, which lowered immigration levels still further. Though President Coolidge and Secretary of State Charles Evans Hughes had opposed many sections of it, particularly the total ban on Japanese immigration, public pressure, the upcoming election cycle, and a number of other issues led them to eventually acquiesce.

This system would remain in place until 1965, when a new immigration act removed all quotas that favored certain nations and radically altered the demographics of the nation. Interestingly, public health played a far different role in this process. Efforts by the U.S., other first world nations, and the UN to eradicate diseases around the planet and improve public health had led to a general decline in deaths by illness around the globe. Arguably, many of these efforts were as driven by altruism as they were by personal concerns over the spread of pandemics. As births began to dramatically outpace deaths, populations skyrocketed in Africa, Asia, and Latin America. Economic growth tended not to keep pace with these growing numbers, poverty and dissatisfaction quickly set in. The changing of immigration laws to the U.S. had as much to do with ethical and moral concerns over equality and fairness and the need to attract labor and talent as they did fears of Malthusian traps that would encourage the spread of communism and Soviet influence.[15]

With the surge in illegal immigration from the 1980s to the 2020s, disease has once again become either a concern or a trope for those who seek to stem its flow. Some of the earliest concerns during this time period were of the importation of AIDS, a topic that will be dealt with in chapter XIV. More recent concerns have focused on diseases carried in across the southern border with Mexico.

After decades of declining cases and a surge in vaccination campaigns, the CDC announced that measles had largely been eliminated from the country by 2000.Yet, beginning in 2010, cases began to increase, especially in California. By 2014, 667 episodes were recorded, while in 2019, the number climbed to over 700. As previously discussed, while the causes of this had to do with vaccine hesitancy and increased Middle Eastern immigration, most focused their attention and blame on the southern border. This became a frequent talking point among Republican candidates during the 2016 campaign cycle as they sought to challenge President Obama's ineffectiveness in fully securing the border.

Dr. Ben Carson, as early as February of 2015, stressed that the surge was being caused by "a combination of noncompliance [with vaccine requirements] and introduction into our society of people who perhaps haven't been well screened."[16] While technically accurate in his logic, left-leaning media outlets such as BET and *The Hill* ran articles on his ideas with such titles as "Carson Blames Measles on Immigrants," ignoring his equal attack on those not getting vaccinated. A few months later, Donald Trump likewise seized upon the issue. In July of 2015 while discussing the problems of the drug trade, he noted, "Tremendous infectious disease is pouring across the border" as well.[17] Trump would occasionally make reference back to these ideas during his presidency, writing on Twitter in

XIII. Immigration and Illness in the 20th Century

December of 2018 that moves by Democrats to push for "Open Borders … brings large scale crime and disease."[18]

The 20th century saw dramatic changes to immigration and the demographics of America. The country alternated between vast importations of people and restrictive laws aimed at stemming these flows. While arguments for or against immigration centered on a variety of topics and ideas, the one constant was a fear of the arrival of deadly diseases in the bodies of those who eventually made it to the shore of the United States. Some argued that America was a country built by immigrants, while others feared it could just as easily be destroyed by illness.

Chapter XIV

The AIDS Epidemic?

"AIDS Worse than the Black Death." The title of a 2002 article written by Daniel DeNoon nicely encapsulates the view of many concerning this pandemic that first arose in the 20th century. At the time of its publication, the author stated that world fatalities had already surpassed 25 million, while another 40 million were most likely infected, with only a bleak future predicted for the planet. However, it was around this same time that the epidemic was actually peaking, with both deaths and infections starting to dramatically decline thanks to new treatments and better education campaigns, among a number of other factors. Yet, at its height, the disease represented one of the most feared contagions in human history. This was due in part to both the mysteries that surrounded it as well as the vast politicization of the illness.

Research over the past two decades has continuously pushed back the origins of HIV and the paths by which it spread around the world. This research now places the beginnings of the virus to between 1888 and 1928 somewhere in southern Cameroon.[1] Between 1901 and 1916, the region was a German possession before being acquired by the French after World War I. For the next several decades, the territory was utilized by Paris to both produce food as well as to serve as a connection point between the Atlantic coast and its territories further inland. To aid in these goals, the French expanded upon the infrastructure accomplishments of the Germans, building a rail line across the colony. The work involved forced labor in some of the most disease-infested parts of the continent, producing frightful death rates. Yet, a far deadlier disease was also emerging at the time in the area.

HIV developed from SIV, a similar disease that was endemic in chimpanzees in the region. At some point before 1930, the disease jumped from its animal host to a local human. From there it spread through the villages and towns of the region, most likely following the path of the railroad. Workers brought in from throughout central Africa, including sex workers, then spread it further afield. This would only increase in the period

XIV. The AIDS Epidemic?

around World War II when French medical services brought into the colony in a bid to help the locals most likely inadvertently made things worse by using contaminated needles and blood.

The disease proceeded to spread throughout Africa, with its slow incubation period and hidden nature contributing to its silent expansion. At some point in the 1950s, Haitians who had been living and working in Africa returned to their home country and brought it back with them. Others likewise brought the illness out of Africa, with it reaching the U.S. sometime around 1970. Despite previously held theories about its arrival in America, the disease most likely appeared in New York City at this time, eventually spreading across the nation to California.

The disease was first noticed in the United States in 1981. In June of that year, Dr. Michael Gottlieb published a study in the CDC's Morbidity and Mortality Weekly Report on five cases of *Pneumocystis carinii* pneumonia among gay men in Los Angeles. The rarity of this fungal infection, except in cases of severe immunosuppression, began to attract attention from researchers. A month later, another article in the CDC publication reported a dramatic uptick in cases of Kaposi's sarcoma among homosexual men in both New York and California. Both of these diseases were almost unheard of in the decade before and led the CDC to form a task force to address the seeming rise in opportunistic infections.

By 1982, amid further cases of rare opportunistic disease deaths and with increased research, it had become clear that a new disease was emerging as the root cause of these problems. Originally referred to as GRID, or Gay Related Immune Deficiency, and later 4H, Homosexuals, Haitians, Heroin, and Hemophiliacs, the disease was soon renamed AIDS by the fall of that year. In 1983 and 1984, researchers in both France and the United States identified the virus responsible, with it eventually being renamed HIV in 1986.

The disease quickly became politicized, much along the same lines that cholera had been in the 19th century. Whereas the earlier disease was viewed as solely confined to immigrants, the poor, the filthy, and those who led "immoral" lives, this new epidemic was seen as largely confined to homosexuals and drug addicts, both of whom were cast in a similarly negative light. Much of this had to do with the contemporary social changes that had been taking place for the previous few decades.

The 1960s and 1970s witnessed a cultural revolution in America that saw challenges to social, sexual, religious, and behavioral norms. American culture became largely polarized into a traditional group and a more radical and modern segment. Drug use, homosexuality, "free love," and the bohemian "hippie" lifestyle were embraced by many in the nation. As the disease initially struck this latter group almost entirely, some saw it as a judgment on the social revolution. For some conservatives, AIDS represented a consequence of behavior, while for some liberals, it represented something that must be either embraced or quickly solved lest their actions and choices be seen as having consequences.

In a 1995 interview with David Sheff for *Playboy*, Camille Paglia nicely sums up the view of many concerning the AIDS epidemic.

> AIDS is a price paid for sins committed in the Sixties, and by gay men who took free love to extremes throughout the Seventies and had unrestrained, decadent, pagan sex. I support paganism in all its forms, but a price must be paid. I believed in free love, too, but we were wrong. It wasn't the Pope who was the problem. It wasn't the struggle with old-fashioned moral codes that was the problem. It was nature.[2]

The extremes of the 1960s produced a backlash in the 1980s. To these more conservative or puritanical elements, AIDS was a consequence of what they had been shouted down for warning about two decades prior.

Perhaps no single group epitomized this more than the Moral Majority. Founded by the Baptist minister Jerry Falwell, Sr., in 1979, it aimed to organize conservative Christians in the South and make their views heard in politics. Though initially supportive of Jimmy Carter in his 1976 election, many of these voters had become disenfranchised with his performance and, by the 1980s, had largely swung toward the Republican Party in national elections. Falwell quickly became an outspoken advocate for linking the disease to "sinful" behaviors, claiming, during a 1983 debate with the Rev. Troy Perry, "God hates sin."[3] That same year, the group's main periodical, *The Moral Majority Report*, carried on its cover an image of a "traditional" American family all wearing medical masks. The image was subtitled "Homosexual Disease Threatens American Families."

Falwell campaigned vigorously for not only a return to traditional social norms but also specifically focused on an effort to close down the bathhouses of San Francisco and New York City. These establishments had been around for decades, functioning largely as areas for promiscuous and anonymous sex for gay men. A study done at the time revealed that 65 percent of men in the Los Angeles region reported having more than 1,000 sexual partners in their lifetime.[4] A lack of safe sex practices among these men, combined with the presence of illicit drug use as well, provided for both a breeding ground for infection as well as an ample population for its rapid spread.

This view of AIDS as a disease resulting from "impure" lifestyles, which targeted homosexuals, was also pushed by some in the gay community itself. As early as 1981, activist Bobbi Campbell was writing some of the first articles on the disease in local and national newspapers, referring to it often as the "gay cancer."[5] He had previously used the term in a poster he had created and hung in the front window of the local Walgreens on Castro Street in San Francisco. The next year, as Campbell and other activists met to form what would eventually become the People with AIDS Movement, two individuals emerged who sought to confront what they saw as their group's part in the emergence of the disease. Richard Berkowitz and Michael Callen began to speak out against the promiscuous and unsafe sex practices of gay men over the previous several decades. Their ideas and solutions were eventually appeared in a pamphlet titled *How to Have Sex in an Epidemic*, released in 1983. The work proved highly controversial at the time, partially for its view that AIDS was caused by a multifactorial model but largely due to its related insistence that gay men partake in safer and less risky activities. Callen, Berkowitz, and others were attacked as reactionaries and self-loathing homosexuals. "This panic could never have set in so quickly and so deeply if within the hearts of Gay men there weren't already a persistent anti-sexual sense of guilt, ready to be tapped."[6] The Denver Principles, which eventually emerged from the People with Aids meeting in 1982, carried a compromise position of both sides. Likewise, an August 1983 edition of *Newsweek* magazine carried Bobbi Campbell and Bobby Hilliard on the cover with the title "Gay America: Sex, Politics, and the Impact of AIDS." Though a gay couple gracing the cover was a first for the periodical, it only reinforced the notion among many that AIDS was simply a "gay disease." Campbell's subsequent embracing of his status as the "AIDS poster boy" did little to stop this. Around the same time, Larry Kramer also emerged as a prominent voice in the community who fought to both solve the AIDS crisis and attack the "overly-sexualized gay culture of excess."[7]

On the opposite end of the spectrum, some moved to exaggerate the risks of the illnesses in non-homosexual and nondrug using populations as a way to both destigmatize the disease and increase funding to find a cure. For many in the community, AIDS was something to be used as a human rights issue, inseparable from the gay rights battles that had been taking place.[8] Thus, the case of Ryan White was feverishly seized upon by many. White was a young hemophiliac who had frequently received blood transfusions to help keep him alive. In 1984, following a particularly severe bout of pneumonia, he was diagnosed with AIDS. The current confusion and misinformation that surrounded the illness led to a protracted legal battle as to whether he could return to school. Despite White winning his appeals, the frequent discrimination that he suffered resulted in the family relocating to a more welcoming town.

White went on to become a poster boy for the impact of the illness on the nongay community. Celebrities and politicians rushed to embrace

White, he routinely appeared on television shows, and in 1989 ABC aired a television movie about his life. His funeral in 1990 was attended by former president Reagan, Elton John, Donald Trump, and Michael Jackson. The former president stated at the time:

> We owe it to Ryan to make sure that the fear and ignorance that chased him from his home and his school will be eliminated. We owe it to Ryan to open our hearts and our minds to those with AIDS. We owe it to Ryan to be compassionate, caring, and tolerant toward those with AIDS, their families, and friends. It's the disease that's frightening, not the people who have it.[9]

His fame and death led to the creation of dozens of new charities that went on to raise millions of dollars a year. His family's own foundation raised hundreds of thousands of dollars a year between 1992 and 2000. Likewise, in 1990, Congress passed the Ryan White CARE Act, which provided funding for programs that helped HIV-positive individuals. Beginning at $220 million in 1991, by the year 2020 it was providing $2.39 billion to individuals and programs in the United States.

The plight of hemophiliacs was recognized as early as 1982, when the CDC began to receive reports of several patients developing *P. carinii*. In fact, the discovery of AIDS among hemophiliacs and drug users around this time helped push the CDC toward investigating it as a possible bloodborne illness. Yet, at a meeting which it called of various groups to discuss ways to limit and monitor blood donations, members of the blood industry and gay rights groups vehemently opposed these suggestions. "It was thought that singling out homosexuals for exclusion would unnecessarily stigmatize them without evidence that they were indeed transmitting the disease. The blood industry, threatened by losing a large donor pool, strongly supported the position of the gay groups on this."[10] Donor screening based on sexual preference was roundly rejected by both gay interest groups and many in the blood industry. It would take another two years of debates, the identification of HIV itself, and further deaths before the blood industry sided with the CDC and moved to screen donors. "Tragically, during the period 1981 to 1984, more than 50% of the population of hemophilic patients in the USA had already become infected, these individuals would continue to present clinical symptoms of AIDS during the next decade and many would die."[11]

With the revelation that Hollywood actor Rock Hudson had AIDS in 1985, the disease took on a whole new level of interest for the American public. Though the famed actor was homosexual, his fame and name recognition brought the disease directly into the living rooms of Americans. As *People* magazine reported in late 1985, "Since Hudson made his announcement, more than $1.8 million in private contributions (more than double the amount collected in 1984) has been raised to support AIDS research and to care for AIDS victims (5,523 reported in 1985 alone)."[12] Hudson's death was followed by those of supermodel Gia Carangi and Perry Ellis in 1986 and Liberace in 1987, and though all contracted AIDS through homosexuality or drug use, it brought about a change in how many in Hollywood viewed the illness. This process was dramatically accelerated in 1991 when basketball legend Magic Johnson announced his diagnosis with the disease. Americans began to both accept that the disease was one of the general public and began to fear its spread. Oprah Winfrey, whose every statement commanded the attention of tens of millions at the time, stated in 1987, "Research studies now project that one in five—listen to me, hard to believe—one in five heterosexuals could be dead from AIDS at the end of the next three years. That's by 1990. One in five. It is no longer just a gay disease. Believe me." AIDS had finally gained the national attention that many of its earliest advocates had pushed for, but the attention was accompanied by abject fear.

This fear also quickly pushed states to enact harsh laws for knowingly spreading the disease. From 1986 to 2017, 34 states and the federal government passed legislation that either required notifying partners of HIV status or criminalized certain practices. This process was helped along by the Ryan White Act of 1990, which tied federal funding for AIDS patients to the criminalization of its spread. This represents possibly the first attempt in American history to specifically penalize the spreading of an epidemic. Yet, many civil rights groups and medical professionals questioned the ethical or scientific value of such laws. Beginning with Texas in 1994, however, several states began to slowly overturn their laws. In 2013, a bill was introduced into Congress titled the REPEAL HIV Discrimination Act, which sought to push for commonsense legislation rather than punitive attacks, but it ultimately stalled.

Yet, as scientists and policy makers began to get a better handle on the nature of the disease and the size of the outbreak, it became apparent that it was not the harbinger of doom that many portrayed it to be. Dr. Stephen Carl Joseph had been appointed as the Health Commissioner for New York City in 1986 and began to aggressively confront the disease. One of his aims was to get an accurate count on the number of infected individuals, as most media outlets and activists routinely claimed the total to be around 400,000 but with little proof. After careful analysis, Dr. Joseph dropped the city's official count to 200,000 in July of 1988, a number that was actually still twice as high as reality. Almost immediately, the Commissioner's office was flooded with complaints and accusations of homophobia and bigotry as victims and their supporters feared a concurrent cut in funding. Dr. Joseph required police protection as the group

ACT UP proceeded to undertake sit-ins outside of his office and later protested outside of and vandalized his home. Hundreds of death threats were recorded against him as well.[13] Fed up with the constant barrage of harassment, Dr. Joseph finally stepped down in 1990.

AIDS activists focused much of their anger, in fact, upon local and federal government for what they saw on one hand as indifferent inaction and on the other as antigay measures. Moves by first San Francisco and then New York City to close bathhouses in 1984 led to protests and accusations across the communities. Meanwhile, the seemingly complete inaction of the White House was met with anger by many. As early as 1982, Lester Kinsolving peppered Reagan's press secretary, Larry Speakes, with questions about the president's view on the epidemic. Speakes' reliance on humor and his lack of knowledge of official policy infuriated victims and their supporters. Yet, the White House largely saw the issue as a matter for individuals or one to be addressed by states first.

As has been seen, the government was aggressively involved through the CDC since the earliest days of the disease becoming identified. Yet, the information it had was limited and its conclusions and policy suggestions were often very inaccurate. In 1983, the organization stated that the disease could be spread through casual contact, food, air, or even tears. This only led to further alienation of both patients and the gay community. During an interview that Bobbi Campbell gave to CBS in 1983, he was placed behind a glass screen and the crew refused to place a microphone on him.

Dr. Anthony Fauci took over the National Institute of Allergy and Infectious Diseases in late 1984. He followed a similar path to his predecessor and was subsequently attacked by both sides, with some claiming he was downplaying its seriousness and being inactive, while others saw him as a fear monger. Years later, he claimed that he surreptitiously visited bathhouses and gay bars in order to study the spread of the disease. Yet, to activists like Larry Kramer, he was little more than "a pill-pushing pimp that cooperates with drug companies in forcing dangerous concoctions down the throats of a desperate community that is brainwashed into believing that taking a pill, any pill, will help them."[14] Yet, the Reagan government largely saw its response as a measured one. Apart from approving millions in funding, it moved to regulate blood donations in order to protect hemophiliacs and others. Likewise, in 1987, it approved the adding of AIDS to the list of diseases that would invalidate an immigrant from coming to the country.

The 1990s and 2000s saw a much fuller recognition of the pandemic by the public and government. In the 2000s, President Bush's PEPFAR focused efforts to combat AIDS in Africa, declaring it a national security threat. Over the next two decades, some $90 billion would be spent to lower rates of transmission and provide treatment and care for the afflicted. It was the largest worldwide undertaking of such a scale since the Balmis Expedition. Yet, politics predictably accompanied its launching. The legislation's requirement for an anti-prostitution pledge, as well as abstinence-only education, were opposed by liberals and some activists. It was eventually challenged in court and ruled unconstitutional in a 6–2 decision in 2013. Despite this, the program was an immense success, saving millions of lives and dropping AIDS rates by over 20 percent in Africa, with some areas reporting reductions of 40 percent or higher.[15]

Yet, in retrospect, some argue that the epidemic was more of a pseudo-epidemic. Almost 90 percent of cases occurred due to unsafe sex practices by homosexual men or from intravenous drug use.[16] For those outside of these risky behaviors, the disease did not pose a noticeable threat.[17] As previously seen, estimates of those infected in America as well as the likely number of victims in the future were drastically overestimated. As late as 2007, the WHO admitted to overestimating the number of those infected around the world by six million, an error of nearly 15 percent.[18]

Despite this, money continued to flow into AIDS funding and research. By 2012, the NIH alone was spending $3.1 billion on AIDS, which represented 9 percent of its budget. At the same time, cancer research consumed $5.6 billion while diabetes claimed $1.1 billion. Yet, the country contained around a million AIDS patients, while at the same time there were 13.4 million being treated for cancer and 29 million with diabetes. This disproportionate funding carried over onto the world stage as well, with fundraisers and concerts being hosted by musicians and big-name celebrities for decades.

Several historians have posited the idea of "AIDS Exceptionalism," that for a variety of reasons the disease was treated far differently than others in history.

> Descriptively, exceptionalism posited that in the early years of the HIV epidemic, HIV was considered so different, so "exceptional" in comparison to other communicable diseases that advocates and public health officials agreed that HIV policy should cater to the uniqueness of the epidemic rather than treat it like all other communicable diseases. Supposedly, the argument goes, public fear was so great, the political power of gay men so substantial, and concern over stigmatization so real, that public health authorities abandoned "traditional" approaches to communicable disease control in favor of a civil liberties approach.[19]

Beginning in the 1990s, as the actual smaller magnitude of the epidemic in the West became apparent and transmission and death rates began to fall dramatically, this exceptionalism spread to the international stage as well. As already mentioned, the disease was declared to be a national security threat by both the U.S. and UN. Fears of internal unrest, increased crime, destabilized countries, and delayed democratization were trumpeted by world leaders. Yet, the threats of the disease failed to materialize and money continued to pour into areas to be ineffectively spent. Worse yet, funding that could have gone to more serious issues and fatal diseases instead went into the coffers of AIDS foundations. As one researcher pointed out,

> It is no longer heresy to point out that far too much is spent on HIV relative to other needs and that this is damaging health systems. Although HIV causes 3.7 percent of mortality, it receives 25 percent of international healthcare aid and a big chunk of domestic expenditure.... Until we put HIV in its place, countries will not get the delivery systems they need.[20]

Diseases which were killing far more people in Africa and America were not being cured, and issues far more pressing to people were not being addressed. The spectacle of AIDS dominated the scene.

CHAPTER XV

Moon Fever

The post–World War II period saw several other epidemics and pandemics of note strike the United States. While not as deadly or as contentious as previous episodes of disease, they each contributed in unique ways to the perfect storm of politicization that would accompany the much larger pandemic of 2019. These outbreaks saw the rise of cooperation between the United States government and pharmaceutical companies to fast-track vaccines and began the promotion of the CDC as the public face of epidemic response, yet they tended to lack the extreme partisanship that had accompanied other pandemics. The absence of this latter piece was perhaps a major reason for the lack of panic during the outbreaks, despite the deaths of over 100,000 in several of them.

Post-War Asian Flus

The first of these postwar pandemics occurred in 1957, when a particularly deadly strain of influenza struck the country. Originating most likely in southwestern China, the disease quickly spread over most of the world. Democratic Senator Richard Neuberger demanded action from the surgeon general and warned as early as July of that year, "I understand this is the most virulent epidemic of the influenza since the tragic outbreak which occurred during World War I. Therefore, I have urged the Public Health Service to do everything within its power to prevent any such spread of the disease to our shores."[1]

Yet his warning was already too late, as the first cases in the United States seem to have been connected to sailors in Rhode Island taking part in a naval exercise in June of that year. Only a few weeks later, similar cases were reported in California as well. Vice President Nixon was even hospitalized with the virus for three days and the stock market entered into a downward trend before crashing between July and October, with the S&P losing almost 20 percent of its value. It's estimated that 60 percent of all children contracted influenza that year, with 45 million adults coming down with it between October and November alone. Deaths in the United States ranged from 70,000 to 116,000 out of a total population of 171,000,000.

The uniqueness of this episode lay in the reaction of a few select individuals to the pandemic. While the federal government set aside money and the United States Public Health Service dispatched a surveillance unit to provide information to citizens and track the outbreak, these moves were little different than those that had occurred during previous epidemics. However, one individual who did suggest a new path was Dr. Maurice Hilleman, chief of the department of respiratory diseases at Walter Reed. Dr. Hilleman gathered samples from some of the first infected individuals, quickly realizing the lethal possibilities of this new strain of flu. Bypassing various regulatory agencies, he personally lobbied the medical industry to begin mass producing vaccines. Seizing upon his initiative, the government quickly used these to vaccinate the military. This was considered a necessity due to the current state of the Cold War as well as the perceived limited jurisdiction of the federal government in mandating vaccinations. Vulnerable populations, health-care workers, truck drivers, communications workers, and utility employees were reached out to next in a concentrated effort to push the shots. Finally, 30 million more doses were offered to the public. Though no mandate existed, seven million citizens eventually received the vaccine, with President Eisenhower eagerly supporting it.[2] Many credited Hilleman with saving hundreds of thousands of lives.

Yet, these efforts were not without controversy. As the fall progressed, schools emptied, workers stayed home, and the New York City subway became a ghost train. Major corporations had put in contracts for vaccinations and received many of the first shipments, causing some in the public to complain that they were being put at risk due to big business. Likewise, rumors abounded that sports stars and celebrities were getting priority doses in order to keep the NFL and Hollywood open.[3] A newspaper reported in the fall how actor Errol Flynn "made a $40 phone call to wife Pat Wymore in Majorca to remind her to get at Asian flu shot before joining him in Hollywood," a luxury not available to most.[4] Even when vaccines finally became available, doubts over their effectiveness, the dangers associated with them, and skepticism that they were merely being pushed to fill the bank accounts of pharmaceutical executives led to low vaccination rates. In fact, many drug companies began to sell doses overseas while up to half of those produced were eventually returned to manufacturers. Instead, herd immunity most likely brought the disease to an end by early 1958.[5]

Another important outbreak of disease occurred in 1964; this time it was an epidemic of rubella, which sickened millions across the nation. The disease, also known as German Measles, arrived from Europe early in the year. Rubella was not normally a particularly deadly illness, and the media and periodicals, including *Time* magazine, had for years recommended hosting "Rubella Parties" to expose children to the disease. This was thought to be especially important for young girls, as by the 1950s it was evident that if they caught the disease later in life when pregnant, it could lead to birth defects.[6] Yet, by the 1964 outbreak, it had become apparent to the National Institutes of Health and others that this was a dangerous practice as it could potentially spread the virus to pregnant women as well. In that year alone, 20,000 birth defects were reported due to the illness.

It was in the middle of this outbreak that Dr. Stanley Plotkin created a revolutionary vaccine. Using fetal cell lines in a controversial experiment, he was able to create the first ever vaccine to prevent rubella. Yet, far beyond the ethical issues of his process, Plotkin faced a more troubling opponent that would delay the approval of his vaccine for a decade. As the scientist himself would later recount, "One of the competing vaccines was actually developed at the licensing authority, a branch of the FDA. For a pharmaceutical manufacturer, that was very appealing, because it meant that they would get a license for the vaccine because they'd be working with the licensing authority."[7] Politics both in and out of the FDA prevented the adoption of the new vaccine until 1979, causing needless cases and suffering.[8] Thankfully, these types of connections between the FDA, NIH, and private manufacturers were eliminated around this time, paving the way in the future for a more free market approach to vaccination development.

The next wave of Asiatic flu to strike America arrived in late 1968. Known at the time as Hong Kong Flu or Mao Flu, it once again originated in China and proceeded to spread around the world. Carried to America by both travelers and soldiers returning from South Vietnam, it was firmly entrenched in the United States by the winter of 1968. After its initial arrival, a second wave swept across the country later in 1969 as well. Despite a death toll of over 100,000 in America alone, and with the *New York Times* referring to it as "one of the worst in the nation's history," life largely continued unabated. NASA sent the first humans to the moon, Woodstock occurred, and millions continued to protest against the war in Washington, D.C. Some people took precautions against the spread of the flu by washing their hands or sanitizing equipment more frequently, some schools saw closures due to mass absences, and some airports increased screenings for travelers, but for the most part, people did little to alter their daily routines.

The importance of this episode lay in three particular historical developments. The first involved a much quicker development and roll out of a vaccine to combat the virus. Once again, Dr. Maurice Hilleman led a team that was able to produce a vaccine in a record-breaking two months. Between November and December of 1968, some six million doses were released. Though the pandemic had largely subsided for the season in America, the vaccine proved very beneficial in the Southern Hemisphere and was also able to be used upon its return in 1969.[9]

The second development was the rise in power of the CDC. Established in 1946 as the Communicable Disease Center, it was initially tasked with combating malaria in America. Over the next two decades, other departments of the USPHS, including those focused on biological warfare, epidemiological training, venereal diseases, and tuberculosis, were brought under its wing. By the time of the 1968 Hong Kong Flu outbreak, it was officially renamed the National Communicable Disease Center. The NCDC began to issue most of the government's public statements on the pandemic, quickly overshadowing the traditional role of the surgeon general. This trend of the bureaucratization of pandemic management would continue for the next five decades.

Finally, the government went to extreme lengths to ensure that the pandemic would not harm the first manned mission to the moon in 1969. Some scientists had speculated for years that life either existed on the moon at some point or continued to on a microscopic level. Yet, for the most part, NASA considered this to be a manageable risk. Then, in April of 1963, Senator Margaret Chase Smith of Maine questioned the possibility of a "biological threat" to the planet from space exploration.[10] Her concerns arose from a congressional staff memo that raised concerns that diseases from the moon could bring about "the violence of the venereal disease epidemics that raged through Europe in the Middle Ages or the measles that took a heavy death toll when it was introduced into Polynesia."[11] While most scientists discounted these fears, or were more concerned with organisms from earth contaminating samples from the moon, some did begin to speak out. Most notable among these were a young Carl Sagan and one of the directors of Lockheed who argued, "The Moon has been a vulnerable target in the path of extraterrestrial debris, possibly organic, bacterial, and living—possibly disease carrying."[12] NASA released a report in 1964 warning of the potential of "back contamination," a move that led to the eruption of intergovernmental fighting as dozens of agencies moved to take control over protecting the earth from biological threats.[13] In order to satisfy all concerned, NASA proposed a $9 million Lunar Sample Receiving Laboratory. While many Republicans in Congress were upset with NASA's mismanagement, focusing on building all of its facilities in Texas, and its failure to train female astronauts, they didn't want to go on record as opposing a solution meant to prevent biological threats. As the head of the Office of Manned Space Flight testified, the chance of biological invasion was "one in a hundred million, but this represents a reasonable probability in the views of the bioscience community of contaminating the Earth and their feeling is that this is a real risk."[14]

The arrival of the "Mao Flu" in 1969, while not causing particular concern among Americans for their own safety, produced a visceral response when combined with the proposed moon landing. The concerns of some in NASA and in Congress over "back contamination" began to be noticed by the public, especially following the release of the book *The Andromeda Strain* that year by Michael Crichton. A wildly popular book, it detailed the arrival on earth, aboard a crashed satellite, of an extraterrestrial virus. Thousands of letters from concerned citizens flooded into NASA. Officials feared that should the astronauts contract the ongoing flu before they departed, their sickened state upon their return would fuel fear of a lunar plague. Therefore, Neil Armstrong, Buzz Aldrin, and Michael Collins were placed into quarantine for two weeks before their launch.

Upon their return, all three men were placed into quarantine at the Lunar Sample Receiving Laboratory. Yet, the containment protocols of the facility proved to be anything but secure. Numerous issues of potential contamination arose, and within weeks an additional 16 scientists and employees were forced into quarantine due to fear of exposure. All of this was kept from the public to avoid panic or damage to the image of NASA.

Swine Flu Pandemic of 2009

President Obama had only recently been inaugurated and was attempting to address both the Great Recession as well as his promised healthcare reform when the country was suddenly struck by a once in a generation pandemic. Sometime in late 2008, an outbreak of influenza erupted in Mexico, spreading slowly through the country before crossing the border into California sometime in the late winter or early spring of 2009. On April 15 of that year, the CDC reported the first identified case of the disease in a 10-year-old child in California, with more following shortly afterward.

The particular strain was soon identified as H1N1 or swine flu, the same type that had caused the disastrous pandemic of 1918. Fears began to mount in some sectors of the return of the virus on a large scale after 90 years and Obama was notified of the outbreak only a few days before the WHO declared an emergency. Apart from allowing for the release of medical supplies from the national stockpile, the president initially took a measured approach to the outbreak, urging the sick to stay home. Yet, only a few days later, Vice President Joe Biden gave a television interview in which he stated:

> I would tell members of my family—and I have—I wouldn't go anywhere in confined places now. It's not that it's going to Mexico in a confined aircraft where one person sneezes, that goes all the way through the aircraft. That's me. I would not be, at this point, if they had another way of transportation, suggesting they ride the subway. From my perspective, this relates to mitigation. If you're out in the middle of the field and someone sneezes, that's one thing. If you're in a closed aircraft, a closed container, a closed car, a closed classroom, that's another thing.[15]

His much more alarmist tone and message was quickly attacked by the travel industry, with the spokesman for American Airlines referring to it as "fear mongering."[16] An emergency meeting was called of top officials at the White House to perform damage control for Biden's misstep.

Conservatives likewise jumped on the pandemic, using it to attack what they saw as the open border policy of the Democrats. Such notable right-wing pundits as Michael Savage, Michelle Malkin, and Glenn Beck all attacked the White House for its failure to address the issue of illegal immigration across the Mexican border.[17] Former presidential candidate Pat Buchanan, referring to the disease as the "Obama flu," wrote, "But if he is perceived at having refused to close the border to buses bringing in sick Mexicans, or airports to planes coming in from Mexico City, so as not to offend the open-borders crowd, and a deadly epidemic ensues, full responsibility will be his."[18]

While Obama invited members of the Ford administration who had dealt with a similar influenza epidemic in 1976 into the White House, negotiated with Congress for $8 billion in funding, and followed a strategy known as PTFOTV, or Put Tony Fauci on TV, his actual efforts to mitigate the spread and impact of the disease were less than successful. Only a few weeks after the WHO declared the outbreak to be the first global pandemic in nearly 41 years, the Obama administration called for a halt to testing and tracking for H1N1. While most public and private health officials and practitioners disagreed with the move, the White House defended it by asking, "Why waste resources testing for H1N1 flu when the government has already confirmed there's an epidemic?"[19] Speculation was also made that the move was due to a lack of available tests as well as fears that revealing the true number of infected could cause a panic. At the same time, efforts by the government to speed up the production and distribution of vaccines failed badly as well. Production delays, viral growth issues, and internal debates all served to delay and reduce the vaccine rollout. An initial call for 100 million doses by October was soon dropped to 40 million and then later further revised down to 11 million. As schools opened for the fall and flu season arrived, panic ensued among some parents as the CDC attempted to restrict the shots to the most vulnerable populations. By November, 200,000 were in the hospital and an estimated one in six Americans had become infected.[20]

Luckily for the nation, the pandemic seems to have peaked shortly afterward and then began a steady decline into the new year. While vaccines were finally made available to the majority of the general public in late December, much like with earlier outbreaks in the 1950s and 1960s, the danger of the disease had already largely passed by this point. In the end, an estimated 60 million Americans would come down with the disease, producing over 12,000 deaths. Ron Klain, Joe Biden's chief of staff at the time, later recounted:

> It is purely a fortuity that this isn't one of the great mass casualty events in American history. It had nothing to do with us doing anything right. It just had to do with luck. If anyone thinks that this can't happen again, they don't have to go back to 1918, they just have to go back to 2009, 2010 and imagine a virus with a different lethality, and you can just do the math on that.[21]

This admission was seized upon a decade later by President Trump during his campaign against Joe Biden in 2020. Facing criticism from Democrats over his handling of the pandemic that year, Trump brought up the former vice president's own missteps during the swine flu epidemic. Beginning in March of that year, the president began to launch a series of tweets comparing their two performances. "Sleepy Joe Biden was in charge of the H1N1 Swine Flu epidemic which killed thousands of people. The response was one of the worst on record. Our response is one of the best, with fast action of border closings & a 78% Approval Rating, the highest on record. His was lowest!"[22] These attacks continued until even after the election. A formal press release was even developed by the Republican Party in October that detailed the three major failings of Obama and Biden in 2009.

> FACT: The Obama-Biden Administration left the Strategic National Stockpile in dangerously short supply of N-95 respirator masks after deploying nearly all of them to combat the 2009 swine flu pandemic.
> FACT: The Obama-Biden Administration stopped all swine flu testing in the middle of the 2009 pandemic.
> FACT: The Obama-Biden Administration completely botched the development and deployment of a swine flu vaccine, making several mistakes that delayed production and caused supply shortages.[23]

For their part, Democrats praised Biden's performance, with Obama noting his leading role confronting both the swine flu of 2009 as well as the Ebola outbreak of 2014.

Ebola in America

While the late 20th and early 21st centuries saw the outbreaks of new and particularly deadly contagions in Asia and Africa, notably SARS, MERS, and Ebola, these largely remained isolated to those places and posed little threat to America. The notion that some deadly hemorrhagic fever or other contagion could rage across the United States was confined to such Hollywood productions as *The Andromeda Strain*, *Outbreak*, or *The Stand*. Yet, when an outbreak of Ebola hit West Africa in late 2013, the unthinkable finally occurred.

Beginning in December of 2013, and stretching into June of 2018, the disease ravaged Guinea, Liberia, and Sierra Leone. In total, some 28,000 people were infected, with 11,000 of these succumbing to the disease. International assistance quickly flowed into the region to stem the rapidly spreading illness, including doctors, money, medicine, and supplies from America.

As the outbreak overlapped a surge in illegal immigration across the southern border and came after six years of contentious battles between Republicans and Democrats over the Obama presidency, the idea of Ebola being inadvertently brought to America quickly became a political football. In July of 2014, Representative Phil Gingrey of Georgia wrote a letter to the CDC expressing concern over the administration's failure to secure the border. "As a physician for over 30 years, I am well aware of the dangers infectious diseases pose.... Reports of illegal migrants carrying deadly diseases such as swine flu, dengue fever, Ebola virus and tuberculosis are particularly concerning."[24] Liberals were quick to take him to task for failing to provide any sources for his concern. Yet, Gingrey was not alone in his concerns or politicization of the outbreak. Fox News ran a story the same month about a man who flew from Liberia to Nigeria only to die of the disease after his arrival. The article cautioned that the victim, Patrick Sawyer, had family in Minnesota and had been planning to visit in August. Apart from sensational speculation, however, it did little to show an actual problem.

A few days later, though, an incident occurred that began to radically change the debate. In July of 2014, two American medical personnel working in Monrovia were stricken with the deadly disease. While most of the public had paid little attention to the ongoing outbreak, the incident quickly dominated both the news and social media.[25] The two victims, Kent Brantly and Nancy Writebol, were treated in Liberia before being flown in specially designed isolation units to Emory University Hospital in Georgia in August. The decision to bring them stateside was met with harsh criticism by some. CNN was quick to accuse conservative pundit

Alex Jones of conspiracy fear mongering for opining that the "Feds would exercise draconian emergency powers if Ebola hits U.S."[26] Jones would be proven to be far more right when it came to the subsequent pandemic a few years later. Yet, even some Democrats began to question the White House's policy of bringing back sickened individuals. Representative Alan Grayson, a Democrat from Florida, wrote to Secretary of State John Kerry to demand the imposition of a travel ban against any African country currently experiencing an outbreak of Ebola. In this request, he was even joined by the widow of Patrick Sawyer who cautioned against allowing men like her husband to freely travel here, stating, "I don't want any other families to go through this. Ebola has to stop."[27]

Despite these fears, President Obama decided to launch a military assistance mission to the region only a few weeks later. Known as Operation United Assistance, it involved sending 3,000 personnel to West Africa to coordinate aid efforts, build infrastructure and facilities, and help with disease management. Consistent with the general 20th-century foreign policy of his party, Obama couched the need for intervention in terms of international security. "Faced with this outbreak, the world is looking to us, the United States, and it's a responsibility that we embrace. It's a potential threat to global security if these countries break down, if their economies break down, if people panic. That has profound effects on all of us, even if we are not directly contracting the disease."[28] One of the many outspoken critics of the move was future president Donald Trump. Tweeting frequently about the issue since August of 2014, he wrote shortly after Obama's announcement, "Why are we sending thousands of ill-trained soldiers into Ebola infested areas of Africa! Bring the plague back to U.S.? Obama is so stupid."[29]

The fears of many conservatives that the disease would soon arrive in America came to fruition in late September. On the 30th of that month, the CDC announced that a patient in Dallas, Texas, was being treated for the disease. Thomas Eric Duncan had flown from Liberia six days before, unknowingly carrying the disease in his body. Though he had helped to transport a sickened woman to the hospital while in Africa, he subsequently lied on his customs form in order to bypass airport screening. After falling ill on the 26th, he went to a local hospital only to be given antibiotics and sent home. When his condition worsened, he was finally tested for Ebola and admitted to the hospital, only to die on October 8, 2014. What followed was a massive manhunt for people who may have come into contact with Duncan, including a homeless man with whom he shared an ambulance. It would take until November 7 and the contact tracing of 177 people for Dallas to finally be proclaimed Ebola free. Two nurses who cared for Duncan did contract the illness, though both eventually recovered.

The incident was quickly politicized by both sides. Many questioned why Brantly was provided with life-saving experimental drugs while Duncan was not, with some suggesting racial bias on the part of the Texan hospital.[30] Duncan's family agreed with this narrative and launched a massive lawsuit against the institution, arguing that the care was "incompetent" at best or "racially motivated" at worst. Trump took both Duncan and Obama to task, tweeting on October 4, "This Ebola patient Thomas Duncan, who fraudulently entered the U.S. by signing false papers, is causing havoc. If he lives, prosecute!."[31] The CDC under Tom Frieden sought to place the blame on Texas Presbyterian Hospital and likewise lambasted infected nurse Amber Vinson for traveling after showing symptoms.[32] Yet, later it was revealed that Vinson had contacted the CDC in advance and had been cleared for travel.

Obama soon moved to salvage the rapidly expanding public relations disaster. In late October, nurse Nina Phan was invited to the White House for a photo opportunity with President Obama. Around the same time, prominent lawyer and presidential advisor Ron Klain was chosen to be the "Ebola czar" and coordinate responses to the disease. The choice was almost immediately attacked by conservatives, with Trump tweeting "Obama just appointed an Ebola Czar with zero experience in the medical area and zero experience in infectious disease control. A TOTAL JOKE!"[33] Republicans in Congress launched a series of investigations, with several calling for Frieden's resignation. Even *Forbes*, while defending Frieden personally, sharply criticized the Obama administration.

> There is no dogma when it comes to Ebola. Indeed, if our political leaders had shown more humility on describing the risk, and our ability to contain it, public confidence might not be so badly shaken. If only they had not been so absolute in declaring that there is zero risk of airborne transmission (when we know that there is a risk of "droplet" spread). If only President Obama hadn't taped a weird video for Liberians declaring that you can't get Ebola by sitting next to an infected person on a bus; at the same time U.S. hazmat teams were wrapping a building in plastic over a suspected Ebola case.[34]

Around the same time, New York City reported its first case of the hemorrhagic fever. Craig Spencer, a physician who had worked in West Africa to battle the illness, returned home only to develop symptoms on October 23. The fact that he had traveled extensively around Manhattan in the days before being hospitalized caused large-scale panic among many. It would take until November 11 for Spencer to be released from the hospital, with luckily no other people falling ill. Though Mayor Bill de Blasio copied Obama and embraced Spencer as he left the hospital, proclaiming New York City to be Ebola free, he quickly came under fire when his administration was duped by a con artist into granting a contract for a costly cleanup of the patient's apartment.[35] Senator Charles Schumer, who represented New York, introduced legislation for an "Ebola fund" that would compensate states who had to deal with cases like Spencer's. Congress would eventually go on to appropriate $5.4 billion for a response to the disease in the next budget cycle. Disease management could be lucrative.

While the White House eventually moved to provide for limited screening at airports and port facilities, it failed to move on the issue of mandatory quarantines for those returning from Ebola-stricken countries. In response, several states moved to undertake their own such measures. The first to move was Democratic governor Dannel Malloy of Connecticut, who issued an executive order requiring a 21-day quarantine for anyone returning from the infected West African nations. The move was soon copied by the governors of New York and New Jersey as well. Over the next few weeks California, Pennsylvania, Maine, Illinois, Virginia, Florida, Maryland, and Georgia also joined in, representing both political parties. Despite this, Obama and his wing of the Democratic Party strongly opposed the moves, with the president personally lobbying governors to relax or rescind the requirements. The president and many of his followers claimed that mandatory quarantines would discourage aid workers from going abroad.[36] Despite this, the Army chief of staff, Ray Odierno, issued a similar order for American military personnel as well.

The issue of quarantines became a constitutional question in late October with the return of Kaci Hickox to America. Having worked as a nurse in Sierra Leone to help treat Ebola victims, she had flown back to Newark, New Jersey, in order to return to her home state of Maine. Upon landing, she was recorded to have a slight fever and was immediately quarantined in a hastily constructed tent at University Hospital in the city. While she tested negative for the disease, she was held from October 24 until her release three days later. Many at the time saw Governor Christie's heavy-handed move as an attempt to portray him as a decisive alternative to Obama, an image that would benefit him in the upcoming Republican presidential primary. When asked about the move to detain the nurse, the governor of the Garden State responded, "I have a much greater, bigger responsibility to the people of the public."[37]

Yet, Hickox's ordeal did not end following her release from containment. Escorted by state troopers back to Maine, she quickly announced that she planned to defy the quarantine order of Governor Paul LePage. Hickox even took to biking around her neighborhood, as state police shadowed her every move. Her case quickly pitted conservatives against liberals, as the registered Democrat nurse hired a lawyer from the ACLU and planned to sue both Republican governors. While Republicans attacked her for her self-righteous attitude and general disregard for the rule of law, liberals hailed her as a feminist, working-class hero. Left-wing firebrand Rachel Maddow opined, "Maine's bombastic walking carnival of a governor, Tea Party Republican Paul LePage, has basically now threatened that that nurse may not be safe in Maine."[38]

A Maine judge eventually struck a middle ground between both the nurse and the governor, allowing her to leave her home as long as she monitored herself for any possible symptoms. Once again, LePage's strong response was seen by some on the left as an attempt to court voters for his reelection, which was only a week away. Hickox's boyfriend, when asked by reporters about his thoughts on the election, replied, "We voted yesterday in absentia, and you can guess who we voted for. We encourage all the good people of Maine to join us in returning decency to Blaine house."[39] Though he had previously been down in the polls, LePage won reelection that year, with Hickox's lawyer later saying, "His stance in the case is what led to his reelection: he was constantly on TV and in the media, talking about protecting public health."[40]

The various pandemics and epidemics that struck America in the decades after World War II were important for several reasons. They showed that disease was still a danger to the modern world despite all of our best precautions, science, and practices. These outbreaks exposed the way in which politicians and parties could and would seize upon both minor and major outbreaks in order to win elections and push policies. They showed the role that the media and public notice played in either promoting or allaying fears of contagion. Finally, the various outbreaks continued the creeping, centralized grasp of disease management that had characterized governments since the turn of the century.

Chapter XVI

The "Wuhan" Virus

Perhaps no epidemic or pandemic has been more politicized in American history than the one that erupted at the end of 2019. Coming at the height of the Trump presidency, amidst bitter rancor and a contentious impeachment process, stretching over an election year, and following years of increased governmental management of epidemics, as well as increased mistrust of these measures, the pandemic became a lightning rod for politics. Yet, the politicization that surrounded the virus was more of a culmination of actions and trends that had already been occurring for over two centuries. The political infighting, the resistance to vaccine mandates, the distortions by the media and politicians, and the revolts against heavy-handed government involvement were merely repetitions of what had occurred during various other outbreaks of disease in the country, yet this time they all collided at once.

While the precise time line of the outbreak of the novel SARS-CoV 2 virus in China is still subject to debate, certain assumptions can be drawn. It appears that the virus originated in China around the area of Wuhan at some point in the late summer or early fall of 2019. The first official case to be confirmed by the Chinese government was a man who lived in Wuhan who reported symptoms as early as December 1, 2019. Cases multiplied in the city over the next couple of weeks and, by the end of the month, most major news networks were carrying stories about the epidemic.

China identified a wet market in Wuhan as ground zero for the pandemic, closing it down on January 1, 2020. The disease continued to spread throughout China, with the first official case outside of the country being reported in Thailand on January 13. Over the next few days, additional cases began to emerge in Japan and the United States and the first deaths were reported in China as well. Containment remained relatively nonexistent in China, with many families traveling both domestically and abroad for the lunar new year. As late as January 6, 2020, Beijing was still denying the possibility of person-to-person transmission.

The World Health Organization, a body which had become heavily dominated by Beijing in previous years, proved very slow to act with regards to the virus and more often than not was entirely complicit in China's cover-up. As late as January 23, the WHO was still debating as to whether to declare the outbreak a pandemic, despite the fact that it had already spread to a dozen countries, including the first identified case in America.[1] Its director-general, Tedros Adhanom Ghebreyesus, even said as late as January 30, "The speed with which China detected the outbreak, isolated the virus, sequenced the genome and shared it with WHO and the world are very impressive and beyond words. It is a new standard of outbreak response."[2] Clearly, the messages coming out of both China and the WHO led to a false sense of security on all sides.

As Trump himself was still deep in negotiations over trade issues with China, he likewise sought to portray Beijing's response in a positive light. On January 24, 2020, Trump announced, "China has been working very hard to contain the Coronavirus. The United States greatly appreciates their efforts and transparency. It will all work out well. In particular, on behalf of the American People, I want to thank President Xi!" Yet, behind the scenes Trump understood the dangers that it presented. Only a week after the first reported case in America, the president ordered a ban on all foreign travelers from China from entering the United States. A week later, during a taped interview with Bob Woodward, the president allegedly stated, "It's also more deadly than even your strenuous flu.... This is deadly stuff," showing his already developed understanding of the new illness. Yet, Trump's pronouncements in public were much more measured and upbeat. While later attacked for duplicity, the president himself was quick to point out that maintaining calm for the good of the country was his sole concern. "I want to show a level of confidence, and I want to show strength as a leader, and I want to show our country is going to be fine one way or another."[3] This was little different than similar pronouncements by Obama, Ford, or Eisenhower in previous decades.

The Trump administration followed well-established protocols for how to deal with a potential pandemic. Already by January 17 the CDC dispatched teams to three American airports to monitor international passengers for illness. Three days later, the NIH was already beginning preliminary work on vaccine development. With no deaths yet in the U.S. and few cases arising, most people focused instead on the impeachment trial of the president that was then being carried out in the Senate.

Trump's first expanded action was to issue a travel ban on any passengers entering the United States who had previously been in mainland China. This came on January 31, less than two weeks after the first reported case in the country. The move was quickly seized upon by many Democrats, especially after President Trump broadened it in February to include Italy, South Korea, and other hotspots. Former vice president Joe Biden took to Twitter to denounce travel bans in general: "A wall will not stop the coronavirus. Banning all travel from Europe—or any other part of the world—will not stop it."[4] This statement was issued in spite of most countries implementing similar policies, with many, especially Taiwan and New Zealand, experiencing immense success. A few days later, following a defense by Trump on Twitter of the move, Biden responded with "Stop the xenophobic fear-mongering. Be honest. Take responsibility. Do your job."[5] The politicization of this move was made blatantly clear a year later when Biden enacted his own ban against several African countries following the emergence of the Omicron variant.

The very acknowledgment of the virus' origins and even its naming quickly became a political battle between both parties. Despite the *New York Times* and almost all other major news outlets referring to the virus as the "China virus," "Chinese virus," or "Wuhan virus" as early as mid-January, Democrats quickly began to attack Trump's usage of the phrase.[6] An article published by the *Wall Street Journal* on February 2 titled "China Is the Real Sick Man of Asia," which sought to lay out the weak economic underpinnings of Beijing, was quickly slammed by many as racist. Speaker Nancy Pelosi toured Chinatown in San Francisco in late February, hugging locals and attacking what she saw as the racist response of Trump and others toward the outbreak.[7] Likewise, Trump's use of the terms was taken as a catalyst by liberals for the rise in anti-Asian hate crimes in 2020. Yet, FBI statistics showed that hate crimes increased against all groups in that year, including a rise in identified hate crimes against blacks from 1,930 to 2,871 and against whites from 643 to 869.[8] Crimes in general, including murder, robbery, looting, arson, and assault, all rose precipitously during the protests and unrest that accompanied the summer of 2020. Finally, in most major cities, a disproportionate, if not outright majority, of attacks against Asian Americans were perpetrated by other minorities, hardly the Trump-fueled "white supremacists" as assumed by the media.[9] Meanwhile, the overreaction on the part of the Democrats to the naming of the virus merely encouraged Trump and his supporters to more aggressively label the virus as a Chinese product.

Historically, almost all major diseases received their name from either a distinguishing characteristic, such as smallpox, Dengue, bubonic plague, and whooping cough, or were named after their place of actual or perceived origin, such as German measles, MERS, Ebola, Zika, Lyme disease, West Nile Virus, Hantavirus, Marburg, and Spanish flu. Yet, already by March of 2020, Democrats and many in the media were calling for an end to the use of the terms "China virus" or the more apt "Wuhan virus." CNN opined, "The past has shown naming diseases after places can have negative consequences for nations, economies and people."[10] Over the next year, college professors and others who used one of the terms were quickly targeted.[11] Social media frequently blocked usage of the term as well, or else linked it directly to results they deemed more acceptable. In January of 2021, one of Joe Biden's first moves when in office was to issue a memorandum banning the use of any geographic reference to the disease. "The Federal Government must recognize that it has played a role in furthering these xenophobic sentiments through the actions of political leaders, including references to the COVID-19 pandemic by the geographic location of its origin."[12]

Once the severity of the illness became apparent, Democrats quickly moved to claim that Trump wasn't doing enough to seal off the country. Many on the left began to push for lockdowns, if not on the federal level than certainly within states. California became the first state to do so, with Governor Gavin Newsom issuing an executive order on March 19, 2020, effectively shutting down much of the state and ordering people to stay at home. This move was soon followed by a host of other liberal bastions and Democrat-run states, including Illinois, New Jersey, New York, Connecticut, Oregon, Washington, Louisiana, Delaware, Michigan, New Mexico, Massachusetts, Hawaii, Vermont, and Wisconsin, within the next week. Republican states were much slower to act, with a few issuing stay-at-home orders in late March, while the vast majority didn't move until early April. For his part, President Trump resisted calls for a national mandate, relying on federalism and believing that this was a matter best left up to municipalities and states.[13] The rallying cry among those in favor of even stricter restrictions on travel across the nation became "two weeks to slow the spread," arguing that these were to be brief and temporary measures.

As two weeks stretched into two months, a political divide developed between those who supported continuing the lockdowns and those who wished to end them. Opponents of the measures cited the economic devastation wrought by the move, as well as the many deaths that resulted from suicides, drug overdoses, and other fatal diseases that went undiagnosed due to fear of leaving one's home. Some conservatives began to see a concentrated effort by liberals to either damage Trump politically before the election or else use the emergency as a means by which to acquire more power. In March, dozens of pages and groups began to appear on Facebook calling for an "American Revolution 2.0" and an end to stay-at-home orders. Within weeks, Facebook moved to take down the various pages, a move attacked by conservatives. Beginning in mid–April, protests and rallies took place across the country but especially in the more heavily restricted Democrat-controlled states, against the lockdown orders.

For his part, President Trump took to Twitter, urging his followers to "Liberate Michigan" and "Liberate Minnesota." These moves infuriated Democrats, with Governor Jay Inslee of Washington claiming that the president was "fomenting domestic rebellion."[14] Some, including Niguel Hoskin of Vox, claimed that the protests were fueled by "anti-black racism."[15] Liberals began labeling the protests and contemporaneous Trump rallies as "super spreader events," blaming them for any upticks in case or death numbers in the state, despite a lack of forensic evidence connecting the two. At the same time, the numerous BLM rallies, Antifa protests, and associated riots that took place that summer and fall were excused from both restrictions and from any blame for the spread of illness.[16]

For his part, the president moved on April 16 to issue guidelines for a phased reopening of the states. Once again, he saw the role of the federal government as an organizing force to help the states manage their own solutions and cases, rather than a top-down manager. In keeping with this type of thinking, he authorized the dispatching of the USNS *Mercy* to Los Angeles and the USNS *Comfort* to New York City upon requests from the leaders of those states to handle the much-feared surge in hospitalizations that would occur. Yet, only a month later in early May, both ships returned to their home ports after only seeing a few dozen patients.[17] A similar situation unfolded with regards to ventilators. At the start of the pandemic, Governor Andrew Cuomo of New York, and others, claimed that they were set to experience a massive ventilator shortfall. The leader of New York claimed that the state "needs a minimum of 30,000 additional ventilators within the next two weeks, when the outbreak is expected to peak."[18] The president once again sought to serve as an organizing influence, dispatching ventilators from national reserves, shuffling units between states, and striking deals with GM and Ford to begin producing units. Cuomo lambasted the efforts of Trump, attacking the number of units that were sent as well as the promises of GM and others. For his part, Trump laid blame directly at the feet of Cuomo for not acting sooner following a 2015 state report that claimed that in the event of a severe flu season, New York would be 16,000 units short.[19] In the end, emergency hospitals constructed in New York City went unused and the available supply of ventilators proved to be more than enough. Cuomo, in an effort to save face, claimed that the experts "didn't know how unified New Yorkers can be and how responsible they can be and how caring they are. That's what they couldn't count in those models. They couldn't count the spirit of New Yorkers and the love of New Yorkers to step up and do the right thing. That's what they couldn't figure out on their computers."[20]

Between the protests, court rulings on the unconstitutionality of the measures, the economic devastation, and a belief among many that they had either failed to stem the tide of the pandemic or else had actually accomplished their goals, most states began to remove restrictions by the first week in May. By summer, largely only the solidly Democratic states remained either locked down or with severe restrictions in place. The Republican states of Arkansas, Iowa, Nebraska, North Dakota, and South Dakota never established statewide lockdowns, while Wyoming, Utah, Oklahoma, and South Carolina only had ones in certain, restricted areas. As the governor of South Dakota, Kristi Noem, stated, "The people themselves are primarily responsible for their safety ... [the state and national constitutions] prevent us from taking draconian measures much like the Chinese government has done."[21]

Amidst the pandemic, the age-old belief in miasma theory returned as well. Though science had firmly demonstrated the germ theory a century before, initial uncertainty over how the novel coronavirus spread left many attempting to block all possible vectors. Even once its person-to-person transmission via sneezing and coughing was firmly identified, many continued to insist on a deep cleaning of all possible surfaces. Rules and regulations were passed by businesses, cities, and even whole states, mandating extensive cleaning to prevent the spread of the virus. For the first time ever, the New York City subway was shut down nightly in order to sanitize all train cars. Though bathrooms and counters were cleaner than they ever have been in America, it provided no benefit to the stopping of the pandemic. Many conservative writers and pundits adopted the phrase "hygiene theater" to describe the belief and practice.[22] Yet, this did not stop many from continuing the habit, with the CDC and liberal media outlets like CNN only moving to speak out against it in April of 2021.[23]

Democrats and Republicans began to politically define themselves by their reactions to the pandemic, with both "hygiene theater" and "mask theater" being prime examples of this. The latter proved to be a particularly divisive issue between both sides. Mask mandates became one of the earliest responses by federal, state, and local governments in an attempt to stem the spread of the virus. Yet, some conservatives began to question the science and/or legality of such a move.

The idea of public masking during an epidemic stretches back for a century. Even before this, it was not uncommon during the period of belief in miasma theory for individuals to wear clothes over their mouths or masks over their entire faces to block the noxious fumes that were sought to spread disease. Examples from the 19th-century Edo Period in Japan of masks show that this was also a worldwide phenomenon.[24] The Spanish flu pandemic at the end of World War I, coming shortly after the discovery of the germ theory and at the height of Progressivism, brought mandatory mask wearing to many parts of the United States. Interestingly, a visceral reaction against these rules developed in certain places usually by a small minority of the population, most notably in San Francisco. Here, an Anti-Mask League was even formed, which questioned both the legal and scientific basis for the move. Thanks in part to their pressure, as well as declining cases of influenza, the mandate was lifted in February of 1919. Since that time, scientists have debated the effectiveness of the original law, as the masks were generally only worn outside, were made of thin cloth material, and were not worn in accordance with any strict, medical practice.[25]

As East Asian cultures have a much longer history of sick individuals wearing masks, the initial weeks of the outbreak saw the practice readily adopted in China, the Koreas, Taiwan, Japan, and other countries in the region. The United States, and most Western nations, initially recommended against the practice, in part to prevent a shortage of masks and other equipment for the medical community, as well as doubt over the effectiveness of nonmedical grade versions. In February of 2020, Surgeon General Jerome Adams spoke out against public masking of the uninfected, saying it would be "not effective" in preventing the illness.[26] Dr. Anthony Fauci would reiterate a similar recommendation a few weeks later. Throughout March, both the CDC and WHO continued to push for mask usage only by the medical community or by those who were infected.

Yet, pressure began building in some sectors as people began to actively wear N-95 respirators, surgical masks, cloth masks, and even homemade coverings. As April progressed, the CDC and Dr. Fauci began to soften their views on the practice. At the same time, President Trump approved usage of the Defense Production Act to have 3M, GE, and other companies begin mass-producing N-95 masks. On April 10, 2020, New Jersey became the first state to mandate their wearing when out in all public places. This move was soon followed by most other Democratic states, with Republican ones either refusing to issue statewide mandates or waiting until July or later to do so.

Many scientists and medical professionals questioned the wisdom of these moves. As early as late March 2020, Drs. Lisa Brosseau and Margaret Sietsema wrote an article for the University of Minnesota's Center for Infectious Disease Research and Policy that questioned both the effectiveness of masks and the potential harm in wearing them. The doctors pointed out that cloth masks in particular were ineffective in stopping the minute particles that spread the infection. Not only did no studies exist that could provide data regarding their effectiveness but also the reports that were in circulation suggested "the evidence from ... laboratory filtration studies suggests that such fabric masks may reduce the transmission of larger respiratory droplets. There is little evidence regarding the transmission of small aerosolized particulates of the size potentially exhaled by asymptomatic or presymptomatic individuals with COVID-19."[27] The researchers also suggested that a reliance upon these could deliver a message "that suggests cloth masks or face coverings can replace physical distancing." The symbolic risk reduction of masks could actually lead to riskier behaviors.[28]

Masks and mask mandates became the next politicized component of the pandemic. Democrats seized upon them as an effective tool to end the scourge of coronavirus, while Republicans either tended to see them as ineffective or else were simply opposed to mandates, preferring to leave it up to the individual to decide when and where to wear them. Trump quickly became the target of the wrath of liberals as he refused to wear a mask during most meetings and press conferences. The president often stated, "I think it's a great thing to wear a mask. I've never been against masks, but I do believe they have a time and a place," wearing one when he visited wounded or sick soldiers in hospitals and at manufacturing plants.[29] Yet, he stated that he would not wear one in the Oval Office when meeting with foreign dignitaries, nor during press conferences, preferring instead to not add to the level of fear already embracing the country. It was in this vein that an early plan to use the postal service to deliver free masks to all Americans was cancelled, as the White House did not wish to produce panic.

While some scientists and left-wing media and politicians claimed over the next year that masks helped to reduce the spread of the virus, many studies done in the real-world environment showed otherwise. Studies comparing American states with mask mandates and European nations without showed little statistical difference in case numbers; a study by the CDC itself done in Georgia likewise showed no clear reduction in outbreaks between masked and unmasked students, while a much-heralded large-scale experiment in Bangladesh was denounced by Dr. Martin Kulldorff of Harvard due to the fact that it "does not show a statistically significant difference in the efficacy of cloth masks vs surgical masks. Based on the confidence intervals, both could be around 0% or both could be around 20%."[30] By April of 2021, even CNN was running articles questioning the wisdom of relying on masks in all situations.[31]

While those who followed these contrarian positions rebelled against at least the forced wearing of masks, for supporters of the idea it became almost a religious talisman. Either pushed by pure fear or the notion that a near mystical adherence to its usage could ward off illness, many in the public took to wearing masks in extremely absurd situations. These included when alone at home, when alone in the car, or while isolated in nature. Actions such as these merely exposed and widened the gap between how liberals and conservatives viewed both the pandemic and the other side's reaction to it. Local governments soon resorted to medically unfounded ordinances, such as requiring masks while walking to a table in a restaurant but removing it to then eat once seated, or allowing customers to eat unmasked at a bar but not drink. By May of 2020, some were even calling for the use of "double masking" to help eliminate the virus.

"Mask theater" was soon accompanied by mask shaming. As one journalist opined at the time, "Sneering at people who refuse to wear face coverings has become a particularly viral form of virtue signaling."[22] President Trump and other Republicans were harshly criticized in the media and online due to their refusal to wear masks in public. Later, as the pandemic began to lessen, those who continued to wear masks reported being harassed and shamed as well.[33]

These views were little helped by the hypocrisy of many pro-mask politicians and reporters. Numerous instances were recorded of newscasters wearing a mask to deliver updates on the virus, only to remove it once the camera stopped rolling. Likewise, some reporters would be seen with them, while the cameraman would not be wearing one.[34] An even more blatant example occurred in early September of 2020, when the Democratic Speaker of the House Nancy Pelosi not only violated California law, which had shut down all salons, but also was caught on camera not wearing a mask while getting her hair cut there.[35] Similar incidents occurred with London Breed, the mayor of San Francisco, who was repeatedly caught violating mask mandates at nightclubs in the city.[36] Representative Rashida Tlaib, an ardent opponent of Trump's and a frequent supporter of masks, was even caught on camera in October of 2021 admitting that "I'm just wearing it because I've got a Republican tracker here."[37] The hypocrisy of the proponents of the policies on masking merely reinforced the notion of many that the disease was being politicized.

The shaming of those who refused to wear masks was quickly followed by the shaming of those who fell ill. This tended to be reserved strictly for Republicans and those who opposed mandates. Much as earlier newspapers morally judged those who fell victim to cholera during the 19th century or pointed out the diseased nature of immigrants, now they seized upon reports of infection by any conservative lawmaker as almost divine retribution. The illnesses of Rudy Giuliani, Rick Scott, Greg Abbott, Corey Lewandowski, Stephen Miller, Mike Lee, Kellyanne Conway, and Kayleigh McEnany were all featured in various media outlets and garnered visceral responses on Twitter. *The Atlantic* ran an entire article in March of 2020 attacking Rand Paul following his testing positive for the disease, insisting that he had "turned the world's greatest deliberative body into the nation's highest-profile vector for the spread of the pandemic."[38] Yet, despite these fears and worst-case scenario prognostications, there was no subsequent major outbreaks or death in Congress. In fact, the first congressional victim was Ron White of Texas, who died nearly a year later in February of 2021 and had been battling cancer for years.

Yet, the greatest vitriol and shaming was saved for President Trump. Following his October 2, 2020, announcement that he had tested positive for the virus, newspapers began to not only shame him for not having previously worn a mask but also attempted to dissect his daily movements prior to the announcement and label him a "super spreader." Months later, the *Washington Post* ran an article titled "The Reckless Timeline of Trump's Positive Coronavirus Test."[39] An article written for the student newspaper at Allegheny College titled "Why I feel morally justified laughing at Trump getting COVID-19" represented a common feeling among those on the left.[40] The *Palm Beach Post* carried a similar attack, stating, "In an irony for the ages, President Donald J. Trump has fallen victim to the coronavirus he has so constantly minimized and underestimated."[41] Hundreds of other such examples abound, closely paralleling similar attacks on victims of cholera a century and a half before. Interestingly, little such victim shaming was carried out by the same journals, stations, and papers when Speaker Pelosi and Vice President Harris were infected in 2022.

Even the president's treatment and recovery became political targets for Democrats. The president had frequently come under attack for discussing possible and unproven therapeutics for treating the coronavirus. Some of these products included hydroxychloroquine, chloroquine, azithromycin, and remdesivir. Once stricken, he credited his speedy recovery to remdesivir as well as a cocktail of other drugs. Various opposition media as well as the World Health Organization came out against these claims, either rejecting the efficacy of the treatments or else arguing that due to their costs they should not be pushed as a global response.[42] A team of researchers even blamed Trump's pushing of the drugs as the cause of at least one overdose, implying that more were possible.[43]

Apart from encouraging the exploration of various treatments and therapeutics, Trump pinned much of his hopes on the discovery of a vaccine. As previously stated, work on just such a product was begun as early as January of 2020 by various medical companies in America and Europe. Much as Bush had done with PEPFAR, President Trump moved to use the power of the American government to better organize, fund, and eliminate obstacles to these efforts. Dubbed Operation Warp Speed, it was formally announced by the president on May 15, 2020. The goal was to produce up to seven different vaccines, facilitate their expedited testing and approval, and then utilize the U.S. military to rapidly diffuse them throughout the nation. Trump touted that these efforts would produce a

XVI. The "Wuhan" Virus

vaccine available to the public by the end of the year, tweeting so as early as May 14.[44]

Yet, his political opponents lambasted these claims as either outright lies or wishful naiveté. NBC News even chose to "fact-check" these claims, arguing, "Experts say that the development, testing and production of a vaccine for the public is still at least 12 to 18 months off, and that anything less would be a medical miracle."[45] An article shared by both the *Washington Post* and *Bloomberg* argued, "The U.S. may waste a tremendous amount of taxpayer money preparing to produce failed Covid-19 vaccines."[46] Republicans responded by attacking these accusations, claiming that "the American people need to understand that the media often times are lying to them because they don't want a vaccine, in order to defeat Donald Trump."[47] The creation, approval, production, and delivery of the vaccine by the end of the year became a major component of the presidential debates between Trump and Biden on September 29, 2020. Biden expressed doubt about both its safety and its delivery, stating, "In terms of the whole notion of a vaccine, we're for a vaccine, but I don't trust him at all. Nor do you. I know you don't."[48]

Democrats, in fact, frequently expressed distrust of the proposed vaccine, arguing that Trump was unduly rushing it for political gains and potentially endangering millions. Then vice-presidential candidate Kamala Harris, when asked whether she would trust a vaccine from Trump, replied, "I think that's going to be an issue for all of us. I will say that I would not trust Donald Trump."[49] A few weeks later, she doubled down on this hesitancy during her televised debate with Mike Pence, stating, "If Donald Trump tells us that we should take it, I'm not taking it."[50] The Republican responded, "The fact that you continue to undermine public confidence in a vaccine, if the vaccine emerges during the Trump administration, I think is unconscionable … stop playing politics with people's lives."

Yet, Harris was not alone in her vaccine hesitancy. Democrats frequently expressed doubt about the proposed vaccine. During a speech given on July 28, 2020, Joe Biden questioned the safety of the vaccine. A month and a half later he issued an even more blunt critique, asking, "Who's going to take the shot? Are you going to be the first one to say sign me up?"[51] One of the most outspoken political voices was that of New York governor Andrew Cuomo. On numerous occasions, he questioned Trump's ability to produce and distribute a safe vaccine. At one point he told reporters, "Frankly, I'm not going to trust the federal government's opinion. New York State will have its own review." While during a speech at Riverside Church in New York City in November, he remarked, "Polls say fifty per cent of American people say they will not take the vaccine if it were available today, because they don't trust the way this federal government has politicized the process."[52] Throughout the process, he frequently utilized the Democratic talking point that Trump was pressuring scientific organizations to rush the vaccine and ignore protocols. Despite claims to the contrary, much of the early vaccine hesitancy was among liberals and pushed by their party for political ends.

Beginning in March of 2020, several websites and small businesses began to sell Anthony Fauci devotional candles. While probably initially designed as a gag gift, they soon developed into the cornerstone of a burgeoning niche market in items focused on the man. Ironically, the medical bureaucrat who had been the acclaimed enemy of the left in the 1980s, now attained an almost cult status. Democrats began to view Fauci as a foil to Trump, while Republicans lambasted his mercurial advice and his status as an unelected bureaucrat. As one columnist for the *New York Post* wrote:

> We can blame one man above anyone for this parlous state of affairs: Saint Anthony Fauci, the coronavirus czar once hailed as the most trusted man in America for his leadership through the pandemic. He has flip-flopped on every piece of advice, never admits doubt and tells lies with brazen indifference.[53]

Fauci became at the same time pilloried by Donald Trump and Rand Paul while being toasted and praised by Joe Biden and Jimmy Kimmel. While Paul frequently clashed with Fauci over the origins of the plague, as well as conflicting reports over America's involvement in "Gain-of-Function" research at Wuhan, Kimmel praised the doctor in November of 2021, stating, "Thank god there's someone who's educated enough and devoted enough to figure this stuff out for us because we are not going to figure it out ourselves."[54] The battles over Fauci and Fauci's own combative disagreements with other medical professionals were entirely reminiscent of the battles between Kuhn and Rush in 1793.

The politicization of the pandemic in 2020 was caused by a number of factors. Among these were disagreements over science and policy, efforts to garner additional political power to either the party or the federal government, and personal ambition. Yet, perhaps the strongest motive concerned the upcoming presidential election set to take place that year. Disease has often been a dramatic change agent in history, especially in the field of politics, and Democrats seized upon the opportunity that the pandemic presented in 2020.[55]

Despite a visceral hatred of President Trump by the left as personified by his impeachment in January of 2020, he seemed poised to win re-election at that time according to various polls. Based upon his own successes, the strength of the economy, and the weakness of the Democrat field, nearly two-thirds of voters polled by CBS News in February of 2020,

XVI. The "Wuhan" Virus

including over a third of Democrats, felt that he would be re-elected.⁵⁶ In fact, according to Gallup, his approval hovered around 50 percent well into May. Some of the more hypocritical and calculated fights between both sides should be seen through this lens of the Democrats' desperate attempts to reduce the popularity of Trump. As Bill Press of *The Hill* opined in October of that year, "The election is now a referendum on how Trump handled COVID-19."⁵⁷ Biden himself marked the passing of the 200,000 death mark by stating, "Anyone who's responsible for that many deaths should not remain as president of the United States of America."⁵⁸ This remark would in turn be thrown back against him by Republicans in 2022 as the death toll reached one million, a fourfold increase after only just over a year in office.

Democrats were quick to call for either a postponement of the election itself or else a switch to electronic or mail-in voting. Sixteen states postponed primaries, while the DNC pushed back their convention by a month until August. While these were all done under the guise of public health safety, some commentators suggested other reasons tied to the mental and physical health of Joe Biden. Republicans were quick to pounce on the issue of mail-in ballots, citing concerns and evidence of voter fraud as well as the constitutional legitimacy of the move by several states. Trump himself tweeted, "With Universal Mail-In Voting (not Absentee Voting, which is good), 2020 will be the most INACCURATE & FRAUDULENT Election in history. It will be a great embarrassment to the USA."⁵⁹ Mail-in voting would ultimately hang a specter over the entire election, leading to unprecedented challenges to its legitimacy afterward.

For its part, the Democratic Party adopted a "bunker strategy" for candidate Joe Biden. Under the pretense of taking the pandemic seriously, the party's nominee engaged in very few public appearances, instead using prerecorded speeches or streaming live from his home. Many took to calling it a "basement strategy," which sought to prevent the frequent gaffes associated with the former vice president, hide his inability to draw crowds in the same way that Trump could, disguise his cognitive and physical decline, and allow for public health-based attacks on Trump's large rallies, which had proven so successful in 2016.⁶⁰ Even some Democrats questioned the strategy, with one newspaper opining:

> With Trump now starting to travel and the election less than six months away, the Biden campaign faces an added risk: the competing images of a president in action, conversing with voters as he pushes to reopen the economy, and a challenger talking into a camera in an empty room.⁶¹

It would not be mere speculation to state that the pandemic of 2020 proved to be a deciding factor in Biden's eventual winning of the White

House. In fact, exit polls showed that the Democrats carried voters whose number-one concern was the virus by 66 points as well as those who prioritized the virus over the economy.[62] Politicizing the virus and keeping Biden out of the public eye proved to be a winning strategy.

Once in office, President Biden vowed that he was "going to shut down the virus." His strategy was largely just a continuation of Trump's reliance upon pushing the vaccine out to states while leaving issues of lockdowns and mask mandates largely in the hands of governors. The new administration announced on January 26, 2021, that there would be sufficient vaccinations for 300 million Americans by the summer. While many on the left praised the move ("In effect, the President is putting a date on a return of a semblance of normal life"), others questioned his ability to reach that goal.[63] Yet, few seemed to realize the vaccine hesitancy that would erupt on both sides of the aisle.

In a move aimed at rewriting history, the Biden White House began to claim credit for the vaccine and its roll-out, largely erasing or severely restricting the role of the previous administration. During an address delivered in February, the president claimed that the previous White House had "failed to order enough vaccines" and in addition had "no real plan to vaccinate most of the country."[64] A month later he stated, "When I first started the vaccination program and we got all that vaccine, enough for everyone, we were vaccinating 3 million people a day, we were getting very close before things began to slow down."[65] However, various outlets were quick to report the lies inherent in these statements, as not only had the Trump administration contracted for 800 million vaccines but also had a published plan in place in December for their delivery. Even Biden's famous goal of reaching one million vaccinations a day had already been reached weeks before his inauguration.[66]

Therapeutics and treatments for the disease continued to be politicized in 2021. While the left thought to rely largely on vaccinations to stem the tide of the pandemic, many on the right began to explore the use of various treatments to address what they saw as a disease was to become endemic to the world. Many of these drugs and regimens were ones that Trump himself had mentioned while in office or had used to treat his own infection. Perhaps none became more controversial than ivermectin. First discovered in the 1970s, it had by the next decade become the most widely used veterinary medicine on the planet. In the 1990s, it was also utilized for treating river blindness and lymphatic filariasis in humans, a usage that eventually won the Nobel Prize for its discoverers. Ivermectin was declared an essential medicine by the WHO, with millions of dosages being delivered yearly to treat such diverse conditions as West Nile Virus, Venezuelan Equine Encephalitis Virus, and influenza.

Already by early January of 2020, studies and discussions were surfacing about the use of the drug to treat the coronavirus in its early stages.[67] Despite this, most major national and worldwide health organizations spoke out against its usage, as there was little clinical evidence that it was effective. Despite this, some doctors and several notable celebrities and politicians began suggesting its efficacy. While a normal, healthy, academic debate should have ensued regarding the drug, it instead produced anger and mockery on the part of Democrats. Many seized upon its usage as a medicine for animals to lambast those who ventured to try it. The FDA itself tweeted in August, "You are not a horse. You are not a cow. Seriously, y'all. Stop it."[68] Podcaster Joe Rogan, who credited ivermectin and other drugs with his rapid recovery from the disease, was personally and frequently attacked on CNN. The network mocked him for taking a "horse dewormer" and labelled him as an "anti-vaxer." After Rogan, various conservative networks and even a few liberal ones took issue with CNN's portrayal, the station doubled down on its invective. "The issue is that a powerful voice in the media, who by example and through his platform, sowed doubt in the proven and approved science of vaccines while promoting the use of an unproven treatment for covid-19—a drug developed to ward off parasites in farm animals."[69] Reports also spread about increased ivermectin self-poisoning, though only around 500 cases were reported by August, with few being fatal. Finally, a *Rolling Stone* article appeared in early September of 2021, which quoted an Oklahoma doctor who claimed there were "gunshot victims left waiting as horse dewormer overdoses overwhelm Oklahoma hospitals." Yet within days, the hospital was not only denying the story but also revealed that the particular medical practitioner had not worked there in months.[70] By this time, however, the story had already been picked up by every major liberal-leaning station and paper and pushed as an example of the dangers and stupidity of using ivermectin off-label.

A similar situation unfolded with various monoclonal antibody treatments, such as Regeneron, in 2021. The drugs had likewise been touted by Trump and other Republicans as a possible treatment for the disease, with some studies showing significant results. As could be expected, many liberals opposed the treatments, either citing contradictory studies or simply dismissing them out of hand. Yet, unlike with other drugs, no firm move was taken to shut down its distribution. This can perhaps be explained in part by the fact that the company overwhelmingly donated to Biden and other Democrats during the 2020 cycle.[71]

Yet, this lukewarm support for Regeneron suddenly ended in December of 2021. Around this time, the Biden administration unilaterally stopped the distribution of Regeneron and Eli Lilly monoclonal antibodies for treatment of the coronavirus. According to government spokespeople, the drugs were no longer affective against the Omicron variant, which they claimed then accounted for some 73 percent of all new infections. Yet, only a few days later, the CDC clarified these numbers to claim that Omicron only represented 22.5 percent of infections, a dramatic decrease. A local doctor spoke out, furious:

> I don't know how many people throughout the country are dead, dying, in the hospital, or about to be hospitalized because of the mistakes that they just made. It's just the height of bureaucratic arrogance, and it's just, it's horrible. I had to turn friends away, family, people call me, "Oh, my uncle has cancer. Can he get an infusion?" I'm like, "I cannot give you an infusion because I will lose my medical license."[72]

At the same time that Democratic mouthpieces were attacking efforts to seek therapeutics, they were also actively censoring opposing voices and viewpoints. Platforms such as Instagram took to attaching labels or warnings to posts that mentioned the virus. Its parent company, Facebook, had announced in late 2020 that it would begin to censor content that had already been debunked by public health experts. Now, in 2021, it was

> widening the list of banned claims to include posts falsely claiming the virus is man-made or manufactured and that face masks don't prevent the spread of COVID. It's also banning false claims about vaccines in general that have long been in circulation despite being repeatedly debunked: that vaccines are toxic, dangerous or cause autism, that they are not effective, and that it's safer to get a disease than the vaccine meant to prevent it.[73]

At the same time, the company actively pushed pro-vaccine or internally approved public health stories onto its users. One researcher reported, "Facebook has removed 16 million pieces of its content and added warnings to around 167 million. YouTube has removed more than 850,000 videos related to 'dangerous or misleading covid-19 medical information.'"[74]

Obvious concerns over this practice soon arose as it seemed to lean more heavily on political alignment rather than science. In February of 2021, Facebook announced that false claims were being made that "COVID-19 is man-made or manufactured."[75] Yet, a few months later, as more evidence began to emerge that the virus possibly emerged from the Wuhan laboratory, the Biden administration begrudgingly began to investigate its origins. In response, Facebook announced in late May that it would no longer be censoring these posts or banning users who referenced its origins. As previously mentioned, various social media platforms also issued warnings about Republican rallies as "super-spreader events," while not including the phrase for Democratic-aligned protests. Finally, liberal-leaning sites were allowed to continue to publish unscientific opinions regarding the virus or its prevention, including a piece by CNN that linked organic food to efforts to prevent and contain the coronavirus.

Yet, apart from the obvious concerns over freedom of thought and speech associated with these moves, it also led to the stifling of scientific debate. During 2021, many established experts in the field of medicine and science saw their posts flagged, pages removed, or YouTube channels demonetized or banned for presenting contrarian opinions. In November of 2021, the Cochrane Collaboration, a network of 30,000 scientists, had its Instagram page removed for unspecified reasons, perhaps related to its review of data regarding the efficacy of ivermectin and masking.[76] In March of 2021, commentator Steven Crowder had an episode of his show removed by YouTube for violating its policy, "which prohibits content claiming that the death rates of Covid-19 are less severe or equally as severe as the common cold or seasonal flu."[77] This occurred despite the fact that Crowder was quoting from data directly provided by the CDC and WHO, which showed this to be the case for children and certain other groups.[78]

Two of the more notable scientists impacted by these moves were Dr. Brett Weinstein and Dr. Robert Malone. Professor Weinstein, a noted progressive in his politics, came out strongly against vaccinations for the virus and in favor of such treatments as ivermectin. In response, YouTube took down several of his videos and shadow-banned others. In an even more egregious case, Dr. Malone had his Twitter account suspended in December of 2021. Malone had been one of the early pioneers of the research needed to create mRNA vaccines. Yet, in 2020 he came out aggressively against the safety and effectiveness of the various mRNA vaccines being pushed on the public. Malone also attacked what he saw as the government's manipulation of the pandemic to further its own ends.

> ...what the heck happened in Germany in the 20s and 30s. Very intelligent, highly educated population, and they went barking mad. And how did that happen? The answer is mass formation psychosis. When you have a society that has become decoupled from each other, and has free floating anxiety, in a sense that things don't make sense. We can't understand it. And then their attention gets focused by a leader or series of events on one small point, just like hypnosis. They literally become hypnotized and can be led anywhere.[79]

In the end, both Trump and Biden largely relied upon the states to tackle the pandemic at a local level. As such, this allowed for varied experimentation on the best ways to confront the virus. Ideally, this should have been used to then inform and formulate regional or national strategies. Instead, Democrats quickly politicized the actions of various governors, with perhaps the most notable being Ron DeSantis of Florida and

Andrew Cuomo of New York. The states soon began to follow diametrically opposed paths driven as much by politics as by science.

Governor Cuomo, as a Democrat, was quickly embraced by liberal media as the epitome of concerned government response. In early April, ABC News ran an article detailing the day-to-day actions of the New York governor to tackle the virus, comparing it to selective examples of what Democrats claimed to be the inaction of the federal government.[80] Cuomo's administration quickly embraced mass testing; quarantines of entire towns; the shutting down of public gatherings, schools, and religious events; and the adoption of masking requirements. As one political advisor stated, "He's becoming America's daddy and America's son at a time when people's communities and relationships are falling apart. He's become the protector of the people from a bullet they can't see."[81] As part of this, the New York governor began to hold daily briefings that were compared by his supporters and some in the media to the fireside chats of President Roosevelt during the Great Depression.[82] Cuomo frequently attacked the president for what he saw as his failure during the crisis. In mid–March he announced that he was coordinating actions with the leaders of Connecticut and New Jersey. "This is not a war that can be won alone, which is why New York is partnering with our neighboring states to implement a uniform standard.... I have called on the federal government to implement nationwide protocols, but in their absence we are taking this on ourselves."[83]

The praise lavished on the governor continued well after his briefings came to a close in June of 2020. Rumors began to circulate in the spring of that year that he could be drafted as a presidential candidate for the Democratic party to replace the faltering and lackluster Joe Biden. Trump himself even noted that Cuomo would be a far more popular and successful opponent.[84] Speculation on swapping the two men continued well into the summer in both Republican and Democratic circles. Even after it became clear that this would not happen, Cuomo remained the most popular choice among liberals for a potential run in 2024.[85]

In November of 2020, the International Academy of Television Arts and Sciences announced it was an awarding an Emmy to Governor Cuomo for his daily briefings. According to the group's president, "The Governor's 111 daily briefings worked so well because he effectively created television shows, with characters, plot lines, and stories of success and failure. People around the world tuned in to find out what was going on, and *New York tough* became a symbol of the determination to fight back."[86] To conservatives, this merely continued the trend of the politicization of awards that had previously occurred with Al Gore's winning of an Emmy and Obama's Nobel Peace Prize. Cuomo also secured a lucrative $5 million book deal to write about his role as a leader during the pandemic.

At the same time that Cuomo was being praised, the Republican governor of Florida was being tarred and feathered in the media. Initially, Florida's response to the pandemic differed little from other states. Governor DeSantis declared a state of emergency on March 1, 2020, six days before a similar move by Cuomo. Likewise, he closed all bars and restaurants on March 17, only a day after Cuomo issued the same order. In addition, unlike New York, DeSantis early on moved to protect the very vulnerable nursing homes of the state. Despite this, many media outlets were quick to attack him for failing to close down the public beaches of the state, hinting that financial motives during the spring break period were trumping public health needs.[87] At the same time, a scathing editorial was run in the *Miami Herald* that bore the title "Coronavirus is killing us in Florida, Gov. DeSantis. Act like you give a damn."[88] Ironically, while DeSantis had done much to reduce the St. Patrick's Day revelry within the state, parades were still held in New York and New Jersey, with only New York City's famed one being pared down to several dozen unmasked people with a police escort. Also, Florida was one of the first states to enforce quarantines on visitors from out of state, particularly those who arrived from New York, doing so in mid–March. Finally, DeSantis issued a stay-at-home order for the entire state on April 1, only 11 days after a similar move in New York.

Yet, as Republicans quickly began to realize the failure of these measures, Florida and other states moved to abrogate the orders. Starting on May 4, 2020, many counties in Florida began to reopen. Complaints and protests erupted almost immediately. MSNBC's Rachel Maddow covered a group named Indivisible, which left body bags on the steps of the state capitol in protest. Despite this, case rates remained relatively steady until mid–June when a small surge occurred that eventually peaked on July 15. Over the summer and fall, DeSantis also announced the reopening of schools and restaurants, all of which were met by extreme vitriol from Democrats. Fauci opined that the state was "really asking for trouble. Now's the time actually to double down a bit."[89] Yet, despite these fears, Florida's subsequent spike during the fall and early winter of 2020 paralleled those of New York and other states that remained on lockdown, with both large states reaching 15,000-plus cases in early January of 2021. From there, rates largely continued to collapse until another surge in July and August of 2021 as the Delta variant hit the country.

Republican periodicals were quick to tout DeSantis as the model governor for their particular philosophy on the proper way to handle the pandemic. In March of 2021, *Politico* claimed that the governor had "won the pandemic," running an entire article detailing his strategies and successes.[90] The governor gradually moved to present himself as an alternative to the Democratic model of public health management. Florida vaccination rates equaled those of New York, California, and New Jersey both in terms of how quickly they reached over 50 percent of the population, as well as the percentages that they reached in age brackets over 18. At the same time, he took on overzealous local leaders by banning mask mandates and closures. DeSantis' focus on "freedom over Faucism" became a rallying cry for conservatives.[91]

Fears over Florida's actions among Democrats led to radical proposals from their local and national leaders. In mid–March of 2020, President Trump floated the idea of establishing a quarantine around the tristate area. "Some people would like to see New York quarantined because it's a hotspot—New York, New Jersey. I'm thinking about that right now. We might not have to do it, but there's a possibility that sometime today we'll do a quarantine—short-term, two weeks—on New York, probably New Jersey, certain parts of Connecticut."[92] Cuomo responded on March 28 by saying, "I don't even know what that means."[93] In the end, due to legal, economic, and practical considerations, the White House decided not to pursue this action, with the CDC simply recommending people avoid travel to these areas. Ironically, though, the governors of the three states themselves soon set up a system by which to categorize and quarantine people arriving from various other states that they considered to be hot spots. Not surprisingly, these were more often than not Republican states and those with different strategies for containment than New Jersey and New York.

Yet, the numbers of cases and deaths emerging from the two extreme camps told a very different story. By November of 2020, deaths from the virus in Florida stood at around 84 per 100,000 people, while the number in New York was 174 and New Jersey was at 181. Governors Cuomo and Murphy were presiding over the worst results of any state in the nation. It was around this time that Cuomo's heroic narrative also began to fall apart. Only two weeks after Cuomo's declaration of a state of emergency, his Department of Health issued a directive call for nursing homes to readmit patients who had been sent to hospitals due to the coronavirus as soon as they were able to be discharged. This was done purely to free up beds for the feared avalanche of cases that never occurred, and no requirement for testing was included. Even though the *Wall Street Journal* reported on the order only a day later, and quoted a doctor's group which said that the move "represents a clear and present danger to all of the residents of a nursing home," little attention was paid by the media or the public to the decision.[94] The administration clearly recognized the potential danger of the situation as the governor signed into law the budget for that year a week later, which granted increased legal protection to all nursing homes in the state.

By April, with deaths beginning to explode in elderly care facilities, some requested permission to send sick patients to either the makeshift hospital being constructed at the Javits Center in New York City or to the *Comfort* docked in the harbor; both requests were denied by Albany. Though Cuomo began to deny knowledge as questions began to mount, at the same time he publicly stated that nursing homes "don't have the right to object" to accepting back patients from the hospital. The governor went so far as to announce the launching of a probe into these facilities to make sure they were following his orders.[95] At the same time, staff who tested positive but were asymptomatic were told to report to work, further spreading the virus among the elderly. Though Cuomo quietly rescinded the order in early May, he continued to deny any wrongdoing and touted the success and low death numbers in the state.

Yet, over the summer of 2020, Republicans and concerned citizen groups began to challenge the prevailing narrative. While the state continued to report low death totals, independent reporting suggested far higher numbers. Cuomo quickly moved to claim he was either just following CDC protocols or else that any deaths that did occur were due to infected visitors who were not properly screened by the nursing homes.[96] While the state admitted to around 6,000 deaths in July, the Associated Press claimed that it was probably closer to 11,000 only a little over a month later.

In August, the state legislature began holding investigations to determine both the true number of deaths, as well as the extent of Cuomo's fault in the disaster that had secretly unfolded. They were soon joined in this by Trump's Department of Justice, which issued a formal request for documents and reports on August 26. In response to these moves, Cuomo publicly claimed that the president was "politicizing the deaths of people's loved ones."[97] Yet, attempts by both him and his deputies to stonewall the various investigations merely infuriated more New Yorkers.

In January of 2021, as reports of sexual harassment and assault by Cuomo began to surface, the state's attorney general, Letitia James, issued a report that claimed that Albany had undercounted pandemic deaths in the state by over 50 percent. Official tallies were increased to 12,473 and, only a few days later, these were again raised to 13,163. On February 10, 2021, Secretary to the Governor Melissa DeRosa held a closed-door meeting with Democratic lawmakers in which she apologized for the undercounting and stonewalling and raised the total figure still higher to over 15,000 deaths. Worse, though, her explanation was that Cuomo had ordered the undercount due to fears that Trump would use the number as a political weapon. "He starts tweeting that we killed everyone in nursing homes. He starts going after [New Jersey governor Phil] Murphy, starts going after [California governor Gavin] Newsom, starts going after [Michigan governor] Gretchen Whitmer."[98]

The assertion turned even many Democrats against the governor, most notably Assemblyman Ron Kim of Queens. As he publicly called for the governor to be stripped of his emergency powers, Cuomo lashed out, allegedly threatening to "destroy" Kim politically.[99] The Assembly soon moved to consider censuring Cuomo and finally stripped him of all extraordinary powers related to the pandemic on March 5. As further state and federal investigations were launched into both his handling of the pandemic as well as sexual harassment and assault claims, he moved to step down in August of 2021.

With the roll out of vaccination in December of 2020 and the inauguration of Biden the next month, Democrats began to heavily push the inoculations that they had once questioned. Yet, by the summer of 2021 it was becoming clear that resistance to the shot was preventing the full vaccination of the public. Despite this, by early August some 70 percent of the general population had been vaccinated, including 90 percent of those over the age of 65. Yet, Democrats were quick to place the blame for the continuing pandemic on the unvaccinated. Ideas of herd immunity and natural resistance were seen as Republican talking points and rejected for the counter notion of full vaccination of the public.

In December of 2020, president-elect Joe Biden announced that he would not support any mandates for vaccination once he was inaugurated. "No—I don't think it should be mandatory. I wouldn't demand it to be mandatory."[100] Yet, calls for just such a move began to emerge during the spring of 2021. Republican legislatures in various states, most notably Michigan, Wisconsin, and Missouri, quickly moved to prevent their governors from enacting any such mandate. These moves were largely lampooned by Democrats at the time. On March 29, the Biden administration, though, announced that it was investigating the concept of launching vaccine passports for all Americans, an idea that had been floated by some over the previous few months.

Beginning in the spring of 2021, many colleges and universities began to mandate vaccinations for students returning during the upcoming fall semester. In July, many medical groups were pushing for similar requirements for health care workers as well. On July 22, 2021, New York City did just that, requiring health-care workers to either show proof of vaccination or else undergo weekly testing. Within a few days, similar rules were put in place for the 115,000 health-care employees of the Department of Veterans Affairs, as well as all federal workers.

New York City continued to tighten its requirements, with Mayor DeBlasio putting in place the first proof-of-vaccine requirements in August. Now, all adults had to show proof of vaccination to enter public places or private businesses in the five boroughs. California imposed similar legislation with regards to health-care workers on August 6, and Los Angeles likewise imposed vaccine requirements to access all businesses in November.

By August, Fauci, who had previously spoken out against the need for vaccine mandates, now predicted their adoption, even for children.[101] Los Angeles soon did just that, mandating them for all schoolchildren in September. The federal government likewise moved to require vaccinations for all care facilities that received federal money in the way of Medicare or Medicaid, as well as all active duty members of the military. Then, on September 9, 2021, President Biden undertook the most extreme vaccine mandate ever in American history. Relying upon the regulatory powers of OSHA, the administration moved to require all businesses that employ over 100 people to require vaccinations or weekly testing for all workers. In total, this would impact the lives of over 80 million Americans. By December, some Democrats began to call for vaccine mandates and testing for domestic flights as well.

By November, various groups and states had begun to launch lawsuits against these rules. Over the next two months, lower-level courts and circuit courts alternatively struck down or allowed the mandates, culminating in the *NFIB v. OSHA* case before the Supreme Court. Apart from the arguments over the potential dangers involved or the very need for it, conservatives pushed back against the perceived overreach of the executive branch. For many, this was best exemplified by a tweet that was shared by Ron Klain, the White House chief of staff, which said that the OSHA mandate was the "'ultimate work-around for the Federal gov't to require vaccinations."[102] The idea that Democrats were using a government agency to bypass either Congress or the Constitution was too much for many but showed the limits to which fear of disease could be used to increase the power and reach of government. It was for these reasons that the Court subsequently struck down the mandate.

The pandemic of 2020, much like the Great Depression, revealed and expanded stark and fundamental differences between the two major political parties in America. While one resisted calls for government intervention, moved to downplay the dangers, and placed the impetus for action on the states and ultimately individuals, the other moved to nationalize and standardize responses, increase the scope and size of government, and institutionalize these changes for years to come.

Conclusion

In Murray Rothbard's 1974 work *Anatomy of the State*, he argues that the state's existence is predicated on convincing the public that its role is not only legitimate but required. Historically, this has been done through attaching religious, social, or genealogical purpose to the ruling body. The king was needed to satisfy the gods, prevent imminent social disruption, or serve as the only viable choice for a leader due to his pedigree. Modern countries have instead relied upon a combination of economic, social, or political arguments to justify their existence, embracing the notion of a social contract or the doctrine of positive liberty as a justification for their existence. Yet, at the same time, government has often been an expansive organism. Politicians, bureaucrats, and parties have sought to expand both their own power as well as the overall size of the system. Some of this has been due to genuine belief that government is the solution to problems, while much of it can be attributed to greed, a desire for power and influence, and even much more sinister reasons. Justification for this has come from utilizing a number of perceived or actual threats against the state, including foreign invasion, internal rebellion, and climatic change. As this book has shown, another often utilized force is disease. The power of illness and the terror that it often causes in the general public has been used by politicians and parties to push for vast expansions of federal authority. Civilization caused the growth of disease, disease necessitated the growth of civilization, and fears of it has expanded the reach of government.

While not all governmental attempts to increase its power to tackle disease have been negative or self-serving, a narrative does emerge in America's 400-year-long battle with pestilence. The earliest efforts by the government tended to be aimed at reducing the presence and spread of illness through classical means. These included the enforcement of regional quarantines and a reliance upon time-tested methods. Early paternalistic efforts at improving public health arose beginning around the time of the Revolution but still tended to be confined to periods of extreme necessity such as during epidemics or in wartime. Thus, Washington's efforts at variolation in the Continental Army were not meant to be the start of a national trend but merely a calculated and potentially dangerous campaign to prevent a larger disaster during the war. For the first several decades of the country's existence, local governments did their best to limit the danger posed by radical and new scientific ideas in disease management. This can be seen as late as the Civil War when a dispute arose between the surgeon general and army doctors over the use of anesthesia during surgery.

This began to change, though, in the late 19th century. While Radical Republicans did push for some sanitary reforms and internal improvements in the north, the roots of this governmental push toward engaging in disease management tended to be dominated by the Progressive and Democratic Parties. From the early attempts by the Know Nothings in Massachusetts to enact radical legislation to engage in public health management up to the 21st century, the left in America has attempted to use legislative, executive, and judicial power to confront disease and grow the size of government. While some of this was built off of the genuine belief that state and later federal institutions were best positioned to handle epidemics and pandemics, some was purely political in nature.

The problem of the claim by some that the government was simply "following the science" emerges from either a misunderstanding or perversion of the word itself. As Ludwig von Mises and others have famously argued, science tells what is, not what ought. Science presents facts regarding a singular issue, facts that can be challenged and can change over time, facts that do not take into consideration issues of economics, politics, morality, religion, and a host of other topics. Science is merely one variable that should be taken into consideration by a leader when making a decision; it is not meant to be the sole one. Yet, beginning with the rise of Positivism in the 19th century, rule by science has been embraced by many, moving it from the realm of debatable facts to that of dogmatic belief. It has become religion for some and a cudgel for others, a club used to beat back opposition and reduce opponents to submission.

Additionally, what constitutes "scientific fact" can also vary by generation. Today's science can easily become tomorrow's pseudoscience. This can be seen in such formerly popular notions as eugenics and phrenology. Likewise, some in medicine have traditionally utilized it to produce racist myths to help perpetuate social and political beliefs. An example of this was Dr. Samuel Cartwright's work on drapetomania in the 19th century, which sought to label attempts by slaves to flee north as products of mental illness or a physical disease. Scientists themselves can become subservient to political ideology, dependent upon funding, and are not infallible.

Finally, with science often being an arena of competing ideas, the "science" and facts that a political party chooses to follow may not be the only ones out there.

Disease presented a unique opportunity for politicians, particularly those on the political left, to grant themselves additional powers, and they have done so for over a century. Leaders were careful to couch these moves under claims of compassion and being proactive, while casting their opponents as anti-science or uncaring. Debates over government-funded health care in the shape of Medicare, Medicaid, or "Obamacare" would follow similar lines.

Yet, disease did not always produce a political divide between the parties, with perhaps the best example being the Spanish influenza pandemic of 1918. While debate ensued in 1918 and early 1919 over spending bills designed to help combat the outbreak, these were largely typical of political maneuvering. In fact, Congress quickly passed a $1 million aid package in late September of 1918 with little discussion. A month later, as hundreds of members either fell sick or fled the city, including Speaker of the House Champ Clark and Majority Leader Claude Kitchin, a gentlemen's agreement was reached to ignore the lack of quorum in the House in order to establish a Public Health Service Reserve Corps. Only one lone Republican from Massachusetts objected to the blatantly unconstitutional move before being convinced otherwise by his fellow party members. Indeed, two Congressmen would die of the illness over the next few months. Further deaths in the late summer of 1919 would again spur additional bipartisan action by the government as well. As with the yellow fever epidemic of 1793 or the experiences of Jackson and Clay during the cholera pandemic, politicians often discounted with politics when their own lives were threatened by the diseases that they hoped to use for leverage.

More often than not, as this history has shown, it is the party out of power who attempts to politicize disease the most. It is a useful, feared, and effective weapon by which to gain power. Republicans weaponized Ebola and Democrats did Covid; it is only the magnitude that tends to vary. There are no political angels in this history, only lesser degrees of opportunism.

But the dangers of the politicization of disease can clearly be seen over the last two centuries. Perhaps nothing is more feared than uncertain illness and death and, when this is preyed upon by those in power or those seeking power, it becomes a dangerous tool. Time and time again, people have been willing to give up rights and liberties or ignore injustices in the name of safety and protection. The rise of fascism in Europe was predicated in part upon the concept of the diseased, filthy, and different "other" and the need to confront them. A survey conducted in January of 2022 showed Democratic voters favoring harsh policies in order to combat the pandemic. Around half supported fining the unvaccinated, forcibly detaining the unvaccinated, constructing camps for the unvaccinated, tracking them, and the move to "fine or imprison individuals who publicly question the efficacy of the existing COVID-19 vaccines."[1] Almost 30 percent or Democrats also favored stripping parents of custody rights as well if they refused the vaccine. These represent harsh and totalitarian moves that clearly are catalyzed by fear of the disease.

Illness has been used to identify, isolate, and target groups and enemies. History is replete with famous examples of this, with perhaps the most well known being the targeting of Jews during the Black Death. Yet this is far from an ancient problem. America's unique geographic position that sees most epidemics arrive from overseas and its history of immigration has naturally led to outbreaks of illness being accompanied by xenophobic reaction. These connections have continued into the modern era and become intertwined with debates over the southern border. Likewise, Democrats have sought to label and target those who refused vaccines, mandates, or masking during the most recent pandemic. President Biden and others religiously claimed, "This continues to be a pandemic of the unvaccinated," despite all data showing otherwise during the winter of 2021–2022.[2] This is reminiscent of Soviet, state-sponsored doctors claiming that opponents of the regime were at a higher risk of developing mental illness, specifically "sluggish schizophrenia."[3]

The fear of the politicization of disease is not simply a matter of concern for those who hesitate to expand the power of government. The loss of liberty and freedom that occurs in the process is usually nonreversible. Even worse, the terror that is often fomented among the populace can easily lead to exclusion, ostracism, violence, and even mass slaughter. These are hardly new reactions to disease but are deep-seated and somewhat natural responses that have often erupted into practice throughout human history. The politicization of disease can be a dangerous element that awakens primitive and violent reactions to pestilence.

A citizen's best tool against all of the politicization and problems addressed in this book remains knowledge. Accurate and factual information regarding illnesses, human biology, risks, and the proper roles and abilities of government would help to prevent many of the negative outcomes that have occurred or could occur in the country during times of sickness. A proper understanding of the risks inherent in a particular disease would often times serve to reduce the overreaction that allows for and even encourages this politicization.

Disease is a threat to humanity, but like all others, there are ways to approach it and manage it so that the cure does not cause greater destruction than the problem itself. Paracelsus' old adage of "sola dosis facit venenum" (it is only the dosage that makes it venomous) has taken on new meaning in our political landscape where the democratic process is often more poisonous than the disease.

Chapter Notes

Introduction

1. Kristin Harper and George Armelagos, "The Changing Disease-Scape in the Third Epidemiological Transition," *International Journal of Environmental Research and Public Health* 7 (2010): 682.

Chapter I

1. Quoted in Lauren Johnson, *So Great a Prince* (New York: Pegasus, 2017).
2. Donna E. Stewart, "Anorexia Nervosa, Bulimia, and Pregnancy," *American Journal of Obstetrics and Gynecology* 157, no. 5 (Nov. 1987): 1194–1198.
3. Giles Tremlett, "Was Henry VIII's First Wife Anorexic? Catherine of Aragon's Secret Problem," *Daily Mail* (Nov. 5, 2010), and Steven McIntosh, "Charli Howard: Is this really a 'plus-size' model?," *BBC* (March 7, 2018).
4. Noble David Cook, *Born to Die: Disease and New World Conquest* (Cambridge: Cambridge University Press, 1998), 25.
5. See Robert McCaa, "Spanish and Nahuatl Views on Smallpox and Demographic Catastrophe in Mexico," *Journal of Interdisciplinary History* 25, no. 3 (Winter 1995): 397–431, for a full discussion of Spanish sources.
6. Bernal Diaz del Castillo, *The Discovery and Conquest of Mexico 1517–1521* (London: Hatchard and Son, 1864), 332–333.
7. Rodolfo Acuna-Soto et al., "Large Epidemics of Hemorrhagic Fevers in Mexico, 1545–1815," *American Journal of Tropical Medicine and Hygiene* 62, no. 6 (2000): 733–739.
8. Arthur Helps, *The Spanish Conquest in America*, Vol. II (New York: Harper, 1856), 30.
9. James Lockhart, "The Central Areas During and After the Conquest," in John R. Herbert, *An Ongoing Voyage: 1492–1992* (Washington, D.C.: Library of Congress, 1992), 132.
10. Daniel Defoe, *A Journal of the Plague Year* (London: E. Nutt, 1722), 1–2.
11. See René Jara and Nicholas Spadaccini, *Amerindian Images and the Legacy of Columbus* (Minneapolis: University of Minnesota Press, 1992), 711, and John Armstrong Crow, *The Epic of Latin America* (Berkeley: University of California Press, 1992), 237, 279, 535.
12. Crow, *Epic of Latin America*, 279 and 535.
13. Wilcomb E. Washburn, *The Indian in America* (New York: Harper and Row, 1975), 105.
14. Adrienne Mayor, "The Nessus Shirt in the New World: Smallpox Blankets in History and Legend," *Journal of American Folklore* 108, no. 427 (Winter 1995): 54–77.
15. Quoted in Mayor, "Nessus Shirt," 57.
16. Thomas Hariot, *A Brief and True Report of the New Found Land of Virginia* (1588).
17. See Peter B. Mires, "Contact and Contagion: The Roanoke Colony and Influenza," *Historical Archaeology* 28, no. 3 (1994).
18. John Smith, *The General History of Virginia*.
19. Harleian MSS., B.M., 388, fo. 188; *Publications of the Colonial Society of Massachusetts*, VII. 71–72.
20. John S. Marr, "New Hypothesis

for Cause of Epidemic among Native Americans, New England, 1616-1619," *EID Journal: Historical Review* 16, no. 2 (Feb. 2010), http://wwwnc.cdc.gov/eid/article/16/2/09-0276_article.htm.

21. See Charles Manning and Merrill Moore, "Sassafras and Syphilis," *The New England Quarterly* 9, no. 3 (Sept. 1936): 473-475.

22. Cushman's *Discourse* (Dec. 1621), 4.

23. Martha J. Lamb, *History of the City of New York: Its Origin, Rise, and Progress*, Vol. I (New York: A.S. Barnes, 1876), 200.

Chapter II

1. An outbreak of the disease in London in 1720 would kill around 3,000 people out of a population of 600,000, while the 1721 outbreak in Boston would send 850 to their graves from a city of only 11,000.

2. Deer Island was later used for a similar purpose during the Irish migration of the 1840s.

3. David Kales, *The Boston Harbor Islands: A History of an Urban Wilderness* (Charleston: The History Press, 2007), 36-37.

4. Arthur Boylston, "The Origins of Inoculation," *Journal of the Royal Society of Medicine* 105, no. 7 (July 2012): 309-313.

5. "E. Timonius, An account of history, of the procuring the small pox by incision, or inoculation: as it has for some time been practised at Constantinople. Being the extract of a Letter from Emanuel Timonius, Oxon and Patav. M.D. F.R.S, dated at Constantinople, December 1713," *Philosophical Transactions of the Royal Society* 29 (1714): 72-82.

6. Quoted in Boylston, "Origins of Inoculation," 309-310.

7. Cotton Mather, *Diary* (May 26, 1721).

8. William Douglass and Alexander Stuart, *The Abuses and Scandals of Some Late Pamphlets in Favour of Inoculation of the Small Pox* (Boston: James Franklin, 1722), 8.

9. William Douglass, "Anti-Inoculation Letter" by 'W. Philanthroper,'" *New England Courant* (July 17, 1721).

10. William Douglass, "Anti-Inoculation Letter," *New England Courant* (Aug. 14, 1721).

11. Frank Scammony, "Anti-Inoculation Letter," *New England Courant* (Aug. 21, 1721).

12. Wilson George Smillie, *Public Health, Its Promise for the Future*, 25.

13. Cotton Mather, *Diary* (July 16, 1721).

14. William Douglass, *The Abuses and Scandals of Some Late Pamphlets in Favour of Inoculation of the Small Pox*, 10-11.

15. Ellen Starr Brinton, "The Rogerenes," *The New England Quarterly* 16, no. 1 (1943): 3-19.

16. Letter from John Adams to Abigail Smith, 13 April 1764 [electronic edition], *Adams Family Papers: An Electronic Archive*, Massachusetts Historical Society, http://www.masshist.org/digitaladams/.

17. Alice Morse Earle wrote of various romances that would spring up among men and women during these periods of inoculation-induced isolation and revelry in her *Customs and Fashions in Old New England* (1893).

18. John Smith was a second-cousin of George Washington, himself an ardent supporter of the process.

19. Hippocrates, *The Law*.

20. Anne R. Davis, "Distempers and Physic Virginia's Health in the Eighteenth Century," *Northern Neck of Virginia Historical Society* 66 (2016): 8285.

21. Suzanne Shultz, "Epidemics in Colonial Philadelphia," *Early American Review* (Winter/Spring 2007).

22. Benjamin Franklin, "On the Death of His Son," *The Pennsylvania Gazette* (Dec. 30, 1736) in *The Papers of Benjamin Franklin*, vol. 2, *January 1, 1735, through December 31, 1744*, ed. Leonard W. Labaree (New Haven: Yale University Press, 1961), 154.

23. Davis, "Distempers and Phisic," 8285.

24. "From Thomas Jefferson to George C. Jenner, 14 May 1806," *Founders Online*, National Archives, https://founders.archives.gov/documents/Jefferson/99-01-02-3718.

25. "Meeting Minutes of University of Virginia Board of Visitors, 3-7 April 1826, 3 April 1826," *Founders Online*, National Archives, https://founders.archives.gov/documents/Jefferson/98-01-02-6013.

26. George Washington to President of Congress (Dec. 19, 1775).

27. Archibald Cary to R.H. Lee (Dec. 24, 1775).

28. George Washington, as quoted by Shaul G. Massry et al., "History of Nephrology," *The American Journal of Nephrology* 17 (1997), 233–240.
29. George Washington to William Shippen (Jan. 6, 1777).
30. The operation only took in one child, with the other needing three attempts at a good amount of wine to speed along the process.
31. "Bill concerning Inoculation for Smallpox (27 December 1777)," *The Papers of Thomas Jefferson*, vol. 2, *1777–18 June 1779*, ed. Julian P. Boyd (Princeton: Princeton University Press, 1950), 122–124.
32. Johann David Schoepff, *The Climate and Diseases of America* (Boston: Houghton, 1875).
33. "From Alexander Hamilton to Daniel Jackson, 14 June 1799," *Founders Online*, National Archives, https://founders.archives.gov/documents/Hamilton/02-01-02-0516.
34. "John Quincy Adams to Thomas Boylston Adams, 2 September 1792,' in *The Adams Papers*, Adams Family Correspondence, vol. 9, *January 1790–December 1793*, ed. C. James Taylor (Cambridge: Harvard University Press, 2009), 303–304.

Chapter III

1. Harlow G. Unger, *John Hancock: Merchant King and American Patriot* (New York: Wiley, 2000), 66–68.
2. William M. Fowler, *The Baron of Beacon Hill: A Biography of John Hancock* (Boston: Houghton Mifflin, 1980), 170.
3. "From John Adams to Timothy Pickering, 6 August 1822," *Founders Online*, National Archives, https://founders.archives.gov/documents/Adams/99-02-02-7674.
4. See Donald J. Proctor, "John Hancock: New Soundings on an Old Barrel," *The Journal of American History* 64, no. 3 (Dec. 1977): 669–670, for a full treatment of this claim.
5. "To George Washington from John Hancock, 25 October 1777," *The Papers of George Washington*, Revolutionary War Series, vol. 11, *19 August 1777–25 October 1777*, ed. Philander D. Chase and Edward G. Lengel (Charlottesville: University Press of Virginia, 2001), 614–615.

6. *Boston Gazette* (Aug. 15, 1774).
7. Alden Bradford, *History of Massachusetts* (Boston: Wells and Lilly, 1825), 19.
8. John Quincy Adams to Abigail Adams (Aug. 27, 1785).
9. Henry Knox to George Washington (Oct. 23, 1786).
10. "From James Madison to James Madison, Sr., 1 April 1787," *The Papers of James Madison*, vol. 9, *9 April 1786–24 May 1787 and supplement 1781–1784*, ed. Robert A. Rutland and William M.E. Rachal (Chicago: University of Chicago Press, 1975), 358–361.
11. "The Federalist No. 21 [12 December 1787]," *The Papers of Alexander Hamilton*, vol. 4, *January 1787–May 1788*, ed. Harold C. Syrett (New York: Columbia University Press, 1962), 396–401.
12. Alfred Owen Aldridge, *Benjamin Franklin: Philosopher and Man* (Philadelphia: Lippincott, 1965), 400.
13. Donald R. Hopkins, *The Greatest Killer: Smallpox in History* (Chicago: University of Chicago Press, 2002), 243.
14. Rufus King to George Thatcher (Jan. 20, 1788).
15. Rufus King to Henry Knox (Feb. 3, 1788).
16. *Hamlet*, Act I, Scene V.
17. Agence France-Presse, "Doctor Says Yeltsin Faked Illness," *New York Times* (April 24, 1999).
18. Robert E. Gilbert, *The Mortal Presidency: Illness and Anguish in the White House* (Fordham University Press, 1998), 89.
19. "Good Behavior Wins President Sixth Star," *St. Petersburg Times* (Oct. 23, 1955), 1.
20. *St. Petersburg Times* (Oct. 23, 1955), 1.
21. Richard Nixon, *Six Crises* (New York: Doubleday, 1962), 138.
22. "A Timeline of Trump's Battle with COVID-19," *CNN* (Oct. 12, 2020).
23. See J.K. Kar et al., "Vaso-epididymal anastomosis," *Fertility and Sterility*, no. 26 (1975): 743–756; W.H. Ropper et al., "Primary Serofibrinous Pleural Effusion in Military Personnel," *American Review of Tuberculosis*, no. 71 (1955): 616–634; G.J. Gorse et al., "Male Genital Tuberculosis: A Review of the Literature with Instructive Case Reports," *Review of Infectious Disease*, no. 7 (1985): 511–524; and W.I.

Christensen, "Genitourinary Tuberculosis: Review of 102 Cases," *Medicine*, no. 53 (1974): 377–390.
    24. James McHenry to George Washington (March 29, 1789).
    25. Lewis Nicola to George Washington (May 22, 1782).
    26. Francis Lieber, *On Civil Liberty and Self-Government* (Philadelphia: Lippincott, 1874), 257.
    27. George Washington to Lewis Nicola (May 22, 1782).
    28. Ron Chernow, "George Washington: The Reluctant President," *Smithsonian Magazine* (Feb. 2011).

Chapter IV

    1. William Joseph Birken, "The Royal College of Physicians of London and Its Support of the Parliamentary Cause in the English Civil War," *Journal of British Studies* 23, no. 1 (Autumn 1983): 47–62.
    2. John Winthrop, *Journal* (June 1647).
    3. The Rev. Samuel Megapolensis to a Friend (Sept. 7, 1668), in *Documents of the Senate of the State of New York*, Vol. 14 (Albany: J.B. Lyon, 1902), 597.
    4. "Minutes of the Executive Council of the Province of New York: Administration of Francis Lovelace, 1668–1673" (Albany: State of New York, 1910), 21.
    5. James Madison, *Federalist No. 10*.
    6. One of these ships, the *Hankey*, became notorious for allegedly bringing yellow fever from the coast of West Africa to the Caribbean the previous year. From there both it and other ships then spread the disease around the region. See Billy G. Smith, *Ship of Death: A Voyage That Changed the Atlantic World* (New Haven: Yale University Press, 2013), for a full account of the *Hankey*.
    7. Isaac Cathrall, *A Medical Sketch of the Synochus Maligna* (Philadelphia: T. Dobson, 1794), 1–2.
    8. Thomas Jefferson to Thomas Mann Randolph Jr. (Sept. 2, 1793).
    9. Mathew Carey, *A short account of the malignant fever, lately prevalent in Philadelphia: with a statement of the proceedings that took place on the subject, in different parts of the United States, to which are added, accounts of the plague in London and Marseilles, and a list of the dead from August 1, to the middle of December, 1793*, 17–19.
    10. Joanna Brooks, *American Lazarus: Religion and the Rise of African-American and Native American Literatures* (Oxford: Oxford University Press, 2003), 168.
    11. Mathew Carey would go on to publish in his famous tract on the outbreak accusations that these local black Philadelphians had profiteered off of the disease and had even robbed the homes of those who were ill. Absalom Jones would himself publish a reply titled *A Narrative of the Proceedings of the Black People*.
    12. Carey, *A short account of the malignant fever*, 19.
    13. George Washington to Henry Knox (Sept. 9, 1793).
    14. George Washington to Lear (Sept. 10, 1793).
    15. Carey, *A short account of the malignant fever*, 32.
    16. Rush, 199.
    17. *Ibid.*, 195.
    18. Jacquelyn Miller, "The Body Politic and the Body Somatic: Benjamin Rush's Fear of Social Disorder and His Treatment of Yellow Fever," in Janet Moore Lindman, *A Centre of Wonders: The Body in Early America* (Ithaca: Cornell University Press, 2001), 61–65.
    19. Timothy Dwight to Oliver Wolcott (Oct. 26, 1794).
    20. Rush, 211.
    21. *Ibid.*, 328.
    22. Clements E. Markham, *Peruvian Bark: A Popular Account of the Introduction of Chinchona Cultivation into British India 1860–1880* (London: John Murray, 1880), 54–55.
    23. Carey, *A short account of the malignant fever*, 16–17.
    24. Thomas Jefferson to James Madison (Sept. 1, 1793).
    25. See Martin Pernick's "Politics, Parties, and Pestilence: Epidemic Yellow Fever in Philadelphia and the Rise of the First Party System" for a statistical treatment of this idea.
    26. Timothy Pickering to George Washington (Oct. 21, 1793).
    27. A notable exception was the former mayor, Samuel Powel, who died from the illness after tending to the sick.

28. Carey, "A short account of the malignant fever," 60.
29. Philip Freneau, 'Pestilence."

Chapter V

1. Wallabout Committee, *An Account of the Internment of the Remains of 11,500 American Seamen, Soldiers, and Citizens, who Fell Victims to the Cruelties of the British On Board their Prison Ships at the Wallabout* (New York: Frank, White, and Co. for the Tammany Society, 1808), 86.
2. From Robert Sheffield as quoted in John Warner Barber, *Connecticut Historical Collections, Containing a General Collection of Interesting Facts, Traditions, Biographical Sketches, Anecdotes, Etc. Relating to the History and Antiquities of Every Town in Connecticut* (New Haven: Durrie and Peck, 1945), 286–287.
3. As reported in the *Boston Gazette* in August of 1781.
4. Philip Morin Freneau, *An Historical Sketch, to the End of the Revolutionary War, of the Life of Silas Talbot* (New York: G. & R. Waite, 1803), 107.
5. Philip Freneau, "The Prison Ship."
6. "From Thomas Jefferson to Pierre Samuel Du Pont de Nemours, 14 July 1807," *Founders Online,* National Archives, https://founders.archives.gov/documents/Jefferson/99-01-02-5960.
7. Philip Freneau, "The Prison Ship."
8. "To Thomas Jefferson from Benjamin Romaine, 11 January 1808," *Founders Online,* National Archives, https://founders.archives.gov/documents/Jefferson/99-01-02-7185
9. Wallabout Committee, *An Account of the Internment,* 50.
10. Ibid., 54 and 57.
11. "To James Madison from Morgan Lewis, 7 September 1808," *Founders Online,* National Archives, https://founders.archives.gov/documents/Madison/99-01-02-3502.
12. Orren Chalmer Hormell, "The Attitude of the Federalist Party Toward the War of 1812," thesis (June 1905), 62.
13. *The Enquirer* (Jan. 14, 1813), 1.
14. *The Portland Gazette and Maine Advertiser* (Nov. 2, 1812), 3.
15. *The Enquirer* (Jan. 9, 1813), 2.
16. Ibid.

17. *New York Evening Post* (Jan. 4, 1813), 4.
18. *New York Evening Post* (Jan. 13, 1813), 1.
19. *Ontario Repository* (Jan. 19, 1813), 3.
20. *The Enquirer* (Jan. 14, 1813), 1.
21. *The Buffalo Gazette* (Feb. 2, 1813), 3.
22. *New York Evening Post* (Feb. 2, 1813), 2.
23. *The Buffalo Whig* (Feb. 17, 1813).
24. *Centinel* (Dec. 17, 1813).

Chapter VI

1. James Fenimore Cooper to William Gore Ouseley (July 23, 1832), in James Franklin Beard, ed., *The Letters and Journals of James Fenimore Cooper,* Vol. II (Boston: Belknap, 1960), 278–279.
2. *Rhode Island Republican* (July 19, 1831), 2.
3. *Phenix Gazette* (Alexandria) (Feb. 7, 1832), 3.
4. Ibid. (Jan. 19, 1832), 2.
5. *Plattsburgh Republican* (Jan. 28, 1832), 2.
6. *Constitutional Whig* (May 29, 1832), 1.
7. *Phenix Gazette* (May 31, 1832), 3.
8. *Plattsburgh Republican* (Jan. 28, 1832), 2.
9. *Constitutional Whig* (May 15, 1832), 2.
10. *Phenix Gazette* (May 21, 1832), 3.
11. See *Plattsburgh Republican* (June 16, 1832), 2, and *Long Island Farmer, and Queens County Advertiser* (July 10, 1832), 4, for two early examples.
12. Charles E. Rosenberg, *The Cholera Years: The United States in 1832, 1849, and 1866* (Chicago: University of Chicago Press, 1962), 79.
13. *Evening Post* (New York) (Feb. 3, 1832).
14. Ibid. (June 16, 1832).
15. Ashleigh R. Tuite, "Cholera, Canals, and Contagion: Re-discovering Dr. Beck's Report," *Journal of Public Health Policy* 32, no. 3 (Aug. 2011), 320–333.
16. Richard Adler, *Cholera in Detroit* (Jefferson, NC: McFarland, 2013), 22.
17. *New York Evening Post* (1832), as quoted in John Noble Wilford, "How

Epidemics Helped Shape the Modern Metropolis," *New York Times* (April 15, 2008).

18. Jon Meacham, *American Lion: Andrew Jackson in the White House* (New York: Random House, 2009), 216. Jackson's inclusion of the term "irregular habits" showed his belief in the standard medical theories of the time as to the vectoring of cholera.

19. *Rhode Island Republican* (Aug. 28, 1832), 3.

20. *Columbia Gazetteer* (Oct. 19, 1793).

21. Addison A. to Sanford Ferguson (July 18, 1832), in *The Ferguson-Jayne Papers, 1826–1938*, ed. Mary S. Briggs (Interlaken, NY: Heart of the Lakes Publishing, 1981), 80.

22. Quoted in Philip Hamburger, *Separation of Church and State* (Cambridge: Harvard University Press, 2004), 185.

23. Andrew Jackson to the Synod of the Reformed Church, June 12, 1832, reprinted in John Spencer Bassett, ed. *Correspondence of Andrew Jackson*, Vol. IV (Washington, D.C.: Carnegie Institution, 1929), 447.

24. Adam Jortner, "Cholera, Christ, and Jackson: The Epidemic of 1832 and the Origins of Christian Politics in Antebellum America," *Journal of the Early Republic* 27, no. 2 (Summer 2007), 27.

25. Henry Clay Remarks in the Senate (June 25, 1832), in *The Papers of Henry Clay, Vol. 8* (Lexington: University of Kentucky Press, 2015), 545.

26. *Richmond Enquirer* (July 27, 1832), 4.

27. Peter Bragdon, "The Bottle on the Hill: Times—and People—Have Changed," *LA Times* (March 12, 1989).

28. Henry Clay to James Brown (Oct. 23, 1832), in *The Papers of Henry Clay, Vol. 8*, 587.

29. Henry Clay to James Brown (Oct. 23, 1832), in *The Papers of Henry Clay, Vol. 8*, 587.

30. Henry Clay to Alexander Coffin (June 11, 1834), in *The Papers of Henry Clay, Vol. 8*, 725.

31. *The Corrector* (Sept. 8, 1832), 2.

32. *Plattsburgh Republican* (Sept. 1, 1832), 2.

33. *Rhode Island Republican* (Aug. 7, 1832), 2.

Chapter VII

1. *Alexandria Daily Advertiser* (Nov. 27, 1804), 2.
2. *Portland Gazette and Maine Advertiser* (Feb. 22, 1808), 3.
3. *The Enquirer* (April 23, 1813), 1.
4. *Daily Madisonian* (Dec. 12, 1837), 2.
5. *Mississippi Democrat* (April 8, 1846), 3.
6. *The New York Herald* (Dec. 31, 1842), 5.
7. *Daily Madisonian* (June 28, 1843), 2.
8. *New York Daily Tribune* (June 29, 1843), 2.
9. *Richmond Enquirer* (July 14, 1843), 2.
10. *Sunbury American Journal* (July 29, 1843), 2.
11. Henry Clay to John M. Berrien (Sept. 4, 1843).
12. *Alexandria Gazette* (July 22, 1843), 3.
13. *New York Daily Tribune* (July 24, 1843), 2, and *Brooklyn Daily Eagle* (July 17, 1843), 2.
14. *Auburn Journal* (July 19, 1843), 3.
15. *Richmond Daily Whig* (Dec. 20, 1843), 2.
16. *Jeffersonian Republican* (Sept. 14, 1843), 2.
17. *Cecil Whig* (April 13, 1844), 1.
18. *Cecil Whig* (Nov. 9, 1844), 1.
19. *Delaware Gazette* (June 25, 1845), 1.
20. *Weekly Hawk-eye and Telegraph* (June 24, 1857), 1.
21. *Richmond Palladium* (Nov. 14, 1867), 3.
22. *The Wheeling Daily Intelligencer* (April 4, 1871), 4.
23. "The Tyler Grip," *Los Angeles Daily Herald* (Dec. 29, 1889), 8.
24. "The World Wide Influenza," *Johnstown Weekly Democrat* (Jan. 10, 1890), 4.
25. Benson Lossing, ed., *The Diary of George Washington: 1789–1791* (New York: Richardson and Co., 1860), 35.
26. *The Sun* (Sept. 20, 1918), 6.
27. *Evening Capital* (March 5, 1885), 1.
28. *The Hillsdale Whig Standard* (May 8, 1849), 2.
29. *Wilmington Journal* (Aug. 17, 1849), 2.
30. *The Spirit of Democracy* (Aug. 18, 1849), 3.
31. *Southern Sentinel* (Sept. 12, 1849), 2.
32. *The Daily Union* (Sept. 25, 1849), 3.

33. *New York Herald* (Aug. 9, 1850), 1.
34. *The Eastern Clarion* (April 27, 1859), 2.
35. *The Bedford Gazette* (April 20, 1855), 1.
36. "Lament of a Know Nothing," *The Independent Press* (June 29, 1855), 2.
37. *True American* (Aug. 22, 1855), 2.
38. "Pelosi Calls Coronavirus the 'Trump virus,'" *The Hill* (July 21, 2020), https://thehill.com/homenews/house/508449-pelosi-refers-to-coronavirus-as-the-trump-virus.
39. Mehdi Hasan on "The Reidout," *MSNBC* (Sept. 20, 2020).

Chapter VIII

1. Farley Grubb, "Morbidity and Mortality on the North Atlantic Passage: Eighteenth-Century German Immigration," *The Journal of Interdisciplinary History* 17, no. 3 (Winter 1987): 568; and Frank Diffenderffer, "The German Immigration into Pennsylvania Through the Port of Philadelphia," *Proceedings of the Pennsylvania-German Society*, Vol. 10 (Lancaster, PA, 1900), 260.
2. Billy G. Smith, "Death and Life in a Colonial Immigrant City: A Demographic Analysis of Philadelphia," *The Journal of Economic History*, Vol. 37, No. 4 (May 2010): 872n.
3. Grubb, "Morbidity and Mortality," 574.
4. Ibid., 579.
5. Ibid., 581.
6. "Pennsylvania Assembly: Reply to the Governor, 15 May 1755," *The Papers of Benjamin Franklin*, vol. 6, *April 1, 1755, through September 30, 1756*, ed. Leonard W. Labaree (New Haven: Yale U P, 1963), 38–41.
7. Ibid.
8. Ben Franklin, "Observations Concerning the Increase of Mankind, 1751," *The Papers of Benjamin Franklin*, vol. 4, *July 1, 1750, through June 30, 1753*, ed. Leonard W. Labaree (New Haven: Yale U P, 1961), 234.
9. "Introduction to John Pringle's Account of Gaol Fever, 4 September 1755," *The Papers of Benjamin Franklin*, vol. 6, *April 1, 1755, through September 30, 1756*, ed. Leonard W. Labaree (New Haven: Yale U P, 1963), 178–179.
10. *Delaware Journal* (July 3, 1827), 1.
11. Quoted in *The Constitutional Whig* (June 16, 1831), 2.
12. *New York Herald* (June 4, 1847), 1.
13. *The Northern Galaxy* (June 15, 1847), 2
14. *Hillsdale Whig and Standard* (Aug. 7, 1849), 2.
15. *Southern Sentinel* (Oct. 5, 1850), 2.
16. *Louisville Chronicle* (Nov. 1851), as carried in *The National Era* (Nov. 13, 1851), 4, and the *Washington Sentinel* (Feb. 5, 1854), 2.
17. Oscar Handlin, *Boston's Immigrants* (Cambridge: Harvard U P, 1959),114.
18. 1847 American Republican Address to the Fayette County Congressional District, American Party Broadsides, 1844–1855, FHS.
19. *The New York Daily Tribune* (May 7, 1846), 1.
20. Keith Runyon, "The specter of George Prentice is not welcome here anymore," *Courier Journal* (Aug. 20, 2018).
21. Dave Wang, "The US Founders and China," *Education About Asia*, Vol. 16, Number 2 (Fall 2011): 5–6.
22. *The Morals of Confucius: A Chinese Philosopher, Who Flourished above Five Hundred Years before the Coming of our LORD and Saviour JESUS CHRIST Being One of the Choicest Pieces of that Nation*, 2nd ed (London: Printed for T. Horne, 1691), 55.
23. "From Benjamin Franklin to Court de Gébelin, 7 May 1781," *The Papers of Benjamin Franklin*, vol. 35, *May 1 through October 31, 1781*, ed. Barbara B. Oberg (New Haven: Yale U P, 1999), 34–36.
24. "An Account of the New Invented Pennsylvanian Fire-Places, [15 November 1744]," *The Papers of Benjamin Franklin*, vol. 2, *January 1, 1735, through December 31, 1744*, ed. Leonard W. Labaree (New Haven: Yale U P, 1961), 419–446.
25. "Notes on Reading an Account of Travel in China, [1762?]," *The Papers of Benjamin Franklin*, vol. 10, *January 1, 1762, through December 31, 1763*, ed. Leonard W. Labaree (New Haven: Yale U P, 1959), 182–183.
26. "From Benjamin Franklin to Cadwalader Evans, 7 September 1769," *The Papers of Benjamin Franklin*, vol. 16, *Janu-*

ary 1 through December 31, 1769, ed. William B. Willcox (New Haven: Yale U P, 1972), 198–201.

27. "From Benjamin Franklin to Thomas Percival, 15 October 1773," *The Papers of Benjamin Franklin*, vol. 20, *January 1 through December 31, 1773*, ed. William B. Willcox (New Haven: Yale U P, 1976), 442–445.

28. "Poor Richard Improved, 1750," *The Papers of Benjamin Franklin*, vol. 3, *January 1, 1745, through June 30, 1750*, ed. Leonard W. Labaree (New Haven: Yale U P, 1961), 437–456.

29. *New York Herald* (Sept. 17, 1842), 2.

30. *Herald of the Times* (Oct. 27, 1842), 3.

31. James Harvey Young, *The Toadstool Millionaires: A Social History of Patent Medicines in America before Federal Regulation* (Princeton: Princeton U P, 1961), 174.

32. Ibid.

33. Christopher Hoolihan, *An Annotated Catalogue of the Edward C. Atwater Collection of American Popular Medicine and Health Reform*, Vol. 3 (Rochester: U of Rochester P, 2008), 114.

34. *Southern Banner* (Aug. 13, 1841), 3.

35. Robert B. Shaw, "History of the Comstock Patent Medicine Business and Dr. Morse's Indian Root Pills," *Smithsonian Studies in History and Technology*, no. 22 (1972).

36. *The Daily Union* (Oct. 21, 1851), 2.

37. *Alexandria Gazette* (Nov. 10, 1851), 2.

38. *Polynesian* (June 28, 1856), 30.

39. *The Weekly Caucasian* (Feb. 23, 1867), 1.

40. "California," *Chicago Tribune* (May 24, 1870), 1.

41. *The Daily Intelligencer* (June 6, 1876), 2.

42. *Pioche Daily Record* (Oct. 26, 1876), 3.

43. *The Daily Phoenix* (Feb. 28, 1873), 1.

44. "San Francisco," *Chicago Daily Tribune* (June 30, 1873), 2.

45. *Daily National Democrat* (April 3, 1860), 2.

46. *Polynesian* (Aug. 4, 1860), 1.

47. *The Weekly Butte Record* (Nov. 23, 1861), 1.

48. *Middletown Transcript* (Nov. 28, 1868), 2.

49. *Daily Kennebec Journal* (June 6, 1873), 2.

50. "City Leprosy Scare," *Weekly Trinity Journal* (June 21, 1873), 4.

51. "Right Action," *Sacramento Daily Record-Union* (March 12, 1884), 2.

52. "Two Chinese Lepers Expected," *The Sun* (July 12, 1884), 3.

53. "'Frisco Chinamen," *The Canton Advocate* (Jan. 2, 1878), 2.

54. "A Pessimistic View," *The Daily Astorian* (Jan. 8, 1882), 2.

55. John Kuo Wei Tchen, *New York before Chinatown: Orientalism and the Shaping of American Culture, 1776–1882* (Baltimore: Johns Hopkins U P, 1999), 281.

56. Eithne Luibhéid, *Denied Entry: Controlling Sexuality at the Border* (Minneapolis: U of Minnesota P, 1998), 35–37.

57. Ibid., 31.

58. "Cholera," *The Salt Lake Herald* (Sept. 11, 1881), 13.

59. Zachary Gussow, *Leprosy, Racism, and Public Health: Social Policy in Chronic Disease Control* (New York: Routledge, 2021), 121.

60. *The Morning Call* (Aug. 30, 1892), 8.

61. Ibid.

62. Ibid.

63. *The Morning Call* (Aug. 31, 1892), 4.

64. "Only Four Suspects," *Waterbury Evening Democrat* (Sept. 21, 1892), 1.

65. "Danger from Immigrants," *Morning Journal and Courier* (Sept. 2, 1892), 2.

66. *Mower County Transcript* (July 20, 1892).

67. "Plague in Hong Kong," *The Evening World* (June 12, 1894), 1.

68. *Los Angeles Herald* (June 19, 1894).

69. *Capital Journal* (June 14, 1894).

70. *Los Angeles Herald* (June 19, 1894).

71. *San Francisco Morning Call* (June 22, 1894).

72. "The Chinese," *Daily Capital Journal* (Nov. 26, 1898), 1.

73. "The Facts Suppressed," *El Paso Daily Herald* (Nov. 26, 1898), 1.

74. "San Francisco Scared," *The Salt Lake Herald* (Nov. 27, 1898), 7.

75. *Omaha Daily Bee* (June 30, 1899).

76. "Frisco's Deadly Danger," *Waterbury Evening Democrat* (June 29, 1899), 5.

77. "Coming Events Foretold," *The Scranton Tribune* (Nov. 1, 1899), 2.

78. "President Dole's Views," *The Hawaiian Star* (Dec. 12, 1899), 1.

79. *The Record-Union* (Dec. 29, 1899), 8.
80. *The Pacific Commercial Advertiser* (Jan. 18, 1900), 2.
81. *The Hawaiian Star* (Jan. 20, 1900), 1.
82. "Two Million Dollar Blaze Razes Honolulu's Chinatown," *The San Francisco Call* (Feb. 1, 1900), 4.
83. Ibid.
84. *The San Francisco Call* (March 7, 1900).
85. *The San Francisco Call* (March 8, 1900), 6.
86. Ibid., 3.
87. *The San Francisco Call* (March 11, 1900), 18.
88. A.J. Viseltear, "The Pneumonic Plague Epidemic of 1924 in Los Angeles," *Yale Journal of Biology and Medicine* 47, no. 1 (1974): 40–54.
89. Jason Davis, "Gov. Ron DeSantis Accuses President Biden of Making Pandemic Worse with Lax Border Security," *WPTV* (Aug. 4, 2021), https://www.wptv.com/news/state/gov-ron-desantis-accuses-president-biden-of-making-pandemic-worse-with-lax-border-security.

Chapter IX

1. David Hosack and John Wakefield Francis, *The American Medical and Philosophical Register, Vol 1* (New York: Van Winkle, 1814), 329.
2. *Commercial Advertiser* (Dec. 2, 1797), 2.
3. *New York Mercury* (July 18, 1832).
4. Charles Dickens, *American Notes for General Circulation*.
5. "The Undrained Swamps Under the City and Their Consequences," *New York Herald* (Feb. 2, 1859), 4.
6. *New York Herald* (Sept. 17, 1849), 2.
7. Dorothea Dix, *Remarks on Prisons and Prison Discipline in the United States*, 2nd ed. (Philadelphia: Kite and Co., 1845), 36.
8. Dorothea Dix, "Memorial of Miss D. Dix in Relation to the Illinois Penitentiary" (1847) and Dorothea Dix, "Memorial of Miss D. Dix to the Hon. the General Assembly in Behalf of the Insane of Maryland" (1852).
9. Stephen Smith, *The City That Was* (Carlisle: Applewood Books, 1911), 37–39.
10. Ibid., 40–42.
11. "Dr. Richardson, of Essex, on the Health Bill," *New York Evening Post* (Oct. 18, 1865), 1.
12. *New York Times* (Nov. 23, 1865).
13. *New York Times* (Jan. 25, 1866).
14. "The Health Bill," *The Brooklyn Daily Eagle* (Feb. 3, 1866), 2.
15. *NY Times* (Feb. 16, 1866), 4.
16. *Evening Courier & Republic* (Feb. 17, 1866), 2.
17. *New York World* (May 18, 1866), 4.
18. "Advertising the Health Code," *Brooklyn Daily Eagle* (May 2, 1866), 2.
19. Charles Rosenberg, *The Cholera Years* (Chicago: University of Chicago Press, 1962), 210–212.
20. "Cuba's Other Scourge," *The Sun* (Jan. 20, 1897), 2.
21. Ibid.
22. "Cabinet at Loggerheads," *The Houston Daily Post* (March 25, 1898), 2.
23. *Anaconda Standard* (Jan. 11, 1898), 4.
24. "War Department Sluggishness," *Salt Lake Herald* (June 8, 1898), 4.
25. "Alger Replies to Pingree," *Kansas City Journal* (June 29, 1898), 2.
26. "More Alger Meat Ordered," *Lexington Gazette* (July 12, 1899), 2.
27. *People's Voice* (July 21, 1898), 5.
28. "Out From the Jaws of Death," *The Herald* (Aug. 29, 1898), 6.
29. "Officers Make Protest," *The Herald* (Aug. 4, 1898), 1.
30. "Time to Call a Halt," *Democratic Advocate* (Aug. 20, 1898), 1.
31. "Mr. Sherman's Opinion," *Evening News* (Aug. 26, 1898), 1.
32. "Alger and Roosevelt," *Dallas Daily Chronicle* (Aug. 10, 1898), 2.
33. "Story of Santiago," *Evening Star* (Dec. 21, 1898), 2.
34. *State Democrat* (Dec. 30, 1898), 1.
35. "Nelson Miles: Testimony before the Dodge Commission (1898), Excerpt." *World at War: Understanding Conflict and Society*, ABC-CLIO, 2021, worldatwar2-abc-clio-com.ezproxy1.apus.edu/Search/Display/1456482. Accessed Sept. 30, 2021.
36. "Gen. Eagan's Attacks," *El Paso Daily Herald* (Jan. 13, 1899), 1.
37. *Coeur d'Alene Press* (May 13, 1899), 2.
38. *Arizona Weekly Journal Miner* (March 8, 1899), 1.

39. *Indianapolis Journal* (March 11, 1899), 4.
40. *Times of Washington* (April 2, 1899), 6.
41. *Kansas City Journal* (April 4, 1899), 4.
42. *Wichita Daily Eagle* (April 8, 1900), 1.
43. "Bryan Pauses to Greet the Brave," *San Francisco Call* (April 8, 1900), 23.
44. *Chicago Eagle* (Jan. 27, 1906), 1.
45. Upton Sinclair, *The Jungle* (New York: Doubleday, Page, 1906), 90.
46. "Much Raking, and Big Sticking," *Spokane Press* (June 1, 1906), 2.
47. *Florida Star* (June 23, 1905), 3.
48. *Commoner* (June 15, 1906), 4.
49. "Neill Makes Protest," *Evening Star* (June 8, 1906), 8.

Chapter X

1. Erich Fromm, *Escape from Freedom* (London: Routledge & Kegan Paul, 1942), 26–27.
2. "Preface to Dr. Heberden's Pamphlet on Inoculation, 16 February 1759," *The Papers of Benjamin Franklin*, vol. 8, *April 1, 1758, through December 31, 1759*, ed. Leonard W. Labaree (New Haven: Yale University Press, 1965), 281–286.
3. Robert Kumamoto, *The Historical Origins of Terrorism in America:1644–1880* (New York: Routledge, 2013), 29.
4. "From Thomas Jefferson to Martha Jefferson Randolph, 16 July 1801," *The Papers of Thomas Jefferson*, vol. 34, *1 May–1 July 1801*, ed. Barbara B. Oberg (Princeton: Princeton University Press, 2007), 580.
5. "To James Madison from James Smith, 26 February 1813," *The Papers of James Madison*, Presidential Series, vol. 6, *8 February–24 October 1813*, ed. Angela Kreider et al. (Charlottesville: University of Virginia Press, 2008), 72.
6. *Richmond Enquirer* (Feb. 2, 1822), 1.
7. *Ibid*. (April 2, 1822), 2.
8. *American Watchman and Delaware Advertiser* (May 3, 1822), 3.
9. Samuel Bayard Woodward, "The Story of Smallpox in Massachusetts," *New England Journal of Medicine* 206, no. 23 (1932): 1181–1191.
10. "The Vaccination of Pupils," *Brooklyn Daily Eagle* (Nov. 7, 1873), 3.
11. "The Board of Education," *Brooklyn Daily Eagle* (Nov. 10, 1875), 2.
12. "Personal Rights and Compulsory Vaccination in the Public Schools," *Brooklyn Daily Eagle* (Nov. 23, 1875), 2.
13. *Ibid*.
14. "Vaccination: A Grand Assault on the Practice," *Chicago Daily Tribune* (May 3, 1879), 9.
15. "Letter from New York," *Orleans County Monitor* (June 28, 1880), 2.
16. *Indianapolis Journal* (Oct. 30, 1885), 5.
17. "Vaccination Claims Another," *New York Tribune* (Nov. 15, 1901), 1.
18. "Report of Camden Board," *The Sun* (Dec. 2, 1901), 3.
19. "The Small-pox Scare," *Seattle Republican* (Jan. 24, 1902), 4.
20. "The Vaccinated Pug," *Waterbury Democrat* (Nov. 12, 1902), 2.
21. "The Anti-Vaccinationists Triumph," *NY Times* (Aug. 18, 1898), 6.
22. *Washington Herald* (Sept. 9, 1907), 8.
23. "Christian Scientists Vaccinate Children," *Leavenworth Times* (March 7, 1900).
24. L.O. Gostin, "Jacobson v Massachusetts at 100 Years: Police Power and Civil Liberties in Tension," *American Journal of Public Health* 95, no. 4 (2005): 576–581.
25. *New York Times* (Feb. 22, 1905), 6.
26. "East Side Schools Mobbed by Hordes of Parents," *Evening World* (June 27, 1906), 14.
27. Carol Pogash, "As Anti-vaxx Dispute Rages, Attention Turns to California's Waldorf Schools," *Guardian* (May 28, 2019).
28. Tracy A. Lieu, "Geographic Clusters in Underimmunization and Vaccine Refusal," *Pediatrics* 135, no. 2 (Feb. 2015), and B. Baumgaertner, "The Influence of Political Ideology and Trust on Willingness to Vaccinate," *PLoS One* 13, no. 1 (Jan. 25, 2018).
29. George Mills, "Threw Rocks, Eggs In 'Cow War,'" *Des Moines Register* (Sept. 22, 1971), and "Iowa Cattle War Is Ended," *Producers News* (Oct. 2, 1931), 1.
30. *Telegraph Herald and Times Journal* (Sept. 22, 1931).

Chapter XI

1. "Relics of the Scourge," *New York Herald* (Nov. 16, 1878), 3.
2. *Evening Star* (May 9, 1879), 1.
3. "Inland Quarantine," *New Orleans Daily Democrat* (June 26, 1879), 4.
4. "Yellow Fever," *New York Herald* (July 25, 1879), 2.
5. "The Fever Elsewhere," *Memphis Daily Appeal* (Aug. 10, 1879), 1.
6. "Yellow Fever," *Weekly Chillicothe Crisis* (Aug. 21, 1879), 4.
7. "The Essence of Nonsense," *Memphis Daily Appeal* (Oct. 1, 1879), 1.
8. *Memphis Daily Appeal* (Aug. 7, 1883), 2.
9. Thomas R. Gray and Jeffery A. Jenkins, "Yellow Fever and Institutional Development: The Rise and Fall of the National Board of Health," *Journal of Political Institutions and Political Economy* 2, no. 1 (2021): 143–167.
10. "Compulsory Vaccine," *Indianapolis Journal* (May 21, 1894), 4.
11. Ruling of William J. Gaynor, 18 May 1894, In Re Smith (n. 39), 35.
12. "Slashed at the Doctors," *Brooklyn Daily Eagle* (May 8, 1894), 12.
13. George A. Soper, "Mary Mallon," *The Military Surgeon* 45, no. 1 (July 1919).
14. Ibid.
15. "Has New York Many Walking Pesthouses?," *New York Tribune* (July 4, 1909), 5.
16. Ibid.
17. "Willing to Wed 'Typhoid Germ,'" *Belding Banner* (July 29, 1909), 2.
18. Soper, "Mary Mallon."
19. "Paralysis Ends Deadly Career of 'Typhoid Mary' at 70," *Evening Star* (Nov. 12, 1938), A-5.
20. "Case of Early," *Washington Times* (June 4, 1914), 1 and 5.
21. Michael Sistrom, "North Carolinians and the Great War," Documenting the American South, https://docsouth.unc.edu/wwi/soldiersintro.html.
22. "Protect Soldiers from Social Evils," *Pullman Herald* (May 11, 1917), 1.
23. "Honor Shown in East to Western Statesman for Their Patriotism," *Anchorage Weekly Times* (Jan. 24, 1918), 10.
24. "Plague Worse than Leprosy Is Battled," *Washington Herald* (Nov. 17, 1918), 1.
25. Allan M. Brandt, "The Syphilis Epidemic and Its Relation to AIDS," *Science* 239, no. 4838 (January 1988): 377.
26. Col. Leonard P. Ayers, "The War with Germany, a Statistical Summary," Chapter IX (Washington, D.C.: U.S. Printing Office, 1919).
27. John H. Stokes, *The Third Great Plague: A Discussion of Syphilis for Everyday People* (Philadelphia: W.B. Saunders Company, 1920), 26, and Elie Metchnikoff, *The New Hygiene: Three Lectures on the Prevention of Infectious Diseases* (Chicago: W.T. Keener and Company, 1907), 77.
28. "Report of the Sanitary Commission Prostitution," *Annual Report of the Metropolitan Board of Health of the State of New York* (New York: Union, 1868), 305.
29. "Instructions on 1936 Marriages," *Waterbury Democrat* (Nov. 29, 1935), 2.
30. Madelin Blitzstein, "Curtains for the Marriage Mills," *Dayton Forum* (July 2, 1937), 10.
31. "Blood Test Law Booms Marriages," *Waterbury Democrat* (Dec. 7, 1936), 3.
32. Thomas Parran, "Fight on Disease Seeks Plain Talk," *Evening Star* (Aug. 16, 1936), A-3.
33. *Seventh Yearbook of the City Manager's Association* (1921), 151.
34. *The Day Book* (Feb. 12, 1917), 24.
35. "Statement of Objections by the Citizens Medical Reference Bureau," Hearing of the House Committee on Interstate and Foreign Commerce (Washington, D.C.: U.S. Printing Office, 1938), 177.
36. Ibid.
37. Francis Galton, *Essays in Eugenics* (London: Eugenics Education Society, 1909), 68.
38. Alison Bashford and Philippa Levine, eds., *The Oxford Handbook of the History of Eugenics* (Oxford: Oxford University Press, 2010), 5.
39. Harry Laughlin, *Eugenics Record Office: Bulletin 10* (Cold Spring Harbor, 1914), 32.
40. "Wyoming Eugenic Laws," *Bridgeport Times and Evening Farmer* (May 20, 1921), 4.
41. *Brunswick News* (Sept. 15, 1921), 4.
42. Brian C. Wilson, *Dr. John Harvey Kellogg and the Religion of Biologic Living* (Bloomington: Indiana University Press, 2014), 159.
43. Samuel Pennypacker, "Veto Mes-

sage" (March 30, 1907), in Harry Laughlin, *Eugenics Record Office: Bulletin 10* (Cold Spring Harbor, 1914), 32.

44. Adam Cohen, *Imbeciles: The Supreme Court, American Eugenics, and the Sterilization of Carrie Buck* (New York: Penguin, 2016), 16.

45. *Ibid.*, 149.

46. *Buck v. Bell*, 274 U.S. 200 (1927).

47. "Virginia Law Upheld," *Coconino Sun* (May 13, 1927), 4.

48. *Ibid.*

49. Margaret Sanger, *The Case for Birth Control* (1917), 29.

50. *Ibid.*, 30.

51. *Ibid.*, 157.

52. *Ibid.*, 18.

53. *Ibid.*, 47.

54. *Ibid.*, 94 and 176.

55. Margaret Sanger, *The Pivot of Civilization* (1922).

56. Margaret Sanger, *Women and the New Race* (1920), chapter X.

57. Sanger, *The Case for Birth Control*.

58. "Mary Halton Causes Near Riot," *The Sun* (Jan. 5, 1917), 4.

59. "Standing Room Only If Births Continue," *New Britain Herald* (March 27, 1925), 1, and Will Durant, "The Story of Civilization," *Evening Star* (Feb. 26, 1928), 3.

60. "Debate on Birth Control," *Waterbury Democrat* (March 2, 1933), 4.

61. *Indianapolis Times* (June 24, 1926), 2.

62. "Peril in Germs That Infest Mexico," *Birmingham Age-Herald* (May 24, 1914), 40.

63. Cited in Allan M. Brandt, "Racism and Research: The Case of the Tuskegee Syphilis Study," *The Hastings Center Report* 8, no. 6 (1978): 26.

64. *Ibid.*

65. Beth Duff-Brown, "Stanford Researchers Explore Legacy of Tuskegee Syphilis Study Today," *Stanford News* (Jan. 6, 2017).

66. Jim Carlton, "Of Microbes and Mock Attacks: Years Ago, The Military Sprayed Germs on U.S. Cities," *Wall Street Journal* (Oct. 22, 2001).

67. Mark S. Williams et al., "Retrospective Analysis of Pneumonic Tularemia in Operation Whitecoat Human Subjects: Disease Progression and Tetracycline Efficacy," *Frontiers in Medicine* (Oct. 22, 2019).

68. Rachel Nowak, "Killer Mousepox Virus Raises Bioterror Fears," *New Scientist* (Jan. 10, 2001), https://www.newscientist.com/article/dn311-killer-mousepox-virus-raises-bioterror-fears/.

69. Talha Burki, "Ban on Gain-of-Function Research Ends," *Lancet* (Feb. 2018).

70. "Doing Diligence to Assess the Risks and Benefits of Life Sciences Gain-of-Function Research," White House Blog (Oct. 17, 2014), https://obamawhitehouse.archives.gov/blog/2014/10/17/doing-diligence-assess-risks-and-benefits-life-sciences-gain-function-research.

71. Emily Crane, "NIH Admits U.S. Funded Gain-of-Function in Wuhan—Despite Fauci's Denials," *New York Post* (Oct. 21, 2021).

72. "Rubio Joins Marshall and Colleagues in Introducing Legislation to Halt Viral Gain of Function Research" (Oct. 19, 2021), https://www.rubio.senate.gov/public/index.cfm/2021/10/rubio-joins-marshall-and-colleagues-in-introducing-legislation-to-halt-viral-gain-of-function-research.

Chapter XII

1. Nicholson to Gallatin (March 6, 1811), *Papers of Gallatin* [microfilm ed.], reel 22.

2. "To Thomas Jefferson from George Clinton, 20 January 1804," *The Papers of Thomas Jefferson*, vol. 42, *16 November 1803–10 March 1804*, ed. James P. McClure (Princeton: Princeton University Press, 2016), 318–319.

3. "Thomas Jefferson to Benjamin Rush, 17 August 1811," *The Papers of Thomas Jefferson*, Retirement Series, vol. 4, *18 June 1811 to 30 April 1812*, ed. J. Jefferson Looney (Princeton: Princeton University Press, 2007), 87–88.

4. "Dolly Madison" (March 27, 1812), in Allen Culling Clark, *Life and Letters of Dolly Madison* (Washington, D.C.: W.F. Roberts Company, 1914), 130.

5. Herbert L. Abrams, "Presidential Health and the Public Interest: The Campaign of 1992," *Political Psychology* 16, no. 4 (Dec. 1995): 796. William Wirt, the Anti-Masonic candidate for president in 1832, likewise was stricken with the condition, dying of it in 1834.

6. J.E.D. Shipp, *Giant Days: Or, The Life and Times of William H. Crawford* (Americus, GA: Southern Printers, 1909), 174. Following the attack, Crawford was bled by his doctors twenty-three times over the next several weeks. Overall, it is unclear whether the medication caused the attack, was a contributing agent to the onset of another condition, or merely was given at the same time as the occurrence of a more serious medical problem.

7. James Monroe to James Madison (Oct. 17, 1823), in *James Madison Papers, 1723 to 1859: Series 2 Additional General Correspondence, 1780 to 1837*, Library of Congress, https://www.loc.gov/item/mjm022798/.

8. John Quincy Adams to George Washington Adams (Oct. 21, 1823), in *Founders Online,* National Archives, https://founders.archives.gov/documents/Adams/99-03-02-4331.

9. Dumas Malone, *Jefferson and His Time, Vol. VI: The Sage of Monticello* (Boston: Little, Brown, 1981), 432.

10. Thomas Jefferson to William H. Crawford (April 20, 1824), in *Founders Online,* National Archives, https://founders.archives.gov/documents/Jefferson/98-01-02-4204.

11. James C. Klotter, *Henry Clay: The Man Who Would Be President* (Oxford: Oxford University Press, 2018), 113.

12. *National Intelligencer* (Oct. 30, 1822).

13. Henry Shaw to Henry Clay (Feb. 11, 1823), in *The Papers of Henry Clay, Vol. 3*, 372.

14. Thomas Jefferson to Francis Walker Gilmer (Oct. 12, 1824), in *Correspondence of Thomas Jefferson and Francis Walker Gilmer, 1814–1826*, ed. Richard Beale Davis (Columbia: University of South Carolina Press, 1946), 108–109.

15. Two of his brothers had succumbed to disease during the Revolution, largely due to mistreatment by the British. Likewise, his mother Elizabeth appears to have fallen victim to either typhus or dysentery while tending to sick soldiers in Charleston in 1781. Andrew was an orphan by the age of 14 and held a profound hatred for the British that would be reflected in his actions in 1818 in Florida with the Arbuthnot and Ambrister affair. Much of the confusion that resulted from his invasion of Florida was caused by President Monroe's own serious illness. Confined to his bed in 1818, the President was unable to read or approve of the various letters being sent by his commander in the field. Years later Monroe recalled how "I well remember that … I was sick in bed, and could not read it … I never read it until after the conclusion of the war." James Monroe as quoted in Michael P. Riccards, "The Presidency: In Sickness and Health," *Presidential Studies Quarterly* 7, no. 4 (Fall 1977): 219.

16. L.M. Deppisch et al., "Andrew Jackson's Exposure to Mercury and Lead: Poisoned President?," *JAMA* 282, no. 6 (1999): 569–571.

17. Some further evidence of this is shown by the anecdotal improvement in the President's health following the removal of one of the bullets from his body in 1832. Jackson largely then turned against the medical use of lead, describing it as "that potent but pernicious remedy to the stomach." J.S. Bassett, *Correspondence of Andrew Jackson*, Vol. 1 (Washington, D.C.: Carnegie Institute of Washington, 1926), 439.

18. Andrew Jackson to John Coffee (March 22, 1829); Andrew Jackson to John Donelson (June 7, 1829), and see Andrew Jackson to John Christmas McLemore (April 26, 1829), among others.

19. Andrew Jackson to John Coffee (Sept. 21, 1829).

20. George Green Shackelford, "From the Society's Collections: Lieutenant Lee Reports to Captain Talcott on Fort Calhoun's Construction on the Rip Raps," *The Virginia Magazine of History and Biography* 60, no. 3 (July 1952): 467; Andrew Jackson to James Alexander Hamilton (Sept. 11, 1829).

21. William E. Smith, "Francis P. Blair, Pen-Executive of Andrew Jackson," *Journal of American History* 17, no. 4 (March 1931), 554.

22. Jon Meacham, *American Lion: Andrew Jackson in the White House* (New York: Random House, 2009), 110, and see Andrew Jackson to John Coffee (Sept. 21, 1829).

23. John C. Fitzpatrick, ed. *The Autobiography of Martin Van Buren* (Washington, D.C.: U.S. Printing Office, 1920), 326.

24. Henry Clay to Christopher Hughes Jr. (Dec. 8, 1816), in *The Papers of Henry Clay, Vol. 2* (Lexington: University of Kentucky Press, 1961), 259.

25. See Henry Clay to Benjamin Howard (March 12, 1811), in *The Papers of Henry Clay, Vol. 1* (Lexington: University of Kentucky Press, 1959), 548.

26. Henry Clay to William Thornton, Dec. 6, 1817, in *The Papers of Henry Clay, Vol. 2*, 407.

27. Ibid., 592.

28. Adam Jortner, "Cholera, Christ, and Jackson: The Epidemic of 1832 and the Origins of Christian Politics in Antebellum America," *Journal of the Early Republic* 27, no. 2 (Summer 2007): 27.

29. Henry Clay Remarks in the Senate (June 25, 1832), in *The Papers of Henry Clay*, Vol. 8 (Lexington: University of Kentucky Press, 2015), 545.

30. Henry Clay Comments in the Senate (June 28, 1832), in *The Papers of Henry Clay*, 546.

31. Charles E. Rosenberg, *The Cholera Years* (Chicago: University of Chicago Press, 2009), 50.

32. Vermont, which had seen armed bands rushing to secure its borders against the Irish, voted for the Anti-Masonic candidate.

33. Henry Clay to James Brown (Oct. 23, 1832), in *The Papers of Henry Clay*, 587.

34. Henry Clay to James Brown (Oct. 23, 1832), in *The Papers of Henry Clay*, 587.

35. Henry Clay to Alexander Coffin (June 11, 1834), in *The Papers of Henry Clay*, 725.

36. "Roosevelt Rests, Health Improves," *Detroit Evening Times* (Jan. 2, 1944), 1.

37. "Mohammad Reza Shah Pahlavi to Franklin D. Roosevelt, June 17, 1944," Foreign Relations of the U.S.: Diplomatic Papers, 1944, The Near East, South Asia, and Africa, Volume V, Document 340.

38. "President Roosevelt to be Sixty Two Years Old Sunday," *Ypsilanti Daily Press* (Jan. 29, 1944), 1.

39. "President Roosevelt Looks Tired, Worn, Says Visitor," *Ypsilanti Daily Press* (March 29, 1944), 1.

40. "Unwise and Untruthful Meddling," *Detroit Evening Times* (April 1, 1944), 16.

41. "Wheeler Says Roosevelt Will Not Enter Race," *Imperial Valley Press* (April 18, 1944), 1.

42. "Would Be a Catastrophe," *Western News* (June 15, 1944), 2.

43. "FDR Reported Planning to Quit," *Detroit Evening Times* (July 18, 1944), 2-C.

44. Paul Mallon, "Behind the News," *Detroit Evening Times* (July 20, 1944), 12-C.

45. David Lawrence, "Taboo Seen Needed on Campaign Gossip," *Evening Star* (Sept. 28, 1944), A-10.

46. "Hannegan Denies FDR Poor Health," *Wilmington Morning Star* (Oct. 14, 1944), 4.

47. *Imperial Valley Press* (Oct. 27, 1944), 3.

48. James F. King, "Missouri GOP Gaining," *Evening Star* (Oct. 29, 1944), C.

49. David Lawrence, "Possibility of Eisenhower Defeat," *Evening Star* (March 9, 1956), A-15.

50. "The World Today," *Virgin Islands Daily News* (Nov. 17, 1955), 1.

51. Gilbert, *The Mortal Presidency*, 104.

52. Cecil Holland, "Kennedy Backers Blast Issue About His Health," *Evening Star* (July 5, 1960), A-6.

53. Lee Cohn, "Nixon's Health Is 'Excellent' Aide Reports," *Evening Star* (July 7, 1960), A-12.

54. Dallek, "The Medical Ordeals of JFK."

55. See Don Hewitt's *Tell Me a Story: Fifty Years and 60 Minutes in Television* (Public Affairs, 2002) for a good discussion of the debate.

56. Cecil Holland, "Nixon in Good Health, Senator Scott Says," *Evening Star* (Sept. 27, 1960), A-11.

57. Joshua M. Glasser, *The Eighteen Day Running Mate: McGovern, Eagleton, and a Campaign in Crisis* (New Haven: Yale University Press, 2012), 149–150.

58. Joe Garofoli, "Obama Bounces Back—Speech Seemed to Help," *San Francisco Gate* (March 26, 2008).

59. David Lauter, "Reagan Remark Spurs Dukakis Health Report," *LA Times* (Aug. 4, 1988).

60. Dylan Scott, "Smears over a candidate's personal health can work. Just ask Michael Dukakis," *Stat News* (Aug. 26, 2016).

61. Johnson was only one year older than Barry Goldwater but certainly cut a more youthful image.

62. Michael Wines, "Bush in Japan," *New York Times* (Jan. 9, 1992).

63. Richard L. Berke, "Still Running: Is Age Bashing the Way to Beat Bob Dole?" *New York Times* (May 5, 1996).

64. Alan Silverleib, "Analysis: Age an issue in the 2008 campaign?" *CNN* (June 15, 2008).

65. Lawrence Altman, "On the Campaign Trail, Few Mentions of McCain's Bout with Melanoma," *New York Times* (March 9, 2008).

66. "Donald Trump's Weight Problem," *Washington Post* (Sept. 28, 2016).

67. Jacqueline Howard, "Weight bias is bigger problem than you may think, experts say," *CNN* (Sept. 29, 2016).

68. Andrew Feinberg, "Trump's mental state is deteriorating dangerously due to impeachment with potentially 'catastrophic outcomes,' psychiatrists urgently warn Congress," *Independent* (Dec. 4, 2019).

69. Carrie Dann, "Trump's Physician Says His Health is 'Astonishingly Excellent,'" *NBC News* (Dec. 14, 2015).

70. Larry Husten, "Trump's CV Event Risk Seven Times Greater than Clinton's," *MedPageToday* (Oct. 5, 2016).

71. Mary Bruce, "Hillary Clinton Took 6 Months to 'Get Over' Concussion, Bill Says of Timeline," *ABC News* (May 14, 2014).

72. "Dr. Drew Show Cancelled Days After Host's Negative Speculation About Hillary Clinton's Health," *Washington Post* (Aug. 26, 2016).

73. James Hamblin, "When Hillary Clinton Coughs," *The Atlantic* (Sept. 6, 2016).

74. Oliver Darcy, "Video shows Clinton stumble, struggle to walk as she enters van to leave 9/11 memorial event," *Business Insider* (Sept. 11, 2016).

75. "Hillary Clinton may not recover from her pneumonia until late October," *Washington Post* (Sept. 13, 2016).

76. Sebastian Jäckle, "A Catwalk to Congress? Appearance-Based Effects in the Elections to the U.S. House of Representatives 2016," *American Politics Research*, Vol. 48, No. 4 (2020): 427–441, and G. Miller, "Women's Suffrage, Political Responsiveness, and Child Survival in American History," *Q. J. Economics*, Vol. 123, No. 3 (2008): 1287–1327.

77. New York State Woman Suffrage Association, *Women in the Home*, n.d. New-York Historical Society Library.

78. Ellen Dubois, "How LA Suffragists Won the Vote for California Women Years Before the 19th Amendment," *LA Times* (Aug. 17, 2020).

79. Inez Haynes Irwin, *The Story of the Woman's Party* (New York: Harcourt, 1921), 268.

80. *New Orleans Times-Picayune* (Oct. 2, 1918).

81. Virginia Kase Solomon, "Then and Now: How Two Pandemics Tested the Power of Women," *League of Women Voters Blog* (March 30, 2021), https://www.lwv.org/blog/then-and-now-how-two-pandemics-tested-power-women.

Chapter XIII

1. "Disease," *New York Herald* (Dec. 18, 1879), 1.

2. *The Evening World* (March 31, 1891), 2.

3. "Sick Italian Immigrants Detained," *Waterbury Evening Democrat* (April 3, 1891), 1.

4. *The Princeton Union* (Sept. 17, 1871), 6.

5. "People Alarmed," *Fort Worth Gazette* (Sept. 8, 1891), 8.

6. *The Morning News* (Feb. 18, 1892), 1.

7. *The Morning Journal-Courier* (Dec. 17, 1907), 7.

8. "Diseased Immigrants Are Menace to New York," *Los Angeles Herald* (Dec. 12, 1907), 3.

9. "Avoid the Poison Gas," *Dearborn Independent* (Jan. 22, 1921), 4.

10. "Reassuring Mr. Caminetti," *The New York Herald* (Jan. 20, 1921), 12.

11. *The Rock Island Argus* (March 15, 1921), 7.

12. "Cumming to Tell of Typhus Menace," *The Washington Herald* (Feb. 9, 1921), 3.

13. "Aliens Choke up Port for Days in Wretched Huddle," *The New York Herald* (Feb. 28, 1921), 5.

14. "Deadly Typhus," *Yorkville Enquirer* (March 25, 1921), 1

15. *Congressional Record* (June 27, 1952), 8267.

16. Peter Sullivan, "Carson Blames Measles on Immigrants," *The Hill* (Feb. 4, 2015).

17. Rupert Neate, "Donald Trump:

Mexican migrants bring 'tremendous infectious disease' to U.S.," *The Guardian* (July 6, 2015).

18. Donald Trump, Twitter (Dec. 11, 2018).

Chapter XIV

1. Julie Steenhuysen, "Study pushes back origin of AIDS pandemic to 1908," *Reuters* (Oct. 1, 2008).

2. "Camille Paglia," *Playboy* (May 1995).

3. Jerry Falwell, "Falwell and Perry," CBC Television, 1983.

4. David Mills, "How the AIDS Epidemic Actually Began," *Healthline* (April 24, 2020). https://www.healthline.com/health-news/how-aids-epidemic-actually-began.

5. Bobbi Campbell, *San Francisco Sentinel* (Dec. 10, 1981).

6. *Bay Area Reporter*, Vol. 12, No. 50 (Dec. 16, 1982): 16.

7. Ryan Benk et al., "Skepticism of Science in a Pandemic Isn't New. It Helped Fuel the AIDS Crisis," *NPR* (May 23, 2021).

8. Julia H. Smith and Alan Whiteside, "The History of AIDS Exceptionalism," *Journal of the International AIDS Society*, Vol. 13, No. 47 (2010).

9. Ronald Reagan, "We Owe it to Ryan," *Washington Post* (April 11, 1990).

10. B.L. Evatt, "The Tragic History of AIDS in the Hemophilia Population, 1982–1984," *Occasional Papers: World Federation of Hemophilia*, no. 6 (Dec. 2007), 2296.

11. Ibid., 2299.

12. "Rock Hudson: His Name Stood for Hollywood's Golden Age of Wholesome Heroics and Lighthearted Romance–Until He Became the Most Famous Person to Die of Aids," *People Magazine* 24, no. 26 (Dec. 23, 1985).

13. John Tierney, "The Big City in the 80s, Fear Spread Faster than AIDS," *New York Times* (June 15, 2001).

14. Larry Kramer to Dr. Anthony Fauci (June 26, 1988).

15. "Results and Impacts of PEPFAR," https://www.state.gov/results-and-impact-pepfar/.

16. "HIV and AIDS-United States, 1981–2000," CDC MMWR Weekly (June 1, 2001). https://www.cdc.gov/mmwr/preview/mmwrhtml/mm5021a2.htm.

17. Monina Klevens et al. "Is There Really a Heterosexual AIDS Epidemic in the United States? Findings from a Multisite Validation Study, 1992–1995," *American Journal of Epidemiology*, Vol. 149, No. 1 (1999): 75–84.

18. Ed Koch, "Overestimating AIDS?," *The Jerusalem Post* (Nov. 27, 2007).

19. Julia H. Smith and Alan Whiteside, "The history of AIDS exceptionalism," *Journal of the International AIDS Society*, Vol. 13, No. 47 (2010).

20. Roger England, "Writing Is on the Wall for UNAIDS," *British Medical Journal*, Vol. 336, no. 7652 (2008):1072.

Chapter XV

1. "Neuberger Warns of Asiatic Flu," *Evening Star* (July 20, 1957), A-21.

2. The President's News Conference (Aug. 21, 1957).

3. Jen Pinkowski, "The History of the Forgotten Pandemic," *Yale Insights* (Jan. 7, 2021). https://insights.som.yale.edu/insights/the-history-of-the-forgotten-pandemic.

4. Sheilah Graham, "Hollywood," *Evening Star* (Nov. 13, 1957), B-21.

5. Mark Honigsbaum, "The Art of Medicine: Revisiting the 1957 and 1968 Influenza Pandemics," *The Lancet*, Vol. 395 (June 30, 2020):1824–1826.

6. "Measles-Catching Party," *The Pittsburgh Press* (May 4, 1958).

7. Mollie Bloudoff-Indelicato, "The 87-year-old doctor who invented the rubella vaccine now working to fight the coronavirus,' *CNBC* (April 9, 2020).

8. Meredith Wadman, "What the Hard Lessons of Rubella Teach Us About a Zika Vaccine," *Time Magazine* (Feb. 22, 2017).

9. Maurice Hilleman, "The Role of Early Alert and of Adjuvant in the Control of Hong Kong Influenza by Vaccines," *Bulletin of the World Health Organization*, Number 41 (1968):623–628.

10. U.S. Congress, 88th Cong, 1st sess., Senate Committee on Aeronautical and Space Sciences, *NASA Authorization for FY64. Part 1: Scientific and Technical Programs*, S. 1245, April 1963, 598–600.

11. Pam Weintraub, "A Lunar Pan-

demic," *AEON* (Dec. 22, 2020), https://aeon.co/essays/what-can-we-learn-from-the-lunar-pandemic-that-never-was.

12. Carl Sagan, "Indigenous Organic Matter on the Moon," *Proceedings of the National Academy of Science*, Vol. 46, No. 4 (April 1960): 393–396, and *LA Times* (May 2, 1963).

13. Kent Carter, "Moon Rocks and Moon Germs: A History of NASA's Lunar Receiving Laboratory," *Prologue Magazine* (Winter 2001).

14. U.S. Congress, 89th Cong., 2nd sess., *Hearings ... NASA FY1967 Authorization*, H.R. 12718, 1231.

15. Joe Biden, quoted in Huma Khan, "Vice President Joe Biden's Remarks on Swine Flu Draw Criticism," *ABC News* (April 30, 2009).

16. *Ibid*.

17. Eric Alterman, "Conservatives Know the Real Origin of Swine Flu," *AmericanProgress.Org* (April 30, 2009).

18. Patrick Buchanan, "Buchanan: The Obama Flu?," *NBC News* (May 1, 2009).

19. Sharyl Attkisson, "Swine Flu Cases Overestimated?," *CBS News* (Oct. 21, 2009).

20. Thomas Maugh II, "Swine flu has hit about 1 in 6 Americans, CDC says," *LA Times* (Dec. 11, 2009).

21. Natasha Korecki, "Biden has fought a pandemic before. It did not go smoothly," *Politico* (May 4, 2020).

22. Donald Trump, Twitter (March 12, 2020).

23. Donald J. Trump, "Campaign Press Release—FACT: Joe Biden's Swine Flu Response Was an Absolute Disaster" (Oct. 07, 2020), https://www.presidency.ucsb.edu/node/345649.

24. Phil Gingrey to CDC (July 7, 2014).

25. Sophie Kleeman, "One Powerful Illustration Shows Exactly What's Wrong With How the West Talks About Ebola," *Mic* (Oct. 7, 2014), https://www.mic.com/articles/100618/one-powerful-illustration-shows-exactly-what-s-wrong-with-media-coverage-of-ebola.

26. Jason Hanna, "Ebola patient walks into Atlanta hospital; wife sees him through glass," *CNN* (Aug. 3, 2014).

27. Steven Nelson, "Congressman: Close Border to Ebola Countries," *U.S. News* (July 30, 2014).

28. Alexandra Sifferlen, "Obama on Ebola: 'The World Is Looking to Us,'" *Time* (Sept. 16, 2014).

29. Donald Trump, Twitter (Sept. 19, 2014).

30. Grace Ji-Sun Kim, "Ebola Outbreak and Outcry: Saving Thomas Eric Duncan," *Huffington Post* (Oct. 7, 2014), https://www.huffpost.com/entry/ebola-outbreak-and-outcry_b_5943216.

31. Donald Trump, Twitter (Oct. 4, 2014).

32. Chris Perez, "Ebola-stricken nurse was allowed to fly to Ohio by CDC," *New York Post* (Oct. 15, 2014).

33. Donald Trump, Twitter (Oct. 17, 2014).

34. Scott Gottlieb, "In the Ebola Fight, a Defense of Embattled CDC Chief Thomas Frieden," *Forbes* (Oct. 17, 2014).

35. Alex Campbell, "How New York City Hired a Con Artist to Clean Up Ebola," *Buzzfeed* (Nov. 15, 2014).

36. Sally Goldenberg, "Schumer cautiously defends mandatory Ebola quarantine," *Politico* (Oct. 26, 2014).

37. Josh Margolin, "Ebola Nurse Kaci Hickox Will 'Understand' Her Quarantine, New Jersey Governor Says," *ABC News* (Oct. 27, 2014).

38. Justin William Moyer, "Ebola nurse Kaci Hickox: 'Flaming' liberals love her. 'Bully' conservatives hate her," *Washington Post* (Oct. 31, 2014).

39. Sydney Lupkin, "Kaci Hickox Boyfriend Bets 'You Can Guess Who We Voted For,'" *ABC News* (Nov. 4, 2014).

40. Lisa Chedekel, "Recalling the Public Panic in Famous Ebola Court Case," *Boston University Today* (March 21, 2017).

Chapter XVI

1. "World Health Coronavirus Disinformation," *Wall Street Journal* (April 5, 2020).

2. Betsy McCaughey, "Why President Trump is entirely right to give up on WHO," *New York Post* (June 4, 2020).

3. Alana Wise, "Trump Says His Misleading Coronavirus Comments Were Meant to Show 'Strength,'" *NPR* (Sept. 10, 2020).

4. Joe Biden, Tweet (March 12, 2020).

5. Joe Biden, Tweet (March 18, 2020).

6. Chris Stanford, "Democrats, China

Virus, Australian Open: Your Monday Briefing," *New York Times* (Jan. 20, 2020), and Anna Flefield, "China virus: Expert says it can be spread by human-to-human contact, sparking concerns about the massive holiday travel underway," *Washington Post* (Jan. 20, 2020).

7. "Nancy Pelosi Visits San Francisco's Chinatown Amid Coronavirus Concerns," *NBC Bay Area* (Feb. 24, 2020), https://www.nbcbayarea.com/news/local/nancy-pelosi-visits-san-franciscos-chinatown/2240247/.

8. All data from FBI Hate Crime Statistics database, https://crime-data-explorer.fr.cloud.gov/pages/explorer/crime/hate-crime.

9. Zaid Jilani, "When 'white supremacists' aren't even white," *The Spectator World* (Feb. 24, 2021), and C.W. Nevius, "Dirty Secret of Black-on-Asian Violence is Out," *San Francisco Gate* (March 2, 2021).

10. Harmeet Kaur, "Yes, we long have referred to disease outbreaks by geographic places. Here's why we shouldn't anymore," *CNN* (March 28, 2020).

11. Colleen Flaherty, "'Cancelled' for Saying 'China Virus'?," *InsideHigherEd* (Sept. 22, 2021), and Katie Camero, "Professor who Called Covid-19 'China Communist Party Virus' is on Leave from Syracuse," *Miami Herald* (Sept. 2, 2020).

12. Joe Biden, "Memorandum Condemning and Combating Racism, Xenophobia, and Intolerance Against Asian Americans and Pacific Islanders in the United States" (Jan. 26, 2021).

13. Libby Cathey, "Coronavirus government response updates: Trump continues to resist calling for nationwide stay-at-home restrictions," *ABC News* (April 1, 2020), and "Donald Trump Coronavirus Task Force Briefing Transcripts" (April 1, 2020).

14. "Inslee statement on Trump encouraging illegal and dangerous acts" (April 17, 2020), https://www.governor.wa.gov/news-media/inslee-statement-trump-encouraging-illegal-and-dangerous-acts.

15. Niguel Hoskin, "The whiteness of anti-lockdown protests," *Vox* (April 25, 2020).

16. Brittany Bernstein, "De Blasio: Black Lives Matter Protests Exempt from Large-Event Ban," *Yahoo News* (July 10, 2020), and Michael Powell, "Are Protests Dangerous? What Experts Say May Depend on Who's Protesting What," *New York Times* (July 6, 2020).

17. Michael Schwirtz, "The 1,000-Bed Comfort Was Supposed to Aid New York. It Has 20 Patients," *New York Times* (April 2, 2020).

18. Noah Higgins-Dunn, "Gov. Cuomo says New York needs ventilators now, help from GM and Ford 'does us no good,'" *CNBC* (March 24, 2020).

19. Betsy McCaughey, "NY Gov. Cuomo Rejected Buying Recommended 16,000 Ventilators in 2015 for Pandemic, Established Death Panels and Lottery Instead," *Gateway Pundit* (March 22, 2020).

20. Kevin Tampone, "NY projections on beds, ventilators were off: Couldn't model love, spirit, Cuomo says," *Syracuse News* (April 10, 2020), https://www.syracuse.com/coronavirus/2020/04/ny-projections-on-beds-ventilators-were-off-couldnt-model-love-spirit-cuomo-says.html.

21. Trevor J. Mitchell, "Why Gov. Noem won't order a shelter-in-place for South Dakotans," *USA Today* (April 1, 2020).

22. Derek Thompson, "Hygiene Theater Is a Huge Waste of Time," *The Atlantic* (July 27, 2020).

23. Kent Sepkowitz, "Now the CDC wants to shut down 'hygiene theater,'" *CNN* (April 21, 2021).

24. Takuma Suzuki, "From 19th century to modern day: A look at Japan's mask-wearing history," *The Mainichi* (April 17, 2021).

25. Wilfred H. Kellogg, "Influenza, A Study of Measures Adopted for the Control of the Epidemic" (Sacramento: California State Printing Office, Jan. 1919), 11–13.

26. Leah Asmelash, "The surgeon general wants Americans to stop buying face masks," *CNN* (March 2, 2020).

27. Lisa Brousseau and Margaret Sietsema, "COMMENTARY: Masks-for-all for COVID-19 not based on sound data," *CIDRAP* (April 1, 2020), https://www.cidrap.umn.edu/news-perspective/2020/04/commentary-masks-all-covid-19-not-based-sound-data.

28. Shane Neilson, "The surgical mask is a bad fit for risk reduction," *CMAJ*, Vol. 188, No. 8 (May 17, 2016): 606–607.

Notes—Chapter XVI

29. Nicky Robertson, "Trump doesn't think U.S. needs a national mask mandate," *CNN* (July 18, 2020).

30. Martin Kulldorff, Twitter (Sept. 8, 2021); Jon Miltimore, "CDC: Schools With Mask Mandates Didn't See Statistically Significant Different Rates of COVID Transmission From Schools With Optional Policies," *Foundation for Economic Education* (Aug. 25, 2021), https://fee.org/articles/cdc-schools-with-mask-mandates-didn-t-see-statistically-significant-different-rates-of-covid-transmission-from-schools-with-optional-policies/; and Jon Miltimore, "Education secretary touts mask study—gets rebuked by senior author of the study," *Maine Wire* (Oct. 5, 2021), https://www.themainewire.com/2021/10/education-secretary-touts-mask-study-gets-rebuked-by-senior-author-of-the-study/.

31. Zachary Wolf, "Hygiene Theater, Mask Theater, Climate Theater," *CNN* (April 22, 2021).

32. Arwa Mahdawi, "Shaming people who refuse to wear face masks isn't a good look," *The Guardian* (July 22, 2020).

33. Kiara Alfonseca, "Mask shaming ignores COVID-19 fears of immunocompromised people," *ABC News* (July 14, 2021).

34. Jon Levine, "CNN reporter Kaitlan Collins caught removing face mask when she thought camera was off," *New York Post* (May 16, 2020), and Frances Mulraney, "'Half your crew's not wearing masks!' MSNBC reporter trying to shame people for not wearing masks is caught out by bystander," *Daily Mail* (May 26, 2020).

35. "Nancy Pelosi seen without mask inside San Francisco hair salon," *BBC News* (Sept. 3, 2020).

36. Julian Mark, "San Francisco's mayor blasted for dancing maskless at a crowded club. She called her critics the 'fun police,'" *Washington Post* (Sept. 21, 2021).

37. Jordan Boyd, "Rep. Rashida Tlaib Admits Her Mask Is All Theater," *The Federalist* (Oct. 7, 2021).

38. Edward Isaac-Dovere, "Rand Paul Has More than a Cold," *The Atlantic* (March 23, 2020).

39. "The Reckless Timeline of Trump's Coronavirus Test," *Washington Post* (Dec. 1, 2021).

40. Peyton Britt, "Why I feel morally justified laughing at Trump getting COVID-19," *The Campus* (Oct. 8, 2020).

41. The Palm Beach Post Editorial Board, "Coronavirus Florida: Editorial: The president gets COVID-19, we should all be worried," *Palm Beach Post* (Oct. 3, 2020).

42. Robert Hart, "World Health Organization Rejects Remdesivir, The Antiviral Trump Took For Covid-19, Saying There's No Evidence It Helps Recovery Or Survival," *Forbes* (Nov. 20, 2020).

43. Kacper Niburski et al., "Impact of Trump's Promotion of Unproven COVID-19 Treatments and Subsequent Internet Trends: Observational Study," *Journal of Medical Internet Research*, Vol. 22, No. 11 (Nov. 2020): e20044.

44. Donald Trump, Twitter (May 14, 2020).

45. Jane C. Timm, "Fact check: Coronavirus vaccine could come this year, Trump says. Experts say he needs a 'miracle' to be right," *NBC News* (May 15, 2020).

46. Max Nisen, "Operation Warp Speed Needs to Waste Money on Vaccines," *Washington Post* (April 30, 2020).

47. Steve Benen, "HHS podcast raises fresh doubts about 'Operation Warp Speed,'" *MSNBC* (Aug. 5, 2020).

48. Presidential Debate (Sept. 29, 2020).

49. Caroline Kelly, "'I will not take his word for it': Kamala Harris says she would not trust Trump alone on a coronavirus vaccine," *CNN* (Sept. 5, 2020).

50. Vice President Debate (Oct. 7, 2020).

51. Joe Biden (Sept. 3, 2020) in "Q-and-A with former vice president Joe Biden," *WKMG Click Orlando*, https://www.clickorlando.com/news/local/2020/09/03/q-and-a-with-former-vice-president-joe-biden/.

52. Michael Specter, "Trump is Right: Andrew Cuomo Should Accept FDA Approval of a Coronavirus Vaccine," *The New Yorker* (Nov. 16, 2020).

53. Miranda Devine, "'Saint' Fauci a Lying Sinner," *New York Post* (May 19, 2021).

54. Triby Beresford, "Jimmy Kimmel Takes Aim at Dr. Fauci Haters: 'Even Trump Says He Liked Him,'" *The Hollywood Reporter* (Nov. 30, 2021).

55. See David Petriello, *A Pestilence on Pennsylvania Avenue: The Impact of*

Disease on the American Presidency (Staunton, Va.: American History Press, 2016), for a full coverage of the topic.

56. William Cummings, "Nearly two-thirds of voters expect Trump to win reelection in November, poll finds," *USA Today* (Feb. 23, 2020).

57. Bill Press, "Election is now referendum on how Trump handled COVID-19," *The Hill* (Oct. 6, 2020).

58. "Biden: Anyone Responsible for So Many Covid Deaths 'Should Not' Be President," *Barron's* (Oct. 22, 2020).

59. Donald Trump, Twitter (July 30, 2020).

60. "Joe Biden's basement strategy really IS his plan," *Washington Times* (Oct. 27, 2020).

61. Joey Garrison, "Biden in the basement: Can campaigning from home work as Trump starts to travel?," *USA Today* (May 11, 2020).

62. W. James Antle III, "'No Federal Solution': Biden's COVID-19 tone shifts away from shutting down the virus," *The Gazette* (Dec. 27, 2021).

63. Stephen Collinson, "Biden sets bold timeline for a return to normal life," *CNN* (Jan. 27, 2021).

64. Lori Robertson, "Biden's Misleading Vaccine Boasts," *FactCheck.Org* (Feb. 23, 2021).

65. Steven Nelson, "Biden says he 'started the vaccination program' despite Trump rollout," *New York Post* (Oct. 7, 2021).

66. Lori Robertson, "Biden's Misleading Vaccine Boasts," *FactCheck.Org* (Feb. 23, 2021).

67. "Study of efficacy and safety oral ivermectin in the prophylaxis of COVID-19 disease in post-exposed to COVID-19 individuals by close contact or epidemiological nexus," https://clinicaltrials.gov/ProvidedDocs/21/NCT04894721/Prot_000.pdf.

68. FDA, Twitter (Aug. 21, 2020).

69. Quoted in Ronny Reyes, "CNN says it won't apologize for 'bruising the ego' of Joe Rogan by claiming he'd taken 'horse dewormer' ivermectin for COVID infection—despite network Dr Sanjay Gupta groveling on Rogan's podcast," *Daily Mail* (Oct. 22, 2021).

70. Storme Jones, "Oklahoma Doctor at Center of Viral Ivermectin Story Says Report Is Wrong," *News On 6* (Sept. 6, 2021).

71. Jay Hancock, "As Trump Touts His 'Great' COVID Drugs, the Pharma Cash Flows to Biden, Not Him," *KHN* (Oct. 9, 2020).

72. Paul Best, "Maryland doctor says people are 'going to die' after Biden admin uses faulty data to snub antibody treatments," *Fox News* (Dec. 29, 2021).

73. Shannon Bond, "Facebook Widens Ban On COVID-19 Vaccine Misinformation in Push to Boost Confidence," *NPR* (Feb. 8, 2021), https://www.npr.org/2021/02/08/965330755/facebook-widens-ban-on-covid-19-vaccine-misinformation-in-push-to-boost-confidence.

74. Laurie Clark, "Covid-19: Who fact checks health and science on Facebook?," *British Medical Journal*, Issue 373 (2021).

75. Guy Rosen, "An Update on Our Work to Keep People Informed and Limit Misinformation About COVID-19," *Meta* (Feb. 8, 2021), https://about.fb.com/news/2020/04/covid-19-misinfo-update/#removing-more-false-claims.

76. Cameron English, "COVID Misinformation Blunder: Instagram Censors Widely Respected Cochrane Collaboration," *America Council on Science and Health* (Nov. 14, 2021).

77. Nico Grant, "YouTube Removes Steven Crowder Video for Violating Covid Policy," *Bloomberg* (March 17, 2021), https://www.bloomberg.com/news/articles/2021-03-17/youtube-removes-steven-crowder-video-for-violating-covid-policy-kmcz9wy6.

78. Richard Harris, "In Kids, the Risk of COVID-19 and the Flu Are Similar—But the Risk Perception Isn't," *NPR* (May 21, 2021), https://www.npr.org/2021/05/21/999241558/in-kids-the-risk-of-covid-19-and-the-flu-are-similar-but-the-risk-perception-isn.

79. Robert Malone, "Joe Rogan Podcast," Episode #1757 (Dec. 31, 2021).

80. Ella Torres, "A timeline of Cuomo's and Trump's responses to coronavirus outbreak," *ABC News* (April 3, 2020).

81. Susan Milligan, "How Coronavirus Made Andrew Cuomo America's Governor," *U.S. News* (March 23, 2020).

82. Ray Sanchez, "New York governor gives final coronavirus briefing after '111 days of hell,'" *CBS58* (June 19, 2020).

83. Torres, "A timeline of Cuomo's and Trump's responses to coronavirus outbreak."

84. Alisa Wiersema, "'Draft Cuomo 2020' groundswell emerges amid the New York governor's coronavirus response," *ABC News* (March 31, 2020).

85. "Cuomo: 'Shocking' to See Poll Showing Him Leading 2024 Democratic Field," *NBC New York* (Aug. 14, 2020).

86. Colin Dwyer, "Andrew Cuomo to Receive International Emmy for 'Masterful' COVID-19 Briefings," *NPR* (Nov. 21, 2020).

87. Corky Siemaszko, "Florida governor takes heat for state's slow response to coronavirus crisis," *NBC News* (March 24, 2020).

88. *Miami Herald* Editorial Board, "Coronavirus is killing us in Florida, Gov. DeSantis. Act like you give a damn," *Miami Herald* (March 22, 2020).

89. Nicholas Reimann, "Covid Cases Spike in Florida as Bars and Restaurants Reopen at Full Capacity," *Forbes* (Sept. 29, 2020).

90. Michael Kruse, "How Ron DeSantis won the pandemic," *Politico* (March 18, 2021).

91. Michael Putney, "DeSantis criticizes Fauci after e-mail release: Florida 'chose freedom over Faucism,'" *Local 10* (June 4, 2021), https://www.local10.com/news/politics/2021/06/04/desantis-criticizes-fauci-after-e-mail-release-florida-chose-freedom-over-faucism/.

92. Blake Nelson, "Trump announces N.J. travel advisory, backs off coronavirus quarantine proposal," *NJ.com* (March 28, 2020).

93. Torres, "A timeline of Cuomo's and Trump's responses to coronavirus outbreak."

94. Anna Wilde Mathews, "New York Mandates Nursing Homes Take Covid-19 Patients Discharged from Hospitals," *Wall Street Journal* (March 26, 2020).

95. Steve Brown, "Cuomo: Nursing homes 'don't have the right to object' to order requiring admission of COVID-19 patients," *WGRZ* (April 23, 2020) https://www.wgrz.com/article/news/health/coronavirus/cuomo-nursing-homes-dont-have-the-right-to-object-to-order-requiring-admission-of-covid-19-patients-coronavirus/71-370ce285-0a0d-4df1-90c5-b5af508444df.

96. Zak Failla, "COVID-19: Cuomo Blames 'Incompetent Federal Government' After AG Report On Nursing Home Deaths," *Nassau Daily Voice* (Jan. 29, 2021).

97. Nick Reisman, "Cuomo Again Defends Nursing Home Policies During Pandemic," *Spectrum News 1* (Sept. 30, 2020).

98. Bernadette Hogan, "Cuomo aide Melissa DeRosa admits they hid nursing home data so feds wouldn't find out," *New York Post* (Feb. 11, 2021).

99. Joshua Chaffin, "How Ron Kim became Andrew Cuomo's nemesis," *Financial Times* (March 10, 2021).

100. Joe Biden (Dec. 4, 2020), in Tom Porter, "Video shows President-elect Biden saying 10 months ago he wouldn't make vaccines mandatory," *Business Insider* (Sept. 10, 2021).

101. Linda So, 'Fauci backs COVID-19 vaccine mandate for U.S. school children," *Reuters* (Aug. 29, 2021).

102. Stephanie Ruhle, Twitter (Sept. 9, 2021).

Conclusion

1. "COVID-19: Democratic Voters Support Harsh Measures Against Unvaccinated," *Rasmussen Reports* (Jan. 13, 2022), https://www.rasmussenreports.com/public_content/politics/partner_surveys/jan_2022/covid_19_democratic_voters_support_harsh_measures_against_unvaccinated.

2. Gunter Kampf, "COVID-19: stigmatizing the unvaccinated is not justified," *The Lancet*, Vol. 398, Issue 10314 (Nov. 20, 2021).

3. Walter Reich, "The world of Soviet psychiatry," *NY Times* (Jan. 30, 1983).

Bibliography

Abrams, Herbert L. "Presidential Health and the Public Interest: The Campaign of 1992." *Political Psychology* 16. no. 4 (Dec. 1995): 795–820.

Acuna-Soto, Rodolfo, Leticia Calderon Romero, and James H. Maguire. "Large Epidemics of Hemorrhagic Fevers in Mexico, 1545–1815." *American Journal of Tropical Medicine and Hygiene* 62, no. 6 (2000): 733–739.

Adler, Richard. *Cholera in Detroit: A History*. Jefferson, NC: McFarland, 2013.

Aldridge, Alfred Owen. *Benjamin Franklin: Philosopher and Man*. Philadelphia: Lippincott, 1965.

Ayres, Leonard P. *The War with Germany: A Statistical Summary*. Chapter IX. Washington, D.C.: Government Printing Office, 1919.

Barber, John Warner. *Connecticut Historical Collections, Containing a General Collection of Interesting Facts, Traditions, Biographical Sketches, Anecdotes, Etc. Relating to the History and Antiquities of Every Town in Connecticut*. New Haven: Durrie and Peck, 1838.

Bashford, Alison, and Philippa Levine, eds. *The Oxford Handbook of the History of Eugenics*. Oxford: Oxford University Press, 2010.

Bassett, J.S., and D.M. Matteson. *Correspondence of Andrew Jackson*. Vol 1. Washington, D.C.: Carnegie Institute of Washington, 1926.

Baumgaertner, Bert, et al. "The influence of political ideology and trust on willingness to vaccinate." *PLoS One* 13, no. 1 (Jan. 25, 2018).

Birken, William Joseph. "The Royal College of Physicians of London and Its Support of the Parliamentary Cause in the English Civil War," *Journal of British Studies* 23, no. 1 (Autumn 1983): 47–62.

Boylston, Arthur. "The Origins of Inoculation." *Journal of the Royal Society of Medicine* 105, no. 7 (July 2012): 309–313.

Bradford, Alden. *History of Massachusetts*. Boston: Wells and Lilly, 1825.

Brandt, Allan M. 'Racism and Research: The Case of the Tuskegee Syphilis Study." *The Hastings Center Report* 8, no. 6 (1978): 21–29.

Brandt, Allan M. "The Syphilis Epidemic and Its Relation to AIDS." *Science* 239, no. 4838 (January 1988): 375–380.

Brinton, Ellen Starr. "The Rogerenes." *The New England Quarterly* 16, no. 1 (1943): 3–19.

Brooks, Joanna. *American Lazarus: Religion and the Rise of African-American and Native American Literatures*. Oxford: Oxford University Press, 2003.

Campbell, John. *An Account of the Spanish Settlement in America*. Edinburgh: A. Donaldson and J. Reid, 1762.

Cathrall, Isaac. *A Medical Sketch of the Synochus Maligna*. Philadelphia: T. Dobson, 1794.

Clark, Allen Culling. *Life and Letters of Dolly Madison*. Washington, D.C.: W.F. Roberts Company, 1914.

Cohen, Adam. *Imbeciles: The Supreme Court, American Eugenics, and the Sterilization of Carrie Buck*. New York: Penguin, 2016.

Cook, Noble David. *Born to Die: Disease and New World Conquest, 1492–1650*. Cambridge: Cambridge University Press, 1998.

Crow, John Armstrong. *The Epic of Latin*

America. Berkeley: University of California Press, 1992.
Davis, Anne R. "Distempers and Physic Virginia's Health in the Eighteenth Century." *Northern Neck of Virginia Historical Society* 66 (2016): 8285.
Davis, Richard Beale. *Correspondence of Thomas Jefferson and Francis Walker Gilmer, 1814–1826*. Columbia: University of South Carolina Press, 1946.
Defoe, Daniel. *A Journal of the Plague Year*. London: E. Nutt, 1722.
del Castillo, Bernal Diaz. *The Discovery and Conquest of Mexico 1517–1521*. London: Hatchard and Son, 1864.
Deppisch, L.M., et al. "Andrew Jackson's Exposure to Mercury and Lead: Poisoned President?" *JAMA* 282, no. 6 (1999): 569–571.
Diffenderffer, Frank Reid. "The German Immigration into Pennsylvania through the Port of Philadelphia from 1700 to 1775 and the Redemptioners." *Proceedings of the Pennsylvania-German Society*, Vol. 10. Lancaster, 1900.
Dix, Dorothea Lynde. *Remarks on Prisons and Prison Discipline in the United States*. 2nd ed. Philadelphia: Kite and Co., 1845.
Douglass, William, and Alexander Stuart. *The Abuses and Scandals of Some Late Pamphlets in Favour of Inoculation of the Small Pox*. Boston: James Franklin, 1722.
England, Roger. "The Writing Is on the Wall for UNAIDS." *British Medical Journal* 336, no. 7652 (2008): 1072.
Fitzpatrick, John C., ed. *The Autobiography of Martin Van Buren*. Washington, D.C.: U.S. Printing Office, 1920.
Fowler, William M. *The Baron of Beacon Hill: A Biography of John Hancock*. Boston: Houghton Mifflin, 1980.
Freneau, Philip Morin. *An Historical Sketch, to the End of the Revolutionary War, of the Life of Silas Talbot*. New York: G. & R. Waite, 1803.
Fromm, Erich. *Escape from Freedom*. London: Routledge & Kegan Paul, 1942.
Galton, Francis. *Essays in Eugenics*. London: Eugenics Education Society, 1909.
Gilbert Robert E. *The Mortal Presidency: Illness and Anguish in the White House*. New York: Fordham University Press, 1998.
Glasser, Joshua M. *The Eighteen Day Running Mate: McGovern, Eagleton, and a Campaign in Crisis*. New Haven: Yale University Press, 2012.
Gostin, L.O. "Jacobson v Massachusetts at 100 Years: Police Power and Civil Liberties in Tension." *American Journal of Public Health* 95, no. 4 (2005): 576–581.
Gray, Thomas R., and Jeffery A. Jenkins. "Yellow Fever and Institutional Development: The Rise and Fall of the National Board of Health." *Journal of Political Institutions and Political Economy* 2, no. 1 (2021): 143–167.
Grubb, Farley. "Morbidity and Mortality on the North Atlantic Passage: Eighteenth-Century German Immigration." *The Journal of Interdisciplinary History* 17, no. 3 (Winter 1987): 565–585.
Gussow, Zachary. *Leprosy, Racism, and Public Health: Social Policy in Chronic Disease Control*. New York: Routledge, 2021.
Hamburger, Philip. *Separation of Church and State*. Cambridge: Harvard University Press, 2004.
Handlin, Oscar. *Boston's Immigrants, 1790–1865: A Study in Acculturation*. Cambridge: Harvard University Press, 1959.
Harper, Kristin, and George Armelagos. "The Changing Disease-Scape in the Third Epidemiological Transition." *International Journal of Environmental Research and Public Health* 7 (2010): 675–697.
Helps, Arthur. *The Spanish Conquest in America*, Vol. II. New York: Harper, 1856.
Hérbert, John R., Ida Altman, and John Fleming. *An Ongoing Voyage: 1492–1992: The Library of Congress Quincentenary Exhibition*. Washington, D.C.: Library of Congress, 1992.
Honigsbaum, Mark. " Revisiting the 1957 and 1968 Influenza Pandemics." *The Lancet* 395, no. 10240 (June 2020): 1824–1826.
Hoolihan, Christopher. *An Annotated Catalogue of the Edward C. Atwater Collection of American Popular Medicine and Health Reform*, Vol. 3. Rochester: University of Rochester Press, 2008.
Hopkins, Donald R. *The Greatest Killer: Smallpox in History*. Chicago: University of Chicago Press, 2002.
Hosack, David, and John Wakefield Francis. *The American Medical and Philo-*

sophical Register, Vol 1. New York: Van Winkle, 1814.

Irwin, Inez Haynes. *The Story of the Woman's Party.* New York: Harcourt, 1921.

Jackle, Sebastian. "A Catwalk to Congress? Appearance-Based Effects in the Elections to the U.S. House of Representatives 2016." *American Politics Research* 48, no. 4 (2020): 427–441.

Jara, René, and Nicholas Spadaccini. *Amerindian Images and the Legacy of Columbus.* Minneapolis: University of Minnesota Press, 1992.

Johnson, Lauren. *So Great a Prince: England and the Accession of Henry VIII.* New York: Pegasus, 2017.

Jortner, Adam. "Cholera, Christ, and Jackson: The Epidemic of 1832 and the Origins of Christian Politics in Antebellum America." *Journal of the Early Republic* 27, no. 2 (Summer 2007): 233–264.

Kales, David. *The Boston Harbor Islands: A History of an Urban Wilderness.* Charleston: The History Press, 2007.

Kampf, Gunter. "COVID-19: Stigmatising the Unvaccinated Is Not Justified." *The Lancet* 398, no. 10314 (Nov. 20, 2021).

Kellogg, Wilfred H. "Influenza, A Study of Measures Adopted for the Control of the Epidemic." Sacramento: California State Printing Office, Jan. 1919.

Klevens, R.M., et al. "Is There Really a Heterosexual AIDS Epidemic in the United States? Findings from a Multisite Validation Study, 1992–1995." *American Journal of Epidemiology* 149, no. 1 (1999): 75–84.

Klotter, James C. *Henry Clay: The Man Who Would Be President.* Oxford: Oxford University Press, 2018.

Kumamoto, Robert. *The Historical Origins of Terrorism in America:1644–1880.* New York: Routledge, 2013.

Lamb, Martha J. *History of the City of New York: Its Origin, Rise, and Progress.* Vol. I. New York: A.S. Barnes, 1876.

Laughlin, Harry. *Eugenics Record Office: Bulletin 10.* Cold Spring Harbor, 1914.

Lieu, Tracy A., et al. "Geographic Clusters in Underimmunization and Vaccine Refusal." *Pediatrics* 135, no. 2 (Feb. 2015): 280–289.

Lindman, Janet Moore, and Michele Lise Tarter. *A Centre of Wonders: The Body in Early America.* Ithaca: Cornell University Press, 2001.

Luibhéid, Eithne. *Denied Entry: Controlling Sexuality at the Border.* Minneapolis: University of Minnesota Press, 1998.

Malone, Dumas. *Jefferson and His Time,* vol. 6: *The Sage of Monticello.* Boston: Little, Brown, 1981.

Manning, Charles, and Merrill Moore. "Sassafras and Syphilis." *The New England Quarterly* 9, no. 3 (Sept. 1936): 473–475.

Markham, Clements R. *Peruvian Bark: A Popular Account of the Introduction of Chinchona Cultivation into British India 1860–1880.* London: John Murray, 1880.

Marr, John S., and John T. Cathey. "New Hypothesis for Cause of Epidemic among Native Americans, New England, 1616–1619." *EID Journal: Historical Review* 16, no. 2 (Feb. 2010): 281–286.

Massry, Shaul G., et al. "History of Nephrology." *The American Journal of Nephrology* 17 (1997): 233–240.

Matthews, Albert, ed. *Publications of the Colonial Society of Massachusetts, Vol. VII.* Cambridge: Cambridge University Press, 1905.

Mayor, Adrienne. "The Nessus Shirt in the New World: Smallpox Blankets in History and Legend." *Journal of American Folklore* 108, no. 427 (Winter 1995): 54–77.

McCaa, Robert. "Spanish and Nahuatl Views on Smallpox and Demographic Catastrophe in Mexico." *Journal of Interdisciplinary History* 25, no. 3 (Winter 1995): 397–431.

Meacham, Jon. *American Lion: Andrew Jackson in the White House.* New York: Random House, 2009.

Metchnikoff, Elie. *The New Hygiene: Three Lectures on the Prevention of Infectious Diseases.* Chicago: W.T. Keener and Company, 1907.

Miller, G. "Women's Suffrage, Political Responsiveness, and Child Survival in American History." *Q.J. Economics* 123, no. 3 (2008): 1287–1327.

Mires, Peter B. "Contact and Contagion: The Roanoke Colony and Influenza." *Historical Archaeology* 28, no. 3 (1994): 28, 30–38.

Niburski, Kacper. "Impact of Trump's Promotion of Unproven COVID-19 Treatments and Subsequent Internet Trends: Observational Study." *Journal* of *Medical Internet Research* 22, no. 11 (November 2020).

Petriello, David R. *A Pestilence on Pennsylvania Avenue: The Impact of Disease upon the American Presidency*. Staunton, VA: American History Press, 2016.

"Report of the Sanitary Commission Prostitution," *Annual Report of the Metropolitan Board of Health of the State of New York*. New York: Union, 1868.

Riccards, Michael P. "The Presidency: In Sickness and Health." *Presidential Studies Quarterly* 7, no. 4 (Fall 1977): 215–231.

Rosenberg, Charlese E. *The Cholera Years: The United States in 1832, 1849, and 1866*. Chicago: University of Chicago Press, 1962.

Rush, Benhamin. *Medical Inquiries and Observations, Vol. III*. Philadelphia: Carey and Sons, 1818.

Schoepff, Johann David. *The Climate and Diseases of America*. Translated by James Read Chadwick. Boston: Houghton, 1875.

Shackelford, George Green. "From the Society's Collections: Lieutenant Lee Reports to Captain Talcott on Fort Calhoun's Construction on the Rip Raps." *The Virginia Magazine of History and Biography* 60, no. 3 (July 1952): 458–487.

Shaw, Robert B. "History of the Comstock Patent Medicine Business and Dr. Morse's Indian Root Pills." *Smithsonian Studies in History and Technology*, no. 22 (1972): 1–49.

Shipp, J.E.D. *Giant Days: Or, The Life and Times of William H. Crawford*. Americus, GA: Southern Printers, 1909.

Shultz, Suzanne M. "Epidemics in Colonial Philadelphia from 1699–1799 and the Risk of Dying." *Early America Review* 11, no. 1 (Winter/Spring 2007).

Smith, Billy G. "Death and Life in a Colonial Immigrant City: A Demographic Analysis of Philadelphia." *The Journal of Economic History* 37, no. 4 (May 2010): 863–889.

Smith, Billy G. *Ship of Death: A Voyage That Changed the Atlantic World*. New Haven: Yale University Press, 2013.

Smith, Julia H., and Alan Whiteside. "The History of AIDS Exceptionalism." *Journal of the International AIDS Society* 13, no. 47 (2010).

Smith, Stephen. *The City That Was*. New York: Frank Allaben, 1911.

Smith, William E. "Francis P. Blair, Pen-Executive of Andrew Jackson." *Journal of American History* 17, no. 4 (Mar. 1931), 543–556.

Soper, George A. "Mary Mallon." *The Military Surgeon* 45, no. 1 (July 1919).

Stewart, Donna E., et al. "Anorexia Nervosa, Bulimia, and Pregnancy." *American Journal of Obstetrics and Gynecology* 157, no. 5 (Nov. 1987): 1194–1198.

Stokes, John H. *The Third Great Plague: A Discussion of Syphilis for Everyday People*. Philadelphia: W.B. Saunders Company, 1920.

Tchen, John Kuo Wei. *New York before Chinatown: Orientalism and the Shaping of American Culture, 1776–1882*. Baltimore: Johns Hopkins University Press, 1999.

Tuite, Ashleigh R. "Cholera, Canals, and Contagion: Rediscovering Dr. Beck's Report." *Journal of Public Health Policy* 32, no. 3 (Aug. 2011): 320–333.

Unger, Harlow G. *John Hancock: Merchant King and American Patriot*. New York: Wiley, 2000.

Viseltear, A.J. "The Pneumonic Plague Epidemic of 1924 in Los Angeles." *Yale Journal of Biology and Medicine* 47, no. 1 (1974): 40–54.

Wallabout Committee. *An Account of the Internment of the Remains of 11,500 American Seamen, Soldiers, and Citizens, who Fell Victims to the Cruelties of the British On Board their Prison Ships at the Wallabout*. New York: Frank, White, and Co. for the Tammany Society, 1808.

Wang, Dave. "The US Founders and China: The Origins of Chinese Cultural Influence on the United States." *Education About Asia* 16, no. 2 (Fall 2011): 5–6.

Washburn, Wilcomb E. *The Indian in America*. New York: Harper and Row, 1975.

Wilson, Brian C. *Dr. John Harvey Kellogg and the Religion of Biologic Living*. Bloomington: Indiana University Press, 2014.

Woodward, Samuel Bayard. "The Story of Smallpox in Massachusetts." *New England Journal of Medicine* 206, no. 23 (1932): 1181–1191.

Young, James Harvey. *The Toadstool Millionaires: A Social History of Patent Medicines in America before Federal Regulation*. Princeton: Princeton University Press, 1961.

Index

Adams, John 21, 25, 27, 28, 31, 42, 61, 106, 138–140, 142, 189, 213–215, 223
Adenoid Riots 112
AIDS 58, 133, 160, 162–170, 221, 227, 233, 235, 236
American Eugenics Society 126
American Medical Association 83, 123, 131
American Revolution 23–25, 27–29, 36, 45, 50, 52, 56, 64, 106, 186, 206, 223
Anti-vaccination League 109

Biden, Joseph 1, 3, 90, 176, 177, 185, 186, 193–200, 204, 205, 209, 220, 227–230, 232, 233, 231
Black Legend 5, 7, 10
Boston 15, 17–22, 24, 25, 27, 28, 38, 54, 66, 68, 75, 94, 105, 106, 108, 212, 214, 215, 217, 218, 228, 233–236
Boylston, Zabdiel 18–20, 22, 105, 212, 214, 233
Bubonic Plague 5
Buck v. Bell 127, 128, 222, 233
Buffalo Fever 48, 53, 54
Burr, Aaron 91–93
Bush, George W. 33

CDC 134, 135, 160, 163, 166, 168, 171, 174, 175, 177–180, 184, 188–190, 198, 199, 202, 203, 227–230
Chamberlain-Kahn Act of 1918 122
Chesapeake-Leopard Affair 50
China 2, 16, 76–85, 89, 135, 171, 173, 183–185, 189, 218, 228, 229, 237
Chinese Exclusion Act 84
Chinese Immigration 5, 32, 64, 76–90, 156, 183, 185, 188, 218, 219, 237
cholera 3, 45, 56–59, 61–63, 66–70, 74, 75, 79–81, 83–85, 93–97, 118, 123, 140, 142, 163, 191, 192, 208, 219
Cholera Epidemic of 1832 57

Christian Science 111
Clay, Henry 61–63, 65–67, 139–143, 208, 219, 220, 223, 225, 235
Cleveland, Grover 33, 68
Clinton, Hillary 153
Clinton, William Jefferson 22, 33, 52, 137, 138, 150, 152, 153, 222, 225
Columbus, Christopher 7, 8, 10, 211, 235
Connecticut 14, 20, 21, 31, 85, 123, 124, 130, 131, 158, 200, 202, 217, 233
Cortés, Hernan 7
Covid 33, 193, 199, 208, 229–233
Cuba 10, 38, 97–100, 220
Cuomo, Andrew 187, 193, 200–204, 229–231, 233

de Las Casas, Bartolome 7
Democratic Party 58, 63, 65, 68, 76, 83, 95, 96, 101, 118, 145, 146, 148–151, 153, 155, 161, 176–179, 184–188, 190, 192–197, 199–202, 204, 205, 208, 209, 228
DeSantis, Ron 199, 201, 202, 220, 231
Dodge Commission 100, 220
dysentery 23, 38, 48, 53, 57, 79, 100, 223

Ebola 177–181, 185, 208, 227, 228
Eisenhower, Dwight D. 32, 145, 146, 150, 172, 184, 226
Election of 1812 137
Election of 1824 138
Election of 1832 140
Election of 1944 143
Election of 1956 145
Election of 1960 146
Election of 1972 148
Election of 1988 148
Emergency Quota Act 158
England 5, 6, 9, 11–13, 15, 17–19, 21, 23, 27, 29, 30, 37, 50–54, 63, 66, 69, 74, 109, 138, 212, 213, 221, 227, 233–235, 237
eugenics 125–128, 130, 136, 158, 159, 207

Index

Fauci, Anthony 135, 168, 176, 189, 194, 201, 205, 222, 227, 230, 231
Federalists 29, 31, 43, 44, 47, 52, 53, 55, 64, 65, 138
Franklin, Benjamin 19, 22, 30, 31, 73, 76–78, 105, 106, 143, 212, 213, 215, 217–219, 221, 225
Franklin, James 18
French and Indian War 23
Freneau, Philip 47, 49, 51, 217, 234

Gage, General Thomas 24, 89
Germans 71–73, 156, 162
Goldwater, Barry 148, 152, 226
Great Yellow Fever Epidemic of 1793 39

Hamilton, Alexander 25, 30, 34, 39, 41–44, 50, 92, 118, 214, 224
Hancock, John 27–32, 214, 233, 234, 237
Harrison, William Henry 65, 67–69
Hayes, Rutherford B. 83, 116, 118
Henry VIII 6, 211, 235
Hong Kong Flu 173

Immigration Act of 1891 157
influenza 12, 53, 66, 68, 77, 78, 135, 143, 144, 150, 155, 171, 172, 175, 176, 189, 196, 208
Iowa Cow War 114
Irish 39, 58–60, 63, 73–75, 82, 90, 119, 142, 156, 157, 212, 225
Irish Immigration 73

Jackson, Andrew 51, 57, 59, 61–63, 65, 68, 139–143, 148, 166, 208, 214, 219, 224, 225, 233–235, 237
Jacobson v. Massachusetts 112, 128, 222, 234
Jamestown 10–13
Jefferson, Thomas 23, 39, 40, 42, 44, 50–52, 59, 61, 64, 65, 106, 137–139, 142, 150, 213, 214, 216–218, 221–223, 233–235
Jersey, HMS 49
Jewish People 5, 112, 113, 156, 209

Kellogg, John Harvey 126, 127, 221, 229, 235
Know Nothing Party 70, 75, 76, 108, 217
Kuhn, Adam 42–44, 194

La Follette-Bulwinkle Act 124
laudanum 31, 42–44
leprosy 81, 83, 122

Madison, James 30, 31, 39, 42, 44, 52, 53, 61, 107, 137, 138, 215–217, 221–223, 233

Mallon, Mary 119, 120, 221, 226, 237
Marine Hospital Service 116
masks 164, 177, 188–191, 198, 229, 230
Massachusetts 14, 16, 27–31, 33, 38, 45, 75, 107, 112, 128, 139, 146, 149, 186, 207, 208, 213, 221, 233–235, 237
Mather, Cotton 15–20, 22, 105, 111, 212, 213
McCain, John 151, 225
Miles, Nelson 100–102, 220
Mississippi Yellow Fever Outbreak of 1878 117
Morris, Robert 34, 72, 73

National Board of Health 117, 118, 221, 234
Native Americans 7, 10, 212, 235
New York City 17, 38, 41, 45, 48, 58–60, 75, 91–97, 108, 109, 112, 119, 120, 134, 163, 164, 167, 168, 172, 180, 187, 188, 193, 201, 203–205, 228
1957 Asian Flu Pandemic 171
Nixon, Richard 33, 145–148, 150, 171, 215, 226

Obama, Barack 134, 135, 151, 160, 175–181, 184, 200, 226, 227
Onesimus 16, 18

Page Act of 1875 157
Paleolithic Age 1
Paracelsus 36, 37, 210
Pelosi, Nancy 70, 185, 191, 192, 217, 229, 230
Philadelphia 22, 24, 30, 38–41, 43–46, 58, 60, 66, 72, 74, 75, 94, 97, 110, 213, 216, 217, 220, 221, 233, 234, 236, 237
Pilgrims 12, 13
Plymouth 10–13
polio 113, 134
Prince v. Mass. 113
Prison Ship Memorial 52
Progressives 104, 109, 207
Public Health Service 131, 132, 171, 172, 208

Raleigh, Walter 11
Reed, Walter 33, 37, 103, 172
Republican Party 32, 43, 44, 48, 50–55, 57, 58, 62, 83, 84, 89, 96, 101–103, 107, 111, 114, 118, 127, 135, 141, 147–152, 154, 159, 160, 164, 181, 182, 186, 188, 191, 193, 198, 200–202, 204, 208, 218–220, 222
Roanoke 11, 12, 22, 211, 235
Rogerenes 20, 21, 233
Roosevelt, Franklin 32, 99, 102, 124, 143–146, 152, 200, 220, 225
Roosevelt, Theodore 99
rubella 173, 227

Rush, Benjamin 40–44, 138, 194, 216, 222, 236

San Francisco 5, 80–86, 88, 89, 99, 134, 164, 165, 168, 185, 189, 191, 219–221, 227, 229, 230
San Francisco Plague Epidemic 85
Sanger, Margaret 129–131, 222
SARS-CoV 135, 183
Seahorse, HMS 17
smallpox 8–10, 13–27, 31, 34, 48, 54, 70, 80, 81, 98, 106–108, 110–112, 118, 123, 135, 185
Smith, John 12, 22, 83, 95, 106, 107, 118, 174, 211, 213, 216, 217, 220, 221, 224, 227, 236
Spain 5–9, 98
Spanish-American War 97
Spanish Flu Pandemic 134
Swine Flu Pandemic of 2009 175

Taylor, Zachary 68–70, 119, 214
Trump, Donald 33, 70, 135, 148, 151–153, 160, 166, 177, 179, 180, 183–187, 189–197, 199, 200, 202, 203, 215, 217, 225–233, 235

Tuskegee Experiment 132
Tyler, John 65–69, 220
typhoid 48, 53, 98, 119, 120

vaccine 54, 90, 105–115, 160, 172–174, 176, 177, 183, 184, 192–194, 196, 198, 205, 209, 227, 230, 231, 233
variolation 16, 20, 22–26, 80, 105–107, 207

War of 1812 52, 55, 65, 217
Washington, George 3, 23–30, 34, 35, 39, 41, 65, 68, 75, 77, 81, 86, 106, 107, 111, 121, 122, 134, 141, 159, 173, 186, 187, 192, 193, 207, 211, 213–216, 218–227, 229, 230, 232–234
Whigs 58, 59, 65, 94, 96, 142
Wilson, Woodrow 143
World War I 122, 155, 171, 188
Wuhan Virus *see* Covid

yellow fever 23, 36–44, 46–48, 55, 60, 66, 92–94, 117, 118, 131, 216

Zucht v. King 113

www.ingramcontent.com/pod-product-compliance
Ingram Content Group UK Ltd.
Pitfield, Milton Keynes, MK11 3LW, UK
UKHW041941140426
5217IPUK00014B/603